Cancer SOURCEBOOK for Women

Sixth Edition

Health Reference Series

Sixth Edition

Cancer SOURCEBOOK for Women

Basic Consumer Health Information about Gynecologic Cancers and Other Cancers of Special Concern to Women, Including Cancers of the Breast, Cervix, Colon, Lung, Ovaries, Thyroid, and Uterus

Along with Facts about Benign Conditions of the Female Reproductive System, Cancer Risk Factors, Screening and Prevention Programs, Women's Issues in Cancer Treatment and Survivorship, Research Initiatives, a Glossary of Cancer Terms, and a Directory of Resources for Additional Help and Information

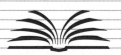

OMNIGRAPHICS

615 Griswold, Ste. 901, Detroit, MI 48226

Bibliographic Note
Because this page cannot legibly accommodate all the copyright notices, the Bibliographic Note portion of the Preface constitutes an extension of the copyright notice.

* * *

OMNIGRAPHICS
Angela L. Williams, *Managing Editor*
***

ISBN 978-0-7808-1630-5
E-ISBN 978-0-7808-1631-2

Library of Congress Cataloging-in-Publication Data

Names: Omnigraphics, Inc., issuing body.

Title: Cancer sourcebook for women: basic consumer health information about gynecologic cancers and other cancers of special concern to women, including cancers of the breast, cervix, colon, lung, ovaries, thyroid, and uterus; along with facts about benign conditions of the female reproductive system, cancer risk factors, screening and prevention programs, women's issues in cancer treatment and survivorship, research initiatives, a glossary of cancer terms, and a directory of resources for additional help and information.

Description: Sixth edition. | Detroit, MI: Omnigraphics, [2018] | Series: Health reference series | Includes bibliographical references and index.

Identifiers: LCCN 2018013236 (print) | LCCN 2018013547 (ebook) | ISBN 9780780816312 (eBook) | ISBN 9780780816305 (hardcover: alk. paper)

Subjects: LCSH: Generative organs, Female--Popular works. | Cancer in women--Popular works.

Classification: LCC RC280.G5 (ebook) | LCC RC280.G5 C34 2018 (print) | DDC 616.99/40082--dc23

LC record available at https://lccn.loc.gov/2018013236

∞

Table of Contents

Part IV: Other Cancers of Special Concern to Women

Part V: Diagnosing and Treating Cancer

Part VI: Coping with the Side Effects of Cancer and Cancer Treatments

Part VII: Women's Issues in Cancer Survivorship

Part VIII: Additional Help and Information

Preface

About This Book

According to the National Cancer Institute (NCI), cancer continues to take a devastating toll. Among women in the United States, cancer is the second-leading cause of death after heart disease. Lung, breast, and colorectal are leading causes of the cancer deaths in women. Medical researchers fighting against cancer have made significant progress, though. In recent years, cancer incidence rates have been stable, and mortality has decreased for 10 of the top 15 cancers in women. With improved cancer screening programs and innovative treatments, women receiving a cancer diagnosis today have a better chance of overcoming their disease than ever before.

Cancer Sourcebook for Women, Sixth Edition offers updated information about gynecologic cancers and other cancers of special concern to women, including breast cancer and cancers of the female reproductive organs. It also explains cancer risks—including lifestyle factors, inherited genetic abnormalities, and hormonal medications—and methods used to diagnose and treat cancer. Practical suggestions for coping with the treatment side effects are provided, and a section on cancer survivorship discusses methods for maintaining quality of life during and after treatment. The book concludes with a glossary of cancer-related terms, a directory of resources, and facts about locating support groups.

How to Use This Book

This book is divided into parts and chapters. Parts focus on broad areas of interest. Chapters are devoted to single topics within a part.

Part I: Understanding Cancer Risks in Women defines what cancer is and what women must know about cancer. It also gives brief insight into common gynecologic conditions that are not cancerous, smoking and cancer risk, human papillomavirus (HPV) and cancer risk, cancer risks associated with hormonal medications, and cancer-causing substances in the environment.

Part II: Breast Cancer begins with statistical data on breast cancer and offers facts about breast cancer including information about risk factors and protective factors. Screening and diagnostic methods, staging, and treatment options are also discussed. Facts about genes associated with breast cancer and pregnancy are also included.

Part III: Gynecologic Cancers discusses cancers of a woman's reproductive organs. Individual chapters include information about symptoms, diagnosis, and treatment of cervical cancer, endometrial cancer, gestational trophoblastic tumors, ovarian cancer, uterine cancer, vaginal cancer, and vulvar cancer.

Part IV: Other Cancers of Special Concern to Women discusses cancers other than gynecologic cancers that have a higher prevalence among women than men or those cancer types responsible for the most cancer-related deaths among women. It provides detailed information on anal cancer, colorectal cancer, gallbladder cancer, bile duct cancer, lung cancer, pancreatic cancer, skin cancer, and thyroid cancer.

Part V: Diagnosing and Treating Cancer covers tests and procedures involved in cancer diagnosis, as well as information about staging and general treatment options including chemotherapy, radiation therapy, biological therapy, biological therapies, stem cell transplant, and other common surgical procedures. It also highlights complementary and alternative medicine (CAM) practices in cancer care. Information on cancer clinical trials are also included.

Part VI: Coping with the Side Effects of Cancer and Cancer Treatments offers practical suggestions for dealing with common adverse effects of various cancer treatments or symptomatic consequences related to the growth of the cancer itself. These side effects include nausea, vomiting, pain, fatigue, gastrointestinal problems, lymphedema, anemia, and neuropathy. It discusses the many side effects of chemotherapy and radiation and how to cope with it. The part concludes with a brief overview of the cognitive-related effects of cancer treatment.

Part VII: Women's Issues in Cancer Survivorship provides supportive information for women who have received a cancer diagnosis. It discusses maintaining the quality of daily life through proper nutrition, exercise, and attention to mental health issues. It also discusses questions about sexual intimacy, fertility, and pregnancy among women who have been treated for gynecologic cancers, and it includes facts about the need for ongoing medical care for long-term well-being.

Part VIII: Additional Help and Information offers a glossary of cancer-related terms, a directory of information resources, and suggestions for finding support groups.

Bibliographic Note

This volume contains documents and excerpts from publications issued by the following government agencies: Centers for Disease Control and Prevention (CDC); Centers for Medicare & Medicaid Services (CMS); *Eunice Kennedy Shriver* National Institute of Child Health and Human Development (NICHD); National Cancer Institute (NCI); National Center for Complementary and Integrative Health (NCCIH); National Institute of Neurological Disorders and Stroke (NINDS); National Institute on Alcohol Abuse and Alcoholism (NIAAA); National Institutes of Health (NIH); National Science Foundation (NSF); Office of Disease Prevention and Health Promotion (ODPHP); Office on Women's Health (OWH); U.S. Department of Veterans Affairs (VA); U.S. Food and Drug Administration (FDA); and U.S. National Library of Medicine (NLM).

It may also contain original material produced by Omnigraphics and reviewed by medical consultants.

About the Health Reference Series

The *Health Reference Series* is designed to provide basic medical information for patients, families, caregivers, and the general public. Each volume takes a particular topic and provides comprehensive coverage. This is especially important for people who may be dealing with a newly diagnosed disease or a chronic disorder in themselves or in a family member. People looking for preventive guidance, information about disease warning signs, medical statistics, and risk factors for health problems will also find answers to their questions in the *Health*

Reference Series. The *Series*, however, is not intended to serve as a tool for diagnosing illness, in prescribing treatments, or as a substitute for the physician/patient relationship. All people concerned about medical symptoms or the possibility of disease are encouraged to seek professional care from an appropriate healthcare provider.

A Note about Spelling and Style

Health Reference Series editors use *Stedman's Medical Dictionary* as an authority for questions related to the spelling of medical terms and the *Chicago Manual of Style* for questions related to grammatical structures, punctuation, and other editorial concerns. Consistent adherence is not always possible, however, because the individual volumes within the *Series* include many documents from a wide variety of different producers, and the editor's primary goal is to present material from each source as accurately as is possible. This sometimes means that information in different chapters or sections may follow other guidelines and alternate spelling authorities. For example, occasionally a copyright holder may require that eponymous terms be shown in possessive forms (Crohn's disease vs. Crohn disease) or that British spelling norms be retained (leukaemia vs. leukemia).

Medical Review

Omnigraphics contracts with a team of qualified, senior medical professionals who serve as medical consultants for the *Health Reference Series*. As necessary, medical consultants review reprinted and originally written material for currency and accuracy. Citations including the phrase, "Reviewed (month, year)" indicate material reviewed by this team. Medical consultation services are provided to the *Health Reference Series* editors by:

Dr. Vijayalakshmi, MBBS, DGO, MD
Dr. Senthil Selvan, MBBS, DCH, MD
Dr. K. Sivanandham, MBBS, DCH, MS (Research), PhD

Our Advisory Board

We would like to thank the following board members for providing initial guidance on the development of this series:

- Dr. Lynda Baker, Associate Professor of Library and Information Science, Wayne State University, Detroit, MI

- Nancy Bulgarelli, William Beaumont Hospital Library, Royal Oak, MI

- Karen Imarisio, Bloomfield Township Public Library, Bloomfield Township, MI

- Karen Morgan, Mardigian Library, University of Michigan-Dearborn, Dearborn, MI

- Rosemary Orlando, St. Clair Shores Public Library, St. Clair Shores, MI

Health Reference Series *Update Policy*

The inaugural book in the *Health Reference Series* was the first edition of *Cancer Sourcebook* published in 1989. Since then, the *Series* has been enthusiastically received by librarians and in the medical community. In order to maintain the standard of providing high-quality health information for the layperson the editorial staff at Omnigraphics felt it was necessary to implement a policy of updating volumes when warranted.

Medical researchers have been making tremendous strides, and it is the purpose of the *Health Reference Series* to stay current with the most recent advances. Each decision to update a volume is made on an individual basis. Some of the considerations include how much new information is available and the feedback we receive from people who use the books. If there is a topic you would like to see added to the update list, or an area of medical concern you feel has not been adequately addressed, please write to:

Managing Editor
Health Reference Series
Omnigraphics
615 Griswold, Ste. 901
Detroit, MI 48226

Part One

Understanding Cancer Risks in Women

Chapter 1

What Women Need to Know about Cancer

Cancer is the name given to a collection of related diseases. In all types of cancer, some of the body's cells begin to divide without stopping and spread into surrounding tissues. Cancer can start almost anywhere in the human body, which is made up of trillions of cells. Normally, human cells grow and divide to form new cells as the body needs them. When cells grow old or become damaged, they die, and new cells take their place.

When cancer develops, however, this orderly process breaks down. As cells become more and more abnormal, old or damaged cells survive when they should die, and new cells form when they are not needed. These extra cells can divide without stopping and may form growths called tumors.

This chapter contains text excerpted from the following sources: Text in this chapter begins with excerpts from "What Is Cancer?" National Cancer Institute (NCI), February 9, 2015; Text beginning with the heading "Factors That Are Known to Increase the Risk of Cancer" is excerpted from "Cancer Prevention Overview (PDQ®)—Patient Version," National Cancer Institute (NCI), August 11, 2017; Text under the heading "Cancer and Women" is excerpted from "Cancer Prevention and Control—Cancer and Women," Centers for Disease Control and Prevention (CDC), May 8, 2017; Text under the heading "Cancer among Women" is excerpted from "Cancer Prevention and Control—Cancer among Women," Centers for Disease Control and Prevention (CDC), June 5, 2017; Text under the heading "A Survivor's Wellness Plan" is excerpted from "Staying Healthy after Cancer Treatment," Centers for Disease Control and Prevention (CDC), April 19, 2018.

Many cancers form solid tumors, which are masses of tissue. Cancers of the blood, such as leukemias, generally do not form solid tumors. Cancerous tumors are malignant, which means they can spread into, or invade, nearby tissues. In addition, as these tumors grow, some cancer cells can break off and travel to distant places in the body through the blood or the lymph system and form new tumors far from the original tumor. Unlike malignant tumors, benign tumors do not spread into, or invade, nearby tissues. Benign tumors can sometimes be quite large, however. When removed, they usually don't grow back, whereas malignant tumors sometimes do. Unlike most benign tumors elsewhere in the body, benign brain tumors can be life-threatening.

Differences between Cancer Cells and Normal Cells

Cancer cells differ from normal cells in many ways that allow them to grow out of control and become invasive. One important difference is that cancer cells are less specialized than normal cells. That is, whereas normal cells mature into very distinct cell types with specific functions, cancer cells do not. This is one reason that, unlike normal cells, cancer cells continue to divide without stopping.

In addition, cancer cells are able to ignore signals that normally tell cells to stop dividing or that begin a process known as programmed cell death, or apoptosis, which the body uses to get rid of unneeded cells.

Cancer cells may be able to influence the normal cells, molecules, and blood vessels that surround and feed a tumor—an area known as the microenvironment. For instance, cancer cells can induce nearby normal cells to form blood vessels that supply tumors with oxygen and nutrients, which they need to grow. These blood vessels also remove waste products from tumors.

Cancer cells are also often able to evade the immune system, a network of organs, tissues, and specialized cells that protects the body from infections and other conditions. Although the immune system normally removes damaged or abnormal cells from the body, some cancer cells are able to "hide" from the immune system.

Tumors can also use the immune system to stay alive and grow. For example, with the help of certain immune system cells that normally prevent a runaway immune response, cancer cells can actually keep the immune system from killing cancer cells.

4

How Cancer Arises

Cancer is a genetic disease—that is, it is caused by changes to genes that control the way our cells function, especially how they grow and divide. Genetic changes that cause cancer can be inherited from our parents. They can also arise during a person's lifetime as a result of errors that occur as cells divide or because of damage to deoxyribonucleic acid (DNA) caused by certain environmental exposures. Cancer-causing environmental exposures include substances, such as the chemicals in tobacco smoke, and radiation, such as ultraviolet (UV) rays from the sun.

Each person's cancer has a unique combination of genetic changes. As the cancer continues to grow, additional changes will occur. Even within the same tumor, different cells may have different genetic changes. In general, cancer cells have more genetic changes, such as mutations in DNA, than normal cells. Some of these changes may have nothing to do with the cancer; they may be the result of the cancer, rather than its cause.

"Drivers" of Cancer

The genetic changes that contribute to cancer tend to affect three main types of genes—proto-oncogenes, tumor suppressor genes, and DNA repair genes. These changes are sometimes called "drivers" of cancer. Proto-oncogenes are involved in normal cell growth and division. However, when these genes are altered in certain ways or are more active than normal, they may become cancer-causing genes (or oncogenes), allowing cells to grow and survive when they should not.

Tumor suppressor genes are also involved in controlling cell growth and division. Cells with certain alterations in tumor suppressor genes may divide in an uncontrolled manner. DNA repair genes are involved in fixing damaged DNA. Cells with mutations in these genes tend to develop additional mutations in other genes. Together, these mutations may cause the cells to become cancerous.

As scientists have learned more about the molecular changes that lead to cancer, they have found that certain mutations commonly occur in many types of cancer. Because of this, cancers are sometimes characterized by the types of genetic alterations that are believed to be driving them, not just by where they develop in the body and how the cancer cells look under the microscope.

When Cancer Spreads

A cancer that has spread from the place where it first started to another place in the body is called metastatic cancer. The process by which cancer cells spread to other parts of the body is called metastasis. Metastatic cancer has the same name and the same type of cancer cells as the original, or primary, cancer. For example, breast cancer that spreads to and forms a metastatic tumor in the lung is metastatic breast cancer, not lung cancer.

Under a microscope, metastatic cancer cells generally look the same as cells of the original cancer. Moreover, metastatic cancer cells and cells of the original cancer usually have some molecular features in common, such as the presence of specific chromosome changes. Treatment may help prolong the lives of some people with metastatic cancer. In general, though, the primary goal of treatments for metastatic cancer is to control the growth of the cancer or to relieve symptoms caused by it. Metastatic tumors can cause severe damage to how the body functions, and most people who die of cancer die of metastatic disease.

Tissue Changes That Are Not Cancer

Not every change in the body's tissues is cancer. Some tissue changes may develop into cancer if they are not treated, however. Here are some examples of tissue changes that are not cancer but, in some cases, are monitored:

Hyperplasia occurs when cells within a tissue divide faster than normal and extra cells build up, or proliferate. However, the cells and the way the tissue is organized look normal under a microscope. Hyperplasia can be caused by several factors or conditions, including chronic irritation.

Dysplasia is a more serious condition than hyperplasia. In dysplasia, there is also a buildup of extra cells. But the cells look abnormal and there are changes in how the tissue is organized. In general, the more abnormal the cells and tissue look, the greater the chance that cancer will form.

Some types of dysplasia may need to be monitored or treated. An example of dysplasia is an abnormal mole (called a dysplastic nevus) that forms on the skin. A dysplastic nevus can turn into melanoma, although most do not.

An even more serious condition is carcinoma in situ. Although it is sometimes called cancer, carcinoma in situ is not cancer because the abnormal cells do not spread beyond the original tissue. That is, they do not invade nearby tissue the way that cancer cells do. But, because some carcinomas in situ may become cancer, they are usually treated.

Factors That Are Known to Increase the Risk of Cancer

Cigarette Smoking and Tobacco Use

Tobacco use is strongly linked to an increased risk for many kinds of cancer. Smoking cigarettes are the leading cause of the following types of cancer:

- Acute myelogenous leukemia (AML)
- Bladder cancer
- Esophageal cancer
- Kidney cancer
- Lung cancer
- Oral cavity cancer
- Pancreatic cancer
- Stomach cancer

Not smoking or quitting smoking lowers the risk of getting cancer and dying from cancer. Scientists believe that cigarette smoking causes about 30 percent of all cancer deaths in the United States.

Infections

Certain viruses and bacteria can cause cancer. Viruses and other infection-causing agents cause more cases of cancer in the developing world (about 1 in 4 cases of cancer) than in developed nations (less than 1 in 10 cases of cancer). Examples of cancer-causing viruses and bacteria include:

- Human papillomavirus (HPV) increases the risk for cancers of the cervix, penis, vagina, anus, and oropharynx
- Hepatitis B and hepatitis C viruses increase the risk for liver cancer
- Epstein-Barr virus increases the risk for Burkitt lymphoma
- *Helicobacter pylori* increases the risk for gastric cancer

Two vaccines to prevent infection by cancer-causing agents have already been developed and approved by the U.S. Food and Drug Administration (FDA). One is a vaccine to prevent infection with hepatitis B virus. The other protects against infection with strains of HPV that cause cervical cancer. Scientists continue to work on vaccines against infections that cause cancer.

Radiation

Being exposed to radiation is a known cause of cancer. There are two main types of radiation linked with an increased risk for cancer:

- UV radiation from sunlight: This is the main cause of nonmelanoma skin cancers.
  - Ionizing radiation including:
    - Medical radiation from tests to diagnose cancer such as X-rays, computed tomography (CT) or computed axial tomography (CAT) scans, fluoroscopy, and nuclear medicine scans
    - Radon gas in our homes

Scientists believe that ionizing radiation causes leukemia, thyroid cancer, and breast cancer in women. Ionizing radiation may also be linked to myeloma and cancers of the lung, stomach, colon, esophagus, bladder, and ovary. Being exposed to radiation from diagnostic X-rays increases the risk of cancer in patients and X-ray technicians. The growing use of CT scans over the last 20 years has increased exposure to ionizing radiation. The risk of cancer also increases with the number of CT scans a patient has and the radiation dose used each time.

Immunosuppressive Medicines after Organ Transplant

Immunosuppressive medicines are used after an organ has been transplanted from one person to another. These medicines stop an organ that has been transplanted from being rejected. These medicines decrease the body's immune response to help keep the organ from being rejected. Immunosuppressive medicines are linked to an increased risk of cancer because they lower the body's ability to keep cancer from forming.

Factors That May Affect the Risk of Cancer

Diet

The foods that you eat on a regular basis make up your diet. Diet is being studied as a risk factor for cancer. It is hard to study the effects of diet on cancer because a person's diet includes foods that may protect against cancer and foods that may increase the risk of cancer.

It is also hard for people who take part in the studies to keep track of what they eat over a long period of time. This may explain why studies have different results about how diet affects the risk of cancer.

Some studies show that fruits and nonstarchy vegetables may protect against cancers of the mouth, esophagus, and stomach. Fruits may also protect against lung cancer.

Some studies have shown that a diet high in fat, proteins, calories, and red meat increases the risk of colorectal cancer, but other studies have not shown this.

It is not known if a diet low in fat and high in fiber, fruits, and vegetables lowers the risk of colorectal cancer.

Alcohol

Studies have shown that drinking alcohol is linked to an increased risk of the following types of cancers in women:

- Oral cancer

- Esophageal cancer

- Breast cancer

Drinking alcohol may also increase the risk of liver cancer and female colorectal cancer.

Physical Activity

Studies show that people who are physically active have a lower risk of certain cancers than those who are not. It is not known if physical activity itself is the reason for this.

Studies show a strong link between physical activity and a lower risk of colorectal cancer. Some studies show that physical activity protects against postmenopausal breast cancer and endometrial cancer.

Obesity

Studies show that obesity is linked to a higher risk of the following types of cancer:

- Postmenopausal breast cancer
- Colorectal cancer
- Endometrial cancer
- Esophageal cancer
- Kidney cancer
- Pancreatic cancer

Some studies show that obesity is also a risk factor for cancer of the gallbladder and liver cancer. It is not known if losing weight lowers the risk of cancers that have been linked to obesity.

Diabetes

Some studies show that having diabetes may slightly increase the risk of having the following types of cancer:

- Bladder cancer
- Breast cancer in women
- Colorectal cancer
- Endometrial cancer
- Liver cancer
- Lung cancer
- Oral cancer
- Oropharyngeal cancer
- Ovarian cancer
- Pancreatic cancer

Diabetes and cancer share some of the same risk factors. These risk factors include the following:

- Being older
- Being obese

- Smoking

- Not eating a healthy diet

- Not exercising

Because diabetes and cancer share these risk factors, it is hard to know whether the risk of cancer is increased more by diabetes or by these risk factors.

Studies are being done to see how medicine that is used to treat diabetes affects cancer risk.

Environmental Risk Factors

Being exposed to chemicals and other substances in the environment has been linked to some cancers:

- Links between air pollution and cancer risk have been found. These include links between lung cancer and secondhand tobacco smoke, outdoor air pollution, and asbestos.

- Drinking water that contains a large amount of arsenic has been linked to skin, bladder, and lung cancers.

Studies have been done to see if pesticides and other pollutants increase the risk of cancer. The results of those studies have been unclear because other factors can change the results of the studies.

Cancer and Women

Every year, cancer claims the lives of more than a quarter of a million women in America. You can lower your cancer risk in several ways.

Fast Facts about Cancer and Women

- The most common kinds of cancer among women in the United States are skin cancer, breast cancer, lung cancer, colorectal cancer, and uterine cancer.

- The HPV vaccine is available for girls and women who are 9–26 years old. It protects against the types of HPV that most often cause cervical and other kinds of cancer.

- Most breast cancers are found in women who are 50 years old or older, but breast cancer also affects younger women.

What You Can Do

- **Don't smoke and avoid secondhand smoke.** More women in the United States die from lung cancer than any other kind of cancer, and cigarette smoking causes most cases.

- **Get recommended screening tests for breast, cervical, colorectal, and lung cancer.** Screening tests are the best way to find these cancers early, when they are easier to treat. Lung cancer screening is recommended only for certain people who are at high risk.

- **Protect your skin from the sun and avoid indoor tanning.** Skin cancer is the most common cancer in the United States. Most cases of melanoma, the deadliest kind of skin cancer, are caused by exposure to UV light from the sun and indoor tanning devices.

- **Stay active and eat healthfully.** Making healthy choices like eating a diet rich in fruits and vegetables, getting regular physical activity, and limiting alcohol consumption can help lower your risk for several kinds of cancer.

Cancer among Women

Three Most Common Cancers among Women

The numbers in parentheses are the rates per 100,000 women of all races and Hispanic* origins combined in the United States.

*Hispanic origin is not mutually exclusive from race categories (white, black, Asian/Pacific Islander, American Indian/Alaska Native).

Breast cancer (123.9)

- First among women of all races and Hispanic* origin populations.

Lung cancer (50.8)

- Second among white, black, Asian/Pacific Islander, and American Indian/Alaska Native women.

- Third among Hispanic* women.

Colorectal cancer (32.8)

- Second among Hispanic* women.

- Third among white, black, Asian/Pacific Islander, and American Indian/Alaska Native women.

Leading Causes of Cancer Death among Women

Lung cancer (34.7)

- First among white, black, Asian/Pacific Islander, and American Indian/Alaska Native women.

- Second among Hispanic* women.

Breast cancer (20.5)

- First among Hispanic* women.

- Second among white, black, Asian/Pacific Islander, and American Indian/Alaska Native women.

Colorectal cancer (11.9)

- Third among women of all races and Hispanic* origin populations.

A Survivor's Wellness Plan

When your treatment is finished, your doctor may tell you that you should get checkups or tests in the future. This is called *follow-up care*. Be sure to follow your doctor's instructions. These tests can help find early signs of a new or the same cancer.

You can lower your risk of getting cancer again or having the cancer come back by making healthy choices like:

- Staying away from tobacco. If you smoke, try to quit, and stay away from other people's smoke.

- Limiting the amount of alcohol you drink

- Protecting your skin from exposure to ultraviolet rays from the sun and tanning beds

- Eating lots of fruits and vegetables

- Keeping a healthy weight

- Being physically active

- Getting a flu shot every year

Chapter 2

Common Gynecologic Conditions That Are Not Indicative of Cancer

Uterine Fibroids

Fibroids are muscular tumors that grow in the wall of the uterus (womb). Fibroids are almost always benign (not cancerous). Not all women with fibroids have symptoms. Women who do have symptoms often find fibroids hard to live with. Some have pain and heavy menstrual bleeding. Treatment for uterine fibroids depends on your symptoms.

This chapter contains text excerpted from the following sources: Text under the heading "Uterine Fibroids" is excerpted from "Uterine Fibroids," Office on Women's Health (OWH), U.S. Department of Health and Human Services (HHS), March 16, 2018; Text under the heading "Endometriosis" is excerpted from "Endometriosis," Office on Women's Health (OWH), U.S. Department of Health and Human Services (HHS), March 16, 2018; Text under the heading "Pelvic Organ Prolapse" is excerpted from "Pelvic Organ Prolapse," Office on Women's Health (OWH), U.S. Department of Health and Human Services (HHS), November 28, 2017; Text under the heading "Ovarian Cysts" is excerpted from "Ovarian Cysts," Office on Women's Health (OWH), U.S. Department of Health and Human Services (HHS), April 28, 2017; Text under the heading "Polycystic Ovary Syndrome (PCOS)" is excerpted from "Polycystic Ovary Syndrome," Office on Women's Health (OWH), U.S. Department of Health and Human Services (HHS), July 26, 2017;

About 20–80 percent of women develop fibroids by the time they reach age 50. Fibroids are most common in women in their 40s and early 50s. Not all women with fibroids have symptoms. Women who do have symptoms often find fibroids hard to live with. Some have pain and heavy menstrual bleeding. Fibroids also can put pressure on the bladder, causing frequent urination, or the rectum, causing rectal pressure. Should the fibroids get very large, they can cause the abdomen (stomach area) to enlarge, making a woman look pregnant.

Endometriosis

Endometriosis happens when the lining of the uterus (womb) grows outside of the uterus. It may affect more than 11 percent of American women between 15 and 44. It is especially common among women in their 30s and 40s and may make it harder to get pregnant. Several different treatment options can help manage the symptoms and improve your chances of getting pregnant.

Endometriosis, sometimes called "endo," is a common health problem in women. It gets its name from the word endometrium, the tissue that normally lines the uterus or womb. Endometriosis happens when this tissue grows outside of your uterus and on other areas in your body where it doesn't belong.

Most often, endometriosis is found on the:

- Ovaries

- Fallopian tubes

- Tissues that hold the uterus in place

- Outer surface of the uterus

Text under the heading "Pelvic Inflammatory Disease (PID)" is excerpted from "Pelvic Inflammatory Disease—CDC Fact Sheet," Centers for Disease Control and Prevention (CDC), December 11, 2015; Text under the heading "Period Problems" is excerpted from "Period Problems," Office on Women's Health (OWH), U.S. Department of Health and Human Services (HHS), March 16, 2018; Text under the heading "Heavy Menstrual Bleeding" is excerpted from "Bleeding Disorders in Women—Heavy Menstrual Bleeding," Centers for Disease Control and Prevention (CDC), December 20, 2017; Text under the heading "Pelvic Pain" is excerpted from "Pelvic Pain," *Eunice Kennedy Shriver* National Institute of Child Health and Human Development (NICHD), January 31, 2017; Text under the heading "Interstitial Cystitis" is excerpted from "Reproductive Health—Common Reproductive Health Concerns for Women," Centers for Disease Control and Prevention (CDC), November 29, 2016.

Other sites for growths can include the vagina, cervix, vulva, bowel, bladder, or rectum. Rarely, endometriosis appears in other parts of the body, such as the lungs, brain, and skin.

Pelvic Organ Prolapse

Pelvic organ prolapse happens when the muscles and tissues supporting the pelvic organs (the uterus, bladder, or rectum) become weak or loose. This allows one or more of the pelvic organs to drop or press into or out of the vagina. Many women are embarrassed to talk to their doctor about their symptoms or think that their symptoms are normal. But pelvic organ prolapse is treatable.

The pelvic muscles and tissues support the pelvic organs like a hammock. The pelvic organs include the bladder, uterus and cervix, vagina, and rectum, which is part of the bowel. A prolapse happens when the pelvis muscles and tissues can no longer support these organs because the muscles and tissues are weak or damaged. This causes one or more pelvic organs to drop or press into or out of the vagina.

Pelvic organ prolapse is a type of pelvic floor disorder. The most common pelvic floor disorders are:

- Urinary incontinence (leaking of urine)

- Fecal incontinence (leaking of stool)

- Pelvic organ prolapse (weakening of the muscles and tissues supporting the organs in the pelvis)

Pelvic floor disorders (urinary incontinence, fecal incontinence, and pelvic organ prolapse) affect one in five women in the United States. Pelvic organ prolapse is less common than urinary or fecal incontinence but affects almost 3 percent of U.S. women. Pelvic organ prolapse happens more often in older women and in white and Hispanic women than in younger women or women of other racial and ethnic groups.

Some women develop more than one pelvic floor disorder, such as pelvic organ prolapse with urinary incontinence.

Ovarian Cysts

Ovarian cysts are fluid-filled sacs in the ovary. They are common and usually form during ovulation. Ovulation happens when the ovary releases an egg each month. Many women with ovarian cysts don't have symptoms. The cysts are usually harmless.

Ovarian cysts are common in women with regular periods. In fact, most women make at least one follicle or corpus luteum cyst every month. You may not be aware that you have a cyst unless there is a problem that causes the cyst to grow or if multiple cysts form. About 8 percent of premenopausal women develop large cysts that need treatment.

Ovarian cysts are less common after menopause. Postmenopausal women with ovarian cysts are at higher risk for ovarian cancer.

At any age, see your doctor if you think you have a cyst. See your doctor also if you have symptoms such as bloating, needing to urinate more often, pelvic pressure or pain, or abnormal (unusual) vaginal bleeding. These can be signs of a cyst or other serious problem.

Polycystic Ovary Syndrome (PCOS)

Polycystic ovary syndrome (PCOS), also known as polycystic ovarian syndrome, is a common health problem caused by an imbalance of reproductive hormones. The hormonal imbalance creates problems in the ovaries. The ovaries make the egg that is released each month as part of a healthy menstrual cycle. With PCOS, the egg may not develop as it should or it may not be released during ovulation as it should be.

PCOS is a health problem that affects one in 10 women of childbearing age. Women with PCOS have a hormonal imbalance and metabolism problems that may affect their overall health and appearance. PCOS is also a common and treatable cause of infertility.

Between 5 percent and 10 percent of women of childbearing age (between 15 and 44) have PCOS. Most often, women find out they have PCOS in their 20s and 30s, when they have problems getting pregnant and see their doctor. But PCOS can happen at any age after puberty.

Women of all races and ethnicities are at risk for PCOS, but your risk for PCOS may be higher if you are obese or if you have a mother, sister, or aunt with PCOS.

Pelvic Inflammatory Disease (PID)

Pelvic inflammatory disease (PID) is an infection of a woman's reproductive organs. It is a complication often caused by some sexually transmitted diseases (STDs), like chlamydia and gonorrhea. Other infections that are not sexually transmitted can also cause PID.

Untreated STDs can cause PID, a serious condition, in women. 1 in 8 women with a history of PID experience difficulties getting pregnant.

Period Problems

Regular periods are a sign that your body is working normally. You should have regular periods unless you are pregnant, breastfeeding, postmenopausal, or have a medical condition that causes your periods to stop. Irregular, painful, or heavy periods may be signs of a serious health problem. Irregular periods also can make it harder to get pregnant. Your doctor can work with you to help get your periods more regular.

Heavy Menstrual Bleeding

Menorrhagia is menstrual bleeding that lasts more than 7 days. It can also be bleeding that is very heavy. How do you know if you have heavy bleeding? If you need to change your tampon or pad after less than 2 hours or you pass clots the size of a quarter or larger, that is heavy bleeding. If you have this type of bleeding, you should see a doctor.

Untreated heavy or prolonged bleeding can stop you from living your life to the fullest. It also can cause anemia. Anemia is a common blood problem that can leave you feeling tired or weak. If you have a bleeding problem, it could lead to other health problems. Sometimes treatments, such as dilation and curettage (D&C) or a hysterectomy, might be done when these procedures could have been avoided.

Heavy bleeding (menorrhagia) is one of the most common problems women report to their doctors. It affects more than 10 million American women each year. This means that about one out of every five women has it.

Pelvic Pain

"Pelvic pain" is a general term used to describe the pain that occurs mostly or only in the region below a woman's belly button. This type of pain is a common reason women seek medical care. The pain can be steady, or it can come and go. Severe pain can interfere with daily living and quality of life.

Researchers are not sure exactly how many women in the United States have chronic pelvic pain.

Because it is often linked to other disorders, such as endometriosis or vulvodynia, chronic pelvic pain may be misdiagnosed as another condition, making it difficult to estimate reliable prevalence rates for pelvic pain. According to one study, about 15 percent of women of

19

childbearing age in the United States reported having pelvic pain that lasted at least 6 months. Worldwide, the rates of chronic pelvic pain for women of childbearing age range from 14–32 percent. Between 13 percent and 32 percent of these women have pain that is severe enough to cause them to miss work.

Interstitial Cystitis (IC)

Interstitial cystitis (IC) is a chronic bladder condition resulting in recurring discomfort or pain in the bladder or surrounding pelvic region. People with IC usually have inflamed or irritated bladder walls that can cause scarring and stiffening of the bladder. IC can affect anyone; however, it is more common in women than men. Some people have some or none of the following symptoms:

- Abdominal or pelvic mild discomfort
- Frequent urination
- A feeling of urgency to urinate
- A feeling of abdominal or pelvic pressure
- Tenderness
- Intense pain in the bladder or pelvic region
- Severe lower abdominal pain that intensifies as the urinary bladder fills or empties

Chapter 3

Does Cancer Run in Your Family?

What Are Gene Families?

A gene family is a group of genes that share important characteristics. In many cases, genes in a family share a similar sequence of DNA building blocks (nucleotides). These genes provide instructions for making products (such as proteins) that have a similar structure or function. In other cases, dissimilar genes are grouped together in a family because proteins produced from these genes work together as a unit or participate in the same process.

Classifying individual genes into families helps researchers describe how genes are related to each other. Researchers can use gene families to predict the function of newly identified genes based on their similarity to known genes. Similarities among genes in a family can also be used to predict where and when a specific gene is active (expressed).

This chapter contains text excerpted from the following sources: Text under the heading "What Are Gene Families?" is excerpted from "What Are Gene Families?" Genetics Home Reference (GHR), National Institutes of Health (NIH), May 1, 2018; Text beginning with the heading "Breast or Ovarian Cancer" is excerpted from "Does Breast or Ovarian Cancer Run in Your Family?" Centers for Disease Control and Prevention (CDC), October 18, 2017; Text beginning with the heading "What Is Genetic Testing?" is excerpted from "Genetic Testing for Hereditary Cancer Syndromes," National Cancer Institute (NCI), April 11, 2013. Reviewed May 2018.

Additionally, gene families may provide clues for identifying genes that are involved in particular diseases.

Sometimes not enough is known about a gene to assign it to an established family. In other cases, genes may fit into more than one family. No formal guidelines define the criteria for grouping genes together. Classification systems for genes continue to evolve as scientists learn more about the structure and function of genes and the relationships between them.

Breast or Ovarian Cancer

If you have close relatives with breast or ovarian cancer, you may be at higher risk for developing these diseases. Does your family health history put you at higher risk? Would you benefit from cancer genetic counseling and testing?

Each year, over 200,000 women in the United States are diagnosed with breast cancer and more than 20,000 are diagnosed with ovarian cancer. About 3 percent of breast cancers (about 6,000 women per year) and 10 percent of ovarian cancers (about 2,000 women per year) result from inherited mutations (changes) in the *BRCA1* and *BRCA2* genes that are passed on in families. Inherited mutations in other genes can also cause breast and ovarian cancer, but *BRCA1* and *BRCA2* are the genes most commonly affected. Knowing your family health history can help you find out if you could be more likely to develop breast, ovarian, and other cancers. If so, you can take steps to prevent cancer or to detect it earlier when it may be more treatable.

Does Your Family Health History Put You at Risk?

Collect your family health history of breast, ovarian, and other cancers and share this information with your doctor. You can inherit *BRCA* and other mutations from your mother or your father, so be sure to include information from both sides of your family. Include your close relatives: parents, sisters, brothers, children, grandparents, aunts, uncles, nieces, nephews, and grandchildren. If you have had breast, ovarian, or other cancers, make sure that your family members know about your diagnosis.

Tell your doctor if you have a personal or family health history of any of the following:

- Breast cancer, especially at a younger age (age 50 or younger)

- Triple negative breast cancer at age 60 or younger in women (Triple negative cancers are a type of breast cancer that lack estrogen receptors, progesterone receptors, and human epidermal growth factor receptor 2.)

- Cancer in both breasts
- Breast cancer in a male relative
- Ovarian, fallopian tube, or primary peritoneal cancer
- Pancreatic cancer or high-grade prostate cancer
- Breast, ovarian, pancreatic, or high-grade prostate cancer among multiple blood relatives
- Ashkenazi (Eastern European) Jewish ancestry
- A known *BRCA* mutation in the family

You can use the *BRCA* tool to collect your family health history information, assess your risk for *BRCA* mutations, and share this information with your doctor. Update your family health history on a regular basis and let your doctor know if any new cases of breast or ovarian cancer occur.

What Can You Do If You Are Concerned about Your Risk?

If your doctor decides that your family health history makes you more likely to get breast, ovarian, and other cancers, he or she may refer you for genetic counseling. Even if your doctor doesn't recommend genetic testing and counseling, your family health history of breast cancer can affect when you start mammography screening. If you are a woman with a parent, sibling, or child with breast cancer, you are at higher risk for breast cancer. Based on current recommendations, you should consider talking to your doctor about starting mammography screening in your 40s.

The genetic counselor can use your family health history information to determine your possible cancer risks and whether you might consider *BRCA* genetic testing to find out if you have a *BRCA1* or *BRCA2* mutation. Genetic testing is most useful if first performed on someone in your family who has had breast or ovarian cancer. If this relative has a *BRCA1* or *BRCA2* mutation, then her close relatives can be offered testing for that mutation. If she does not have a *BRCA1* or *BRCA2* mutation, then her relatives may not need to be tested. Remember that most breast and ovarian cancer is not caused by *BRCA* mutations so most women don't need *BRCA* genetic testing.

The genetic counselor can discuss the pros and cons of testing and what possible test results could mean for you and your family. It is important to note that genetic testing for *BRCA* mutations will not find all causes of hereditary breast or ovarian cancer. In some cases, the genetic counselor might recommend genetic testing using a panel that looks for mutations in several genes in addition to *BRCA1* and *BRCA2*. *BRCA* genetic counseling and testing is often, but not always, covered without cost sharing by many health plans under the Affordable Care Act (ACA).

What Is Genetic Testing?

Genetic testing looks for specific inherited changes (mutations) in a person's chromosomes, genes, or proteins. Genetic mutations can have harmful, beneficial, neutral (no effect), or uncertain effects on health. Mutations that are harmful may increase a person's chance, or risk, of developing a disease such as cancer. Overall, inherited mutations are thought to play a role in about 5–10 percent of all cancers.

Cancer can sometimes appear to "run in families" even if it is not caused by an inherited mutation. For example, a shared environment or lifestyle, such as tobacco use, can cause similar cancers to develop among family members. However, certain patterns—such as the types of cancer that develop, other noncancer conditions that are seen, and the ages at which cancer typically develops—may suggest the presence of a hereditary cancer syndrome.

The genetic mutations that cause many of the known hereditary cancer syndromes have been identified, and genetic testing can confirm whether a condition is, indeed, the result of an inherited syndrome. Genetic testing is also done to determine whether family members without obvious illness have inherited the same mutation as a family member who is known to carry a cancer-associated mutation.

Inherited genetic mutations can increase a person's risk of developing cancer through a variety of mechanisms, depending on the function of the gene. Mutations in genes that control cell growth and the repair of damaged deoxyribonucleic acid (DNA) are particularly likely to be associated with increased cancer risk.

Genetic testing of tumor samples can also be performed, but this chapter does not cover such testing.

Does Someone Who Inherits a Cancer-Predisposing Mutation Always Get Cancer?

No. Even if a cancer-predisposing mutation is present in a family, it does not necessarily mean that everyone who inherits the mutation will develop cancer. Several factors influence the outcome in a given person with the mutation.

One factor is the pattern of inheritance of the cancer syndrome. To understand how hereditary cancer syndromes may be inherited, it is helpful to keep in mind that every person has two copies of most genes, with one copy inherited from each parent. Most mutations involved in hereditary cancer syndromes are inherited in one of two main patterns: autosomal dominant and autosomal recessive.

With autosomal dominant inheritance, a single altered copy of the gene is enough to increase a person's chances of developing cancer. In this case, the parent from whom the mutation was inherited may also show the effects of the gene mutation. The parent may also be referred to as a carrier.

With autosomal recessive inheritance, a person has an increased risk of cancer only if he or she inherits a mutant (altered) copy of the gene from each parent. The parents, who each carry one copy of the altered gene along with a normal (unaltered) copy, do not usually have an increased risk of cancer themselves. However, because they can pass the altered gene to their children, they are called carriers.

A third form of inheritance of cancer-predisposing mutations is X-linked recessive inheritance. Males have a single X chromosome, which they inherit from their mothers, and females have two X chromosomes (one from each parent). A female with a recessive cancer-predisposing mutation on one of her X chromosomes and a normal copy of the gene on her other X chromosome is a carrier but will not have an increased risk of cancer. Her sons, however, will have only the altered copy of the gene and will, therefore, have an increased risk of cancer.

Even when people have one copy of a dominant cancer-predisposing mutation, two copies of a recessive mutation, or, for males, one copy of an X-linked recessive mutation, they may not develop cancer. Some mutations are "incompletely penetrant," which means that only some people will show the effects of these mutations. Mutations can also "vary in their expressivity," which means that the severity of the symptoms may vary from person to person.

What Genetic Tests Are Available for Cancer Risk?

More than 50 hereditary cancer syndromes have been described. The majority of these are caused by highly penetrant mutations that are inherited in a dominant fashion. The list below includes some of the more common inherited cancer syndromes for which genetic testing is available, the gene(s) that are mutated in each syndrome, and the cancer types most often associated with these syndromes.

Hereditary Breast Cancer and Ovarian Cancer Syndrome

- Genes: *BRCA1, BRCA2*
- Related cancer types: Female breast, ovarian, and other cancers

Li-Fraumeni Syndrome

- Gene: *TP53*
- Related cancer types: Breast cancer, soft tissue sarcoma, osteosarcoma (bone cancer), leukemia, brain tumors, adrenocortical carcinoma (cancer of the adrenal glands), and other cancers

Cowden Syndrome (PTEN Hamartoma Tumor Syndrome)

- Gene: *PTEN*
- Related cancer types: Breast, thyroid, endometrial (uterine lining), and other cancers

Lynch Syndrome (Hereditary Nonpolyposis Colorectal Cancer)

- Genes: *MSH2, MLH1, MSH6, PMS2, EPCAM*
- Related cancer types: Colorectal, endometrial, ovarian, renal pelvis, pancreatic, small intestine, liver and biliary tract, stomach, brain, and breast cancers

Familial Adenomatous Polyposis

- Gene: *APC*
- Related cancer types: Colorectal cancer, multiple nonmalignant colon polyps, and both noncancerous (benign) and cancerous tumors in the small intestine, brain, stomach, bone, skin, and other tissues

Retinoblastoma

- Gene: *RB1*
- Related cancer types: Eye cancer (cancer of the retina), pinealoma (cancer of the pineal gland), osteosarcoma, melanoma, and soft tissue sarcoma

Multiple Endocrine Neoplasia Type 1 (Wermer Syndrome)

- Gene: *MEN1*
- Related cancer types: Pancreatic endocrine tumors and (usually benign) parathyroid and pituitary gland tumors

Multiple Endocrine Neoplasia Type 2

- Gene: *RET*
- Related cancer types: Medullary thyroid cancer and pheochromocytoma (benign adrenal gland tumor)

Von Hippel-Lindau Syndrome

- Gene: *VHL*
- Related cancer types: Kidney cancer and multiple noncancerous tumors, including pheochromocytoma

Who Should Consider Genetic Testing for Cancer Risk?

Many experts recommend that genetic testing for cancer risk should be strongly considered when all three of the following criteria are met:

- The person being tested has a personal or family history that suggests an inherited cancer risk condition.
- The test results can be adequately interpreted (that is, they can clearly tell whether a specific genetic change is present or absent).
- The results provide information that will help guide a person's future medical care.

The features of a person's personal or family medical history that, particularly in combination, may suggest a hereditary cancer syndrome include:

- Cancer that was diagnosed at an unusually young age
- Several different types of cancer that have occurred independently in the same person
- Cancer that has developed in a set of paired organs, such as both kidneys or both breasts

- Several close blood relatives that have the same type of cancer (for example, a mother, daughter, and sisters with breast cancer)

- Unusual cases of a specific cancer type (for example, breast cancer in a man)

- The presence of birth defects, such as certain noncancerous (benign) skin growths or skeletal abnormalities, that are known to be associated with inherited cancer syndromes

- Being a member of a racial/ethnic group that is known to have an increased chance of having a certain hereditary cancer syndrome and having one or more of the above features as well

It is strongly recommended that a person who is considering genetic testing speak with a professional trained in genetics before deciding whether to be tested. These professionals can include doctors, genetic counselors, and other healthcare providers (such as nurses, psychologists, or social workers). Genetic counseling can help people consider the risks, benefits, and limitations of genetic testing in their particular situation. Sometimes the genetic professional finds that testing is not needed.

Genetic counseling includes a detailed review of the individual's personal and family medical history related to possible cancer risk. Counseling also includes discussions about such issues as:

- Whether genetic testing is appropriate, which specific test(s) might be used, and the technical accuracy of the test(s)

- The medical implications of a positive or a negative test result

- The possibility that a test result might not be informative—that is, that the information may not be useful in making healthcare decisions

- The psychological risks and benefits of learning one's genetic test results

- The risk of passing a genetic mutation (if one is present in a parent) to children

Learning about these issues is a key part of the informed consent process. Written informed consent is strongly recommended before a genetic test is ordered. People give their consent by signing a form saying that they have been told about, and understand, the purpose of the test, its medical implications, the risks and benefits of the test, possible alternatives to the test, and their privacy rights.

Unlike most other medical tests, genetic tests can reveal information not only about the person being tested but also about that person's relatives. The presence of a harmful genetic mutation in one family member makes it more likely that other blood relatives may also carry the same mutation. Family relationships can be affected when one member of a family discloses genetic test results that may have implications for other family members. Family members may have very different opinions about how useful it is to learn whether they do or do not have a disease-related genetic mutation. Health discussions may get complicated when some family members know their genetic status while other family members do not choose to know their test results. A conversation with genetics professionals may help family members better understand the complicated choices they may face.

How Is Genetic Testing Done?

Genetic tests are usually requested by a person's doctor or other healthcare provider. Although it may be possible to obtain some genetic tests without a healthcare provider's order, this approach is not recommended because it does not give the patient the valuable opportunity to discuss this complicated decision with a knowledgeable professional. Testing is done on a small sample of body fluid or tissue—usually blood, but sometimes saliva, cells from inside the cheek, skin cells, or amniotic fluid (the fluid surrounding a developing fetus).

The sample is then sent to a laboratory that specializes in genetic testing. The laboratory returns the test results to the doctor or genetic counselor who requested the test. In some cases, the laboratory may send the results to the patient directly. It usually takes several weeks or longer to get the test results. Genetic counseling is recommended both before and after genetic testing to make sure that patients have accurate information about what a particular genetic test means for their health and care.

What Do the Results of Genetic Testing Mean?

Genetic testing can have several possible results: positive, negative, true negative, uninformative negative, false negative, variant of unknown significance, or benign polymorphism. These results are described below.

A "positive test result" means that the laboratory found a specific genetic alteration (or mutation) that is associated with a hereditary cancer syndrome. A positive result may:

- Confirm the diagnosis of a hereditary cancer syndrome

- Indicate an increased risk of developing certain cancer(s) in the future

- Show that someone carries a particular genetic change that does not increase their own risk of cancer but that may increase the risk in their children if they also inherit an altered copy from their other parent (that is, if the child inherits two copies of the abnormal gene, one from their mother and one from their father)

- Suggest a need for further testing

- Provide important information that can help other family members make decisions about their own healthcare

Also, people who have a positive test result that indicates that they have an increased risk of developing cancer in the future may be able to take steps to lower their risk of developing cancer or to find cancer earlier, including:

- Being checked at a younger age or more often for signs of cancer

- Reducing their cancer risk by taking medications or having surgery to remove "at-risk" tissue (These approaches to risk reduction are options for only a few inherited cancer syndromes.)

- Changing personal behaviors (like quitting smoking, getting more exercise, and eating a healthier diet) to reduce the risk of certain cancers

A positive result on a prenatal genetic test for cancer risk may influence a decision about whether to continue a pregnancy. The results of preimplantation testing (performed on embryos created by in vitro fertilization) can guide a doctor in deciding which embryo (or embryos) to implant in a woman's uterus.

Finally, in patients who have already been diagnosed with cancer, a positive result for a mutation associated with certain hereditary cancer syndromes can influence how the cancer is treated. For example, some hereditary cancer disorders interfere with the body's ability to repair the damage that occurs to cellular DNA. If someone with one of these conditions receives a standard dose of radiation or chemotherapy to treat their cancer, they may experience severe, potentially life-threatening treatment side effects. Knowing about the genetic disorder before treatment begins allows doctors to modify the treatment and reduce the severity of the side effects.

A "negative test result" means that the laboratory did not find the specific alteration that the test was designed to detect. This result is most useful when working with a family in which the specific, disease-causing genetic alteration is already known to be present. In such a case, a negative result can show that the tested family member has not inherited the mutation that is present in their family and that this person, therefore, does not have the inherited cancer syndrome tested for, does not have an increased genetic risk of developing cancer, or is not a carrier of a mutation that increases cancer risk. Such a test result is called a "true negative." A true negative result does not mean that there is no cancer risk, but rather that the risk is probably the same as the cancer risk in the general population.

When a person has a strong family history of cancer but the family has not been found to have a known mutation associated with a hereditary cancer syndrome, a negative test result is classified as an "uninformative negative" (that is, does not provide useful information). It is not possible to tell whether someone has a harmful gene mutation that was not detected by the particular test used (a "false negative") or whether the person truly has no cancer-predisposing genetic alterations in that gene. It is also possible for a person to have a mutation in a gene other than the gene that was tested.

If genetic testing shows a change that has not been previously associated with cancer in other people, the person's test result may report "variant of unknown significance," or VUS. This result may be interpreted as "ambiguous" (uncertain), which is to say that the information does not help in making healthcare decisions.

If the test reveals a genetic change that is common in the general population among people without cancer, the change is called a polymorphism. Everyone has commonly occurring genetic variations (polymorphisms) that are not associated with any increased risk of disease.

What Are At-Home or Direct-to-Consumer (DTC) Genetic Tests?

Some companies offer at-home genetic testing, also known as direct-to-consumer (DTC) genetic testing. People collect a tissue sample themselves and submit the sample through the mail. They learn about the test results online, by mail, or over the phone. DTC genetic testing is often done without a doctor's order or guidance from a doctor or genetic counselor before the test. Some states in the United States do not allow DTC genetic testing.

Whereas the genetic testing for cancer that is typically ordered by a doctor involves testing for rare major hereditary cancer syndromes, most DTC genetic testing for cancer risk involves the analysis of common inherited genetic variants, called single-nucleotide polymorphisms, that have been shown to be statistically associated with a particular type of cancer. Each individual variant is generally associated with only a minor increase in risk, and even when added together all the known variants for a particular cancer type account for only a small portion of a person's risk of that cancer. Although the identification and study of such variants is an active area of research, genetic tests based on these variants have not yet been found to help patients and their care providers make healthcare decisions and, therefore, they are not a part of recommended clinical practice.

Even when people have DTC genetic tests for known mutations in genes associated with hereditary cancer syndromes, there are potential risks and drawbacks to the use of DTC testing. In particular, without guidance about genetic test results from an informed, genetically knowledgeable healthcare provider, people may experience unneeded anxiety or false reassurance, or they may make important decisions about medical treatment or care based on incomplete information.

Also, although some people may view DTC genetic testing as a way to ensure the privacy of their genetic test results, companies that offer DTC genetic testing do not always tell the consumer the details of their privacy policies. In addition, if people consult their doctor or other healthcare provider about the test results obtained from a DTC testing vendor, the results may become part of the patient's medical record anyway. Also, companies that provide DTC testing may not be subject to current state and federal privacy laws and regulations. It is generally recommended that people considering DTC genetic testing make sure that they have chosen a reputable company.

The Federal Trade Commission (FTC) has details about at-home genetic tests which offers advice for people who are considering such a test. As part of its mission, the FTC investigates complaints about false or misleading health claims in advertisements.

The American Society of Human Genetics (ASHG), a membership organization of genetics professionals, has issued a statement about DTC genetic tests that recommends transparency in such testing, provider education about the testing, and the development of appropriate regulations to ensure test and laboratory quality.

How Are Genetic Tests Regulated?

U.S. laboratories that perform health-related testing, including genetic testing, are regulated under the Clinical Laboratory Improvement Amendments (CLIA) program. Laboratories that are certified under CLIA are required to meet federal standards for quality, accuracy, and reliability of tests. All laboratories that do genetic testing and share results must be CLIA certified. However, CLIA certification only indicates that appropriate laboratory quality control standards are being followed; it does not guarantee that a genetic test being done by a laboratory is medically useful. The Centers for Medicare & Medicaid Services (CMS) has information about CLIA programs. The U.S. National Library of Medicine (NLM) also has information about how genetic testing is regulated and how to judge the quality of a genetic test.

What Research Is Being Done to Improve Genetic Testing for Cancer?

Research to find newer and better ways of detecting, treating, and preventing cancer in people who carry genetic mutations that increase the risk of certain cancers is ongoing. Scientists are also doing studies to find additional genetic changes that can increase a person's risk of cancer.

The National Cancer Institute (NCI) runs an active program of genome-wide association studies (GWAS) through its Cancer Genomics Research Laboratory (CGR). This technique compares the genomes from many different people to find genetic markers associated with a particular observable characteristic or risk of disease. The goal is to understand how genes contribute to the disease and to use that understanding to help develop better prevention and treatment strategies.

Additional NCI research is focused on improving genetic counseling methods and outcomes, the risks and benefits of at-home genetic testing, and the effects of advertising of these tests on patients, providers, and the healthcare system. Researchers are also working to improve the laboratory methods available for genetic testing.

Chapter 4

What Women Need to Know about Smoking and Cancer Risk

Chapter Contents

Section 4.1

Smoking and Cancer

This section contains text excerpted from the following
sources: Text in this section begins with excerpts from
"Smoking and Cancer," Centers for Disease Control and
Prevention (CDC), October 15, 2014. Reviewed May 2018; Text
under the heading "Dangers of Smoking for Women" is excerpted
from "Women and Smoking," Centers for Disease Control and
Prevention (CDC), October 15, 2014. Reviewed May 2018.

One of every three cancer deaths in the United States is linked to
smoking. The Surgeon General's Report (SGR) identifies additional
cancers that are linked to smoking: cancer of the colon and of the rectum (also called colorectal cancer) and liver cancer. Colorectal cancer
causes the second largest number of cancer deaths every year, behind
only lung cancer, and is the fourth most commonly diagnosed cancer in
the United States. About 30,000 new cases of liver cancer are diagnosed
every year in this country; about 20,000 deaths from liver cancer occur.

In all, SGRs from 1964–2014 have identified the following specific
cancers caused by smoking, including cancer of:

- the lungs, trachea, and bronchus

- the oropharynx

- the esophagus

- the larynx

- the stomach

- the bladder

- the kidney and ureter

- the pancreas

- the uterine cervix

- the colon and rectum (colorectal cancer)

- the liver

- acute myeloid leukemia

Lung Cancer

Lung cancer, the first of many deadly diseases to be identified in an SGR as being caused by smoking, is now the nation's most common cancer killer among both men and women. Smoking causes almost 9 out of 10 lung cancers. Even though smoking rates have gone down dramatically, the risk for lung cancer has gone up over the last 50 years.

Three studies tracked cancer risks among U.S. men and women over age 55. The studies showed that in the early 1960s, men who smoked were 12.2 times more likely to develop lung cancer than men who did not smoke; by 2010, that risk had more than doubled, from 12.2–25. Among women smokers, the risk of lung cancer went up even more dramatically. In 1965, women smokers were 2.7 times more likely to develop lung cancer than women nonsmokers; by 2010, the risk for women smokers had jumped to 25.7. Cancer risks went up even though smokers in the 2000–2010, study smoked fewer cigarettes than did smokers in earlier studies.

The 2014 SGR finds that changes in how cigarettes are designed and what they contain have contributed to higher risks of lung cancer in smokers. The evidence suggests that ventilated filters and increased levels of certain chemicals in cigarettes may have played a role.

How Smoking Causes Cancer

Each cigarette puff delivers a mixture of chemicals to the lungs where they are absorbed into the bloodstream and carried to every organ in the body. Many of these chemicals damage deoxyribonucleic acid (DNA), which controls how cells reproduce and direct cells to carry out different tasks. DNA damage can cause cells to mutate and grow uncontrollably, and can start the body on the path to cancer. Tobacco smoke contains more than 7,000 chemicals, at least 70 of which are known to cause cancer.

Smoking Is Dangerous for Cancer Patients and Survivors

Smoking not only causes cancer but also interferes with cancer treatment. Cancer patients and cancer survivors who smoke are at greater risk for their cancer to recur. They are also more likely to die from their primary cancer and from secondary cancer (a cancer that occurs in a different organ). They are more likely to have serious medical issues from their cancer treatment—a condition known as treatment toxicity. They are also at higher risk for death from all other causes, such as pneumonia and infection. Quitting smoking improves the prognosis of cancer patients.

Dangers of Smoking for Women

In the last 50 years, a woman's risk of dying from smoking has more than tripled and is now equal to men's risk. The United States has more than 20 million women and girls who currently smoke cigarettes. Smoking puts them at risk for:

- heart attacks
- strokes
- lung cancer
- emphysema
- other serious chronic illnesses such as diabetes

More than 170,000 American women die of diseases caused by smoking each year, with additional deaths coming from the use of other tobacco products such as smokeless tobacco.

A Target Market

When the first SGR on smoking was released in 1964, it caused a rapid drop in smoking among men. Yet smoking rates among women continued to go up in the years immediately following the report as tobacco companies aggressively marketed to women. Documents from the tobacco industry show that cigarette companies created a line of slimmer cigarettes packaged in pastel colors to appeal to women, and implied that smoking could keep girls and women thin. They also used slogans, advertising, and sports sponsorships to tie their products to the women's rights movement throughout the 1960s and 1970s.

The women most likely to smoke today are among the most vulnerable—those disadvantaged by low income, less education, and mental health disorders. Women in these groups are also less likely to quit smoking when they become pregnant and are more likely to start smoking again after delivery. This worsens the dangerous health effects from smoking on mothers and their children.

Disease and Women Smokers

Many of the findings in the 2014 SGR are especially important for women who smoke. Between 1959 and 2010, lung cancer risk for smokers rose dramatically. While men's risk doubled, the risk among female smokers increased nearly ten-fold. Today, more women die from lung cancer than breast cancer.

Smoking and Pregnancy

Smoking during pregnancy causes premature birth, low birth weight, certain birth defects, and ectopic pregnancy in which the fertilized egg implants somewhere in the abdomen other than the womb. Smoking during pregnancy also causes complications with the placenta, the organ through which nutrients pass from mother to fetus. These complications include placenta previa and placental abruption, conditions that jeopardize the life and health of both mother and child. Women who are pregnant or who are planning a pregnancy should not smoke. It's important to encourage women to quit smoking before or early in pregnancy, when the most health benefits can be achieved, but cessation in all stages, even in late pregnancy, benefits maternal and fetal health.

Respiratory Diseases

Chronic obstructive pulmonary disease (COPD) includes emphysema, chronic bronchitis, and other conditions that damage airways. People with the disease suffer from shortness of breath and lack of oxygen that worsens over time. COPD has no cure. Nearly 9 out of 10 cases of COPD are caused by smoking. Women smokers in certain age groups are up to 38 times more likely to develop COPD than women who have never smoked. More women than men are now dying every year from COPD, and women appear more susceptible to developing severe COPD at younger ages.

Cardiovascular Disease (CVD)

For more than half a century, the evidence that smoking causes cardiovascular disease (CVD) has grown steadily. Women over age 35 who smoke have a slightly higher risk of dying from coronary heart disease than men who smoke. They are also slightly more likely to die from an abdominal aortic aneurysm—a weakened and bulging area of the artery that runs through the abdomen and carries blood to the major organs—than men who smoke.

Cessation

Nicotine addiction can be difficult to overcome, but over half of smokers in the United States have already quit. There are many support programs and cessation tools available to smokers who want to quit, including nicotine replacement products such as patches and gum, prescription medication, and free coaching. Benefits to women's health from quitting smoking are enormous and immediate. Heart attack risks drop dramatically in the first year and within five years, women who have quit smoking can see their stroke risk drop to that of a never smoker. In 10 years, a woman's risk of dying from lung cancer is cut in half. Women who want to quit smoking should ask their doctors for help, call 800-QUIT-NOW (800-784-8669), or visit women.smokefree.gov and www.cdc.gov/tobacco/campaign/tips.

Section 4.2

Women's Health and Smoking

This section contains text excerpted from the following sources:
Text in this section begins with excerpts from "Health Information—Women's Health and Smoking," U.S. Food and Drug Administration (FDA), January 26, 2018; Text under the heading "FAQs on Tobacco and Smoking" is excerpted from "Harms of Cigarette Smoking and Health Benefits of Quitting," National Cancer Institute (NCI), December 19, 2017.

Smoking continues to have a profound impact on the health and well-being of women and their families in the United States.

- About 13.6 percent of all women smoke cigarettes.

- Every day, nearly 1,100 girls under 18 years of age smoke their first cigarette.

- Nearly 7 percent of all high school aged girls smoke cigarettes.

Impacts of Smoking on Women and Their Families

There's abundant research about the many harms of smoking—whether it's the dangerous chemicals, the addictive properties, or the damage smoking causes to the body, these effects can have a profound impact on not only your own body, but also those around you. Here are some facts about smoking's effects on women, families, babies, and pregnant moms.

For Women

- Smoking causes coronary heart disease, cancer, and stroke—the first, second, and fourth leading causes of death for women in the United States.

- Smoking cigarettes causes chronic obstructive pulmonary disease (COPD). People with COPD have trouble breathing and slowly start to die from lack of air. Women who smoke cigarettes are up to 40 times more likely to develop COPD than female nonsmokers.

- Life expectancy for smokers—both male and female—is at least 10 years less than for nonsmokers.

For Families

- Secondhand smoke causes disease and premature death in nonsmoking adults and children.

- The U.S. Surgeon General estimates that living with a smoker increases a nonsmoker's chances of developing lung cancer by 20–30 percent.

- Exposure to secondhand smoke increases children's risk for ear infections, lower respiratory illnesses, more frequent and more severe asthma attacks, and slowed lung growth, and can cause coughing, wheezing, phlegm, and breathlessness.

- Teens are more likely to smoke if they have friends or family who smoke.

For Babies and Pregnant Moms

- Smoking during pregnancy can affect the baby's health.

- Infants born to mothers who smoked during pregnancy are at a higher risk of low birth weight, birth defects like cleft palate,

41

lungs that don't develop in a normal way, and sudden infant death syndrome (SIDS).

FAQs on Tobacco and Smoking

What Harmful Chemicals Does Tobacco Smoke Contain?

Tobacco smoke contains many chemicals that are harmful to both smokers and nonsmokers. Breathing even a little tobacco smoke can be harmful. Of the more than 7,000 chemicals in tobacco smoke, at least 250 are known to be harmful, including hydrogen cyanide, carbon monoxide, and ammonia.

Among the 250 known harmful chemicals in tobacco smoke, at least 69 can cause cancer. These cancer-causing chemicals include the following:

- Acetaldehyde
- Aromatic amines
- Arsenic
- Benzene
- Beryllium (a toxic metal)
- 1,3–Butadiene (a hazardous gas)
- Cadmium (a toxic metal)
- Chromium (a metallic element)
- Cumene
- Ethylene oxide
- Formaldehyde
- Nickel (a metallic element)
- Polonium-210 (a radioactive chemical element)
- Polycyclic aromatic hydrocarbons (PAHs)
- Tobacco-specific nitrosamines
- Vinyl chloride

What Are Some of the Health Problems Caused by Cigarette Smoking?

Smoking is the leading cause of premature, preventable death in this country. Cigarette smoking and exposure to tobacco smoke cause about 480,000 premature deaths each year in the United States. Of those premature deaths, about 36 percent are from cancer, 39 percent are from heart disease and stroke, and 24 percent are from lung disease. Mortality rates among smokers are about three times higher than among people who have never smoked.

Smoking harms nearly every bodily organ and organ system in the body and diminishes a person's overall health. Smoking causes cancers of the lung, esophagus, larynx, mouth, throat, kidney, bladder, liver, pancreas, stomach, cervix, colon, and rectum, as well as acute myeloid leukemia.

Smoking also causes heart disease, stroke, aortic aneurysm (a balloon-like bulge in an artery in the chest), COPD (chronic bronchitis and emphysema), diabetes, osteoporosis, rheumatoid arthritis (RA), age-related macular degeneration (AMD), and cataracts, and worsens asthma symptoms in adults. Smokers are at higher risk of developing pneumonia, tuberculosis, and other airway infections. In addition, smoking causes inflammation and impairs immune function.

Since the 1960s, a smoker's risk of developing lung cancer or COPD has actually increased compared with nonsmokers, even though the number of cigarettes consumed per smoker has decreased. There have also been changes over time in the type of lung cancer smokers develop—a decline in squamous cell carcinomas but a dramatic increase in adenocarcinomas. Both of these shifts may be due to changes in cigarette design and composition, in how tobacco leaves are cured, and in how deeply smokers inhale cigarette smoke and the toxicants it contains.

Smoking makes it harder for a woman to get pregnant. A pregnant smoker is at higher risk of miscarriage, having an ectopic pregnancy, having her baby born too early and with an abnormally low birth weight, and having her baby born with a cleft lip and/or cleft palate. A woman who smokes during or after pregnancy increases her infant's risk of death from SIDS. Men who smoke are at greater risk of erectile dysfunction.

The longer a smoker's duration of smoking, the greater their likelihood of experiencing harm from smoking, including earlier death. But regardless of their age, smokers can substantially reduce their risk of disease, including cancer, by quitting.

What Are the Risks of Tobacco Smoke to Nonsmokers?

Secondhand smoke (also called environmental tobacco smoke, involuntary smoking, and passive smoking) is the combination of "sidestream" smoke (the smoke given off by a burning tobacco product) and "mainstream" smoke (the smoke exhaled by a smoker).

The U.S. Environmental Protection Agency (EPA), the U.S. National Toxicology Program (NTP), the U.S. Surgeon General, and the International Agency for Research on Cancer (IARC) have classified secondhand smoke as a known human carcinogen (cancer-causing agent). Inhaling secondhand smoke causes lung cancer in nonsmoking adults. Approximately 7,300 lung cancer deaths occur each year among adult nonsmokers in the United States as a result of exposure to secondhand smoke. The U.S. Surgeon General estimates that living with a smoker increases a nonsmoker's chances of developing lung cancer by 20–30 percent.

Secondhand smoke causes disease and premature death in nonsmoking adults and children. Exposure to secondhand smoke irritates the airways and has immediate harmful effects on a person's heart and blood vessels. It increases the risk of heart disease by an estimated 25–30 percent. In the United States, exposure to secondhand smoke is estimated to cause about 34,000 deaths from heart disease each year. Exposure to secondhand smoke also increases the risk of stroke by 20–30 percent. Pregnant women exposed to secondhand smoke are at increased risk of having a baby with a small reduction in birth weight.

Children exposed to secondhand smoke are at an increased risk of SIDS, ear infections, colds, pneumonia, and bronchitis. Secondhand smoke exposure can also increase the frequency and severity of asthma symptoms among children who have asthma. Being exposed to secondhand smoke slows the growth of children's lungs and can cause them to cough, wheeze, and feel breathless.

Is Smoking Addictive?

Smoking is highly addictive. Nicotine is the drug primarily responsible for a person's addiction to tobacco products, including cigarettes. The addiction to cigarettes and other tobacco products that nicotine causes is similar to the addiction produced by using drugs such as heroin and cocaine. Nicotine is present naturally in the tobacco plant. But tobacco companies intentionally design cigarettes to have enough nicotine to create and sustain addiction.

The amount of nicotine that gets into the body is determined by the way a person smokes a tobacco product and by the nicotine content and design of the product. Nicotine is absorbed into the bloodstream through the lining of the mouth and the lungs and travels to the brain in a matter of seconds. Taking more frequent and deeper puffs of tobacco smoke increases the amount of nicotine absorbed by the body.

Are Other Tobacco Products, Such as Smokeless Tobacco or Pipe Tobacco, Harmful and Addictive?

Yes. All forms of tobacco are harmful and addictive. There is no safe tobacco product. In addition to cigarettes, other forms of tobacco include smokeless tobacco, cigars, pipes, hookahs (waterpipes), bidis, and kreteks.

- **Smokeless tobacco:** Smokeless tobacco is a type of tobacco that is not burned. It includes chewing tobacco, oral tobacco, spit or spitting tobacco, dip, chew, snus, dissolvable tobacco, and snuff. Smokeless tobacco causes oral (mouth, tongue, cheek and gum), esophageal, and pancreatic cancers and may also cause gum and heart disease.

- **Cigars:** These include premium cigars, little filtered cigars (LFCs), and cigarillos. LFCs resemble cigarettes, but both LFCs and cigarillos may have added flavors to increase appeal to youth and young adults. Most cigars are composed primarily of a single type of tobacco (air-cured and fermented), and have a tobacco leaf wrapper. Studies have found that cigar smoke contains higher levels of toxic chemicals than cigarette smoke, although unlike cigarette smoke, cigar smoke is often not inhaled. Cigar smoking causes cancer of the oral cavity, larynx, esophagus, and lung. It may also cause cancer of the pancreas. Moreover, daily cigar smokers, particularly those who inhale, are at increased risk for developing heart disease and other types of lung disease.

- **Pipes:** In pipe smoking, the tobacco is placed in a bowl that is connected to a stem with a mouthpiece at the other end. The smoke is usually not inhaled. Pipe smoking causes lung cancer and increases the risk of cancers of the mouth, throat, larynx, and esophagus.

- **Hookah or waterpipe** (other names include argileh, ghelyoon, hubble-bubble, shisha, boory, goza, and narghile): A hookah is a device used to smoke tobacco (often heavily flavored) by passing the smoke through a partially filled water bowl before being inhaled by the smoker. Although some people think hookah smoking is less harmful and addictive than cigarette

45

smoking, research shows that hookah smoke is at least as toxic as cigarette smoke.

- **Bidis:** A bidi is a flavored cigarette made by rolling tobacco in a dried leaf from the tendu tree, which is native to India. Bidi use is associated with heart attacks and cancers of the mouth, throat, larynx, esophagus, and lung.

- **Kreteks:** A kretek is a cigarette made with a mixture of tobacco and cloves. Smoking kreteks is associated with lung cancer and other lung diseases.

Is It Harmful to Smoke Just a Few Cigarettes a Day?

There is no safe level of smoking. Smoking even just one cigarette per day over a lifetime can cause smoking-related cancers (lung, bladder, and pancreas) and premature death.

Section 4.3

Smoking Cessation

This section includes text excerpted from "Smoking and
Tobacco Use—Quitting Smoking," Centers for Disease
Control and Prevention (CDC), December 11, 2017.

Tobacco use can lead to tobacco/nicotine dependence and serious health problems, including cancers. Quitting smoking greatly reduces the risk of developing smoking-related diseases. Tobacco/nicotine dependence is a condition that often requires repeated treatments, but there are helpful treatments and resources for quitting. Smokers can and do quit smoking. In fact, today, there are more former smokers than current smokers.

Nicotine Dependence

- Most smokers become addicted to nicotine, a drug that is found naturally in tobacco.

- More people in the United States are addicted to nicotine than to any other drug. Research suggests that nicotine may be as addictive as heroin, cocaine, or alcohol.

- Quitting smoking is hard and may require several attempts. People who stop smoking often start again because of withdrawal symptoms, stress, and weight gain.

- Nicotine withdrawal symptoms may include:

  - Feeling irritable, angry, or anxious

  - Having trouble thinking

  - Craving tobacco products

  - Feeling hungrier than usual

Health Benefits of Quitting

Tobacco smoke contains a deadly mix of more than 7,000 chemicals; hundreds are harmful, and about 70 can cause cancer. Smoking increases the risk for serious health problems, many diseases, and death. People who stop smoking greatly reduce their risk for disease and early death. Although the health benefits are greater for people who stop at earlier ages, there are benefits at any age. You are never too old to quit.

Stopping smoking is associated with the following health benefits:

- Lowered risk for lung cancer and many other types of cancer

- Reduced risk for heart disease, stroke, and peripheral vascular disease (narrowing of the blood vessels outside your heart)

- Reduced heart disease risk within 1–2 years of quitting

- Reduced respiratory symptoms, such as coughing, wheezing, and shortness of breath. While these symptoms may not disappear, they do not continue to progress at the same rate among people who quit compared with those who continue to smoke

- Reduced risk of developing some lung diseases (such as chronic obstructive pulmonary disease, also known as COPD, one of the leading causes of death in the United States)

- Reduced risk for infertility in women of childbearing age. Women who stop smoking during pregnancy also reduce their risk of having a low birth weight baby

Ways to Quit Smoking

Most former smokers quit without using one of the treatments that scientific research has shown can work. However, the following treatments are proven to be effective for smokers who want help to quit:

- Brief help by a doctor (such as when a doctor takes 10 minutes or less to give a patient advice and assistance about quitting)

- Individual, group, or telephone counseling

- Behavioral therapies (such as training in problem-solving)

- Treatments with more person-to-person contact and more intensity (such as more or longer counseling sessions)

- Programs to deliver treatments using mobile phones

Medications for quitting that have been found to be effective include the following:

- Nicotine replacement products

  - Over-the-counter (OTC) (nicotine patch [which is also available by prescription], gum, lozenge)

  - Prescription (nicotine patch, inhaler, nasal spray)

- Prescription nonnicotine medications: bupropion SR (Zyban®), varenicline tartrate Chantix®)

Counseling and medication are both effective for treating tobacco dependence, and using them together is more effective than using either one alone.

- More information is needed about quitting for people who smoke cigarettes and also use other types of tobacco.

Helpful Resources

Quitline Services

Call 800-QUIT-NOW (800-784-8669) if you want help quitting. This is a free telephone support service that can help people who want to stop smoking or using tobacco. Callers are routed to their state quitlines, which offer several types of quit information and services. These may include:

- Free support, advice, and counseling from experienced quitline coaches

- A personalized quit plan

- Practical information on how to quit, including ways to cope with nicotine withdrawal

- The latest information about stop-smoking medications

- Free or discounted medications (available for at least some callers in most states)

- Referrals to other resources

- Mailed self-help materials

Online Help

Get free help online, too.

- For information on quitting, go to the Quit Smoking Resources (www.cdc.gov/tobacco/quit_smoking/how_to_quit/resources/index.htm) page on Centers for Disease Control and Prevention's (CDC) Smoking and Tobacco Use website.

- Read inspiring stories about former smokers and their reasons for quitting at CDC's Tips From Former Smokers (www.cdc.gov/tobacco/campaign/tips) website.

- I'm Ready to Quit! (www.cdc.gov/tobacco/campaign/tips/quit-smoking/?s_cid=OSH_tips_D9170) contains page links to many helpful resources.

Chapter 5

Facts about Human Papillomavirus (HPV) and Cancer Risk

Chapter Contents

Section 5.1

HPV Facts

This section includes text excerpted from "Human
Papillomavirus (HPV)—What Is HPV?" Centers for Disease
Control and Prevention (CDC), December 13, 2016.

Human papillomavirus (HPV) is a group of more than 150 related
viruses. Each HPV virus in this large group is given a number which
is called its HPV type. HPV is named for the warts (papillomas) some
HPV types can cause. Some other HPV types can lead to cancer. Men
and women can get cancer of mouth/throat, and anus/rectum caused
by HPV infections. Men can also get penile HPV cancer. In women,
HPV infection can also cause cervical, vaginal, and vulvar HPV cancers. But there are vaccines that can prevent infection with the types
of HPV that most commonly cause cancer.

How Do People Get HPV?

HPV is transmitted through intimate skin-to-skin contact. You can
get HPV by having vaginal, anal, or oral sex with someone who has the
virus. It is most commonly spread during vaginal or anal sex. HPV is
so common that nearly all men and women get it at some point in their
lives. HPV can be passed even when an infected person has no signs
or symptoms. You can develop symptoms years after being infected,
making it hard to know when you first became infected.

In most cases, HPV goes away on its own and does not cause any
health problems. But when HPV does not go away, it can cause health
problems like genital warts and cancer.

Genital warts usually appear as a small bump or groups of bumps
in the genital area. They can be small or large, raised or flat, or shaped
like a cauliflower. A healthcare provider can usually diagnose warts
by looking at the genital area.

HPV cancers include cancer of the cervix, vulva, vagina, penis, or
anus. HPV infection can also cause cancer in the back of the throat,
including the base of the tongue and tonsils.

The Link between HPV and Cancer

Cancer often takes years, even decades, to develop after a person gets HPV. The types of HPV that can cause genital warts are not the same as the types of HPV that can cause cancers. There is no way to know which people who have HPV will develop cancer or other health problems. People with weak immune systems (including individuals with human immunodeficiency virus infection and acquired immunodeficiency syndrome (HIV/AIDS)) may be less able to fight off HPV and more likely to develop health problems from it.

HPV cancers include cancer of the cervix, vulva, vagina, penis, or anus. HPV infection can also cause cancer in the back of the throat, including the base of the tongue and tonsils (called oropharyngeal cancer). HPV cancer usually does not have symptoms until it is quite advanced, very serious and hard to treat. For this reason, it is important for women to get regular screening for cervical cancer. Cervical cancer screening can find early signs of disease so that problems can be treated early, before they ever turn into cancer. Because there is not screening for the other cancers caused by HPV, it is very important to prevent infection with HPV vaccination.

What Screening Tests Exist for HPV-Related Diseases?

- **Cervical cancer:** Cervical cancer can be detected with routine cervical cancer screening (Pap test) and follow-up of abnormal results. The Pap (Papanicolaou) test can find abnormal cells on the cervix so that they can be removed before cancer develops. Abnormal cells often become normal over time, but can sometimes turn into cancer. These cells can usually be treated, depending on their severity and on the woman's age, past medical history, and other test results. An HPV deoxyribonucleic acid (DNA) test, which can find certain HPV types on a woman's cervix, may also be used with a Pap test in certain cases (called co-testing). Even women who were vaccinated when they were younger need regular cervical cancer screening because the vaccines do not protect against all cervical cancers.

- **Anal and penile cancers:** There is no routinely recommended screening test for anal or penile cancer because more information is still needed to find out if those tests are effective.

- **Cancers of the back of the throat (Oropharynx):** There is no approved test to find early signs of oropharyngeal cancer because more information is still needed to find out if those tests are effective.

While there is no routine screening test for HPV-associated diseases other than cervical cancer, you should visit your doctor regularly for checkups. It is also important to be vaccinated to prevent these cancers; prevention is always better than treatment.

Is There a Treatment for HPV or Related Problems?

HPV vaccination could prevent most cancers and other diseases caused by HPV. There is no treatment for the virus itself, but there are treatments for the problems that HPV can cause:

- Visible genital warts may remain the same, grow more numerous, or go away on their own. The warts can be treated when they appear.

- Abnormal cervical cells (found on a Pap test) often become normal over time, but they can sometimes turn into cancer. If they remain abnormal, these cells can usually be treated to prevent cervical cancer from developing. This may depend on the severity of the cell changes, the woman's age and past medical history, and other test results. It is critical to follow up with testing and treatment, as recommended by a doctor.

- Cervical cancer is most treatable when it is diagnosed and treated early. Problems found can usually be treated, depending on their severity and on the woman's age, past medical history, and other test results. Most women who get routine cervical cancer screening and follow-up as told by their provider can find problems before cancer even develops. Other HPV cancers are also more treatable when diagnosed and treated early. Although there is no routine screening test for these cancers, you should visit your doctor regularly for checkups.

- Laryngeal papillomatosis, also known as recurrent respiratory papillomatosis (RRP), a rare condition in which warts grow in the throat, can be treated with surgery or medicines. It can sometimes take many treatments or surgeries over a period of years.

Section 5.2

HPV Vaccine for
Young Women in the United States

This section contains text excerpted from the following sources: Text beginning with the heading "Why Is the HPV Vaccine Important?" is excerpted from "HPV Vaccine Information for Young Women," Centers for Disease Control and Prevention (CDC), December 28, 2016; Text beginning with the heading "What Kinds of Problems Does HPV Infection Cause?" is excerpted from "Human Papillomavirus (HPV)—Questions and Answers," Centers for Disease Control and Prevention (CDC), November 21, 2016.

Why Is the HPV Vaccine Important?

Genital HPV is a common virus that is passed from one person to another through direct skin-to-skin contact during sexual activity. Most sexually active people will get HPV at some time in their lives, though most will never even know it. HPV infection is most common in people in their late teens and early 20s. There are about 40 types of HPV that can infect the genital areas of men and women. Most HPV types cause no symptoms and go away on their own. But some types can cause cervical cancer in women and other less common cancers— like cancers of the anus, penis, vagina, and vulva and oropharynx. Other types of HPV can cause warts in the genital areas of men and women, called genital warts. Genital warts are not life-threatening. But they can cause emotional stress and their treatment can be very uncomfortable. Every year, about 12,000 women are diagnosed with cervical cancer and 4,000 women die from this disease in the United States. About 1 percent of sexually active adults in the United States have visible genital warts at any point in time.

Which Girls/Women Should Receive HPV Vaccination?

HPV vaccination is recommended for 11 and 12-year-old girls. It is also recommended for girls and women age 13 through 26 years of age who have not yet been vaccinated or completed the vaccine series; HPV vaccine can also be given to girls beginning at age 9 years.

Will Sexually Active Females Benefit from the Vaccine?

Ideally, females should get the vaccine before they become sexually active and exposed to HPV. Females who are sexually active may also benefit from vaccination, but they may get less benefit. This is because they may have already been exposed to one or more of the HPV types targeted by the vaccines. However, few sexually active young women are infected with all HPV types prevented by the vaccines, so most young women could still get protection by getting vaccinated.

Can Pregnant Women Get the Vaccine?

The vaccine is not recommended for pregnant women. Studies show that the HPV vaccine does not cause problems for babies born to women who were vaccinated while pregnant, but more research is still needed. A pregnant woman should not get any doses of the HPV vaccine until her pregnancy is completed.

Getting the HPV vaccine when pregnant is not a reason to consider ending a pregnancy. If a woman realizes that she got one or more shots of an HPV vaccine while pregnant, she should do two things:

- Wait until after her pregnancy to finish any remaining HPV vaccine doses

- Call the pregnancy registry (800-986-8999 for Gardasil and Gardasil 9, or 888-825-5249 for Cervarix)

Should Girls and Women Be Screened for Cervical Cancer before Getting Vaccinated?

Girls and women do not need to get an HPV test or Pap test to find out if they should get the vaccine. However, it is important that women continue to be screened for cervical cancer, even after getting all recommended shots of the HPV vaccine. This is because the vaccine does not protect against all types of cervical cancer.

How Effective Is the HPV Vaccine?

The HPV vaccine targets the HPV types that most commonly cause cervical cancer and can cause some cancers of the vulva, vagina, anus, and oropharynx. It also protects against the HPV types that cause most genital warts. The HPV vaccine is highly effective in preventing the targeted HPV types, as well as the most common health problems caused by them. The vaccine is less effective in preventing HPV-related disease in young women who have already been exposed to one or more HPV types. That is because the vaccine prevents HPV before a person is exposed to it. The HPV vaccine does not treat existing HPV infections or HPV-associated diseases.

How Long Does Vaccine Protection Last?

Research suggests that vaccine protection is long-lasting. Current studies have followed vaccinated individuals for ten years, and show that there is no evidence of weakened protection over time.

What Does the Vaccine Not Protect Against?

The vaccine does not protect against all HPV types—so they will not prevent all cases of cervical cancer. Since some cervical cancers will not be prevented by the vaccine, it will be important for women to continue getting screened for cervical cancer. Also, the vaccine does not prevent other sexually transmitted infections (STIs). So it will still be important for sexually active persons to lower their risk for other STIs.

How Safe Is the HPV Vaccine?

The HPV vaccine has been licensed by the U.S. Food and Drug Administration (FDA). The Centers for Disease Control and Prevention (CDC) has approved this vaccine as safe and effective. The vaccine was studied in thousands of people around the world, and these studies showed no serious safety concerns. Side effects reported in these studies were mild, including pain where the shot was given, fever, dizziness, and nausea. Vaccine safety continues to be monitored by CDC and the FDA. More than 60 million doses of HPV vaccine have been distributed in the United States as of March 2014. Fainting, which can occur after any medical procedure, has also been noted after HPV vaccination. Fainting after any vaccination is more common in adolescents. Because fainting can cause falls and injuries, adolescents and adults should be seated or lying down during HPV vaccination. Sitting or lying down for about 15 minutes after a vaccination can help prevent fainting and injuries.

Why Is HPV Vaccination Only Recommended for Women through Age 26?

HPV vaccination is not currently recommended for women over age 26 years. Clinical trials showed that, overall, HPV vaccination offered women limited or no protection against HPV-related diseases. For women over age 26 years, the best way to prevent cervical cancer is to get routine cervical cancer screening, as recommended.

What Vaccinated Girls/Women Need to Know: Will Girls/Women Who Have Been Vaccinated Still Need Cervical Cancer Screening?

Yes, vaccinated women will still need regular cervical cancer screening because the vaccine protects against most but not all HPV types that cause cervical cancer. Also, women who got the vaccine after becoming sexually active may not get the full benefit of the vaccine if they had already been exposed to HPV.

Are There Other Ways to Prevent Cervical Cancer?

Regular cervical cancer screening (Pap and HPV tests) and follow-up can prevent most cases of cervical cancer. The Pap test can detect cell changes in the cervix before they turn into cancer. The HPV test looks for the virus that can cause these cell changes. Screening can detect most, but not all, cervical cancers at an early, treatable stage. Most women diagnosed with cervical cancer in the United States have either never been screened, or have not been screened in the last 5 years.

What Kinds of Problems Does HPV Infection Cause?

Most people with HPV never develop symptoms or health problems. Most HPV infections (9 out of 10) go away by themselves within two years. But, sometimes, HPV infections will last longer, and can cause certain cancers and other diseases. HPV infections can cause:

- Cancers of the cervix, vagina, and vulva in women

- Cancers of the penis in men

- Cancers of the anus and back of the throat, including the base of the tongue and tonsils (oropharynx), in both women and men. Every year in the United States, HPV causes 30,700 cancers in men and women.

Does HPV Vaccination Offer Similar Protection from Cervical Cancer in All Racial/Ethnic Groups?

Yes. Several different HPV types cause cervical cancer. HPV vaccines are designed to prevent the HPV types that cause most cervical cancers, so HPV vaccination will provide high protection for all racial/ethnic groups.

All three licensed HPV vaccines protect against types 16 and 18, which cause the majority of cervical cancers across racial/ethnic groups (67% of the cervical cancers among whites, 68% among blacks, and 64% among Hispanics). The 9-valent HPV vaccine protects against seven HPV types that cause about 80 percent of cervical cancer among all racial/ethnic groups in the United States.

Teens and young adults who haven't completed the HPV vaccine series should make an appointment to get vaccinated. To protect against cervical cancer, women age 21–65 years should get screened for cervical cancer at regular intervals and get follow-up care as recommended by their doctor or nurse.

What Are the Possible Side Effects of HPV Vaccination?

Vaccines, like any medicine, can have side effects. Many people who get HPV vaccine have no side effects at all. Some people report having very mild side effects, like a sore arm. The most common side effects are usually mild. Common side effects of HPV vaccine include:

- Pain, redness, or swelling in the arm where the shot was given
- Fever
- Headache or feeling tired
- Nausea
- Muscle or joint pain

Brief fainting spells and related symptoms (such as jerking movements) can happen after any medical procedure, including vaccination. Sitting or lying down while getting a shot and then staying that way for about 15 minutes can help prevent fainting and injuries caused by falls that could occur from fainting.

On very rare occasions, severe (anaphylactic) allergic reactions may occur after vaccination. People with severe allergies to any component of a vaccine should not receive that vaccine.

HPV vaccine does not cause HPV infection or cancer. HPV vaccine is made from one protein from the virus, and is not infectious, meaning that it cannot cause HPV infection or cancer. Not receiving HPV vaccine at the recommended ages can leave one vulnerable to cancers caused by HPV.

There are no data that suggest getting HPV vaccine will have an effect on future fertility for women. In fact, getting vaccinated and protecting against HPV-related cancers can help women and families have healthy pregnancies and healthy babies.

Not getting HPV vaccine leaves people vulnerable to HPV infection and related cancers. Treatments for cancers and precancers might include surgery, chemotherapy, and/or radiation, which might cause pregnancy complications or leave someone unable to have children.

Chapter 6

Cancer Risks Associated with Hormonal Medications

Chapter Contents

Section 6.1

Oral Contraceptives and Cancer Risk

This section includes text excerpted from "Oral Contraceptives and Cancer Risk," National Cancer Institute (NCI), February 22, 2018.

What Are Oral Contraceptives?

Oral contraceptives (birth control pills) are hormone-containing medications that are taken by mouth to prevent pregnancy. They prevent pregnancy by inhibiting ovulation and also by preventing sperm from penetrating through the cervix. By far the most commonly prescribed type of oral contraceptive in the United States contains synthetic versions of the natural female hormones estrogen and progesterone. This type of birth control pill is often called a combined oral contraceptive. Another type of oral contraceptive, sometimes called the mini pill, contains only progestin, which is a man-made version of progesterone.

What Is Known about the Relationship between Oral Contraceptive Use and Cancer?

Nearly all the research on the link between oral contraceptives and cancer risk comes from observational studies, both large prospective cohort studies and population-based case-control studies. Data from observational studies cannot definitively establish that an exposure—in this case, oral contraceptives—causes (or prevents) cancer. That is because women who take oral contraceptives may differ from those who don't take them in ways other than their oral contraceptive use, and it is possible that these other differences—rather than oral contraceptive use—are what explains their different cancer risk.

Overall, however, these studies have provided consistent evidence that the risks of breast and cervical cancers are increased in women who use oral contraceptives, whereas the risks of endometrial, ovarian, and colorectal cancers are reduced.

- **Breast cancer:** An analysis of data from more than 150,000 women who participated in 54 epidemiologic studies showed that, overall, women who had ever used oral contraceptives had a slight (7%) increase in the relative risk of breast cancer compared with women who had never used oral contraceptives. Women who were currently using oral contraceptives had a 24 percent increase in risk that did not increase with the duration of use. Risk declined after use of oral contraceptives stopped, and no risk increase was evident by 10 years after use had stopped.

A 2010 analysis of data from the Nurses' Health Study (NHS), which has been following more than 116,000 female nurses who were 24–43 years old when they enrolled in the study in 1989, also found that participants who used oral contraceptives had a slight increase in breast cancer risk. However, nearly all of the increased risk was seen among women who took a specific type of oral contraceptive, a "triphasic" pill, in which the dose of hormones is changed in three stages over the course of a woman's monthly cycle. An elevated risk associated with specific triphasic formulations was also reported in a nested case-control study that used electronic medical records to verify oral contraceptive use.

In 2017, a large prospective Danish study reported breast cancer risks associated with more recent formulations of oral contraceptives. Overall, women who were using or had recently stopped using oral combined hormone contraceptives had a modest (about 20%) increase in the relative risk of breast cancer compared with women who had never used oral contraceptives. The risk increase varied from 0–60 percent, depending on the specific type of oral combined hormone contraceptive. The risk of breast cancer also increased the longer oral contraceptives were used.

- **Cervical cancer:** Women who have used oral contraceptives for 5 or more years have a higher risk of cervical cancer than women who have never used oral contraceptives. The longer a woman uses oral contraceptives, the greater the increase in her risk of cervical cancer. One study found a 10 percent increased risk for less than 5 years of use, a 60 percent increased risk with 5–9 years of use, and a doubling of the risk with 10 or more years of use. However, the risk of cervical cancer has been found to decline over time after women stop using oral contraceptives.

- **Endometrial cancer:** Women who have ever used oral contraceptives have a lower risk of endometrial cancer than women who have never used oral contraceptives. Risk is reduced by at least 30 percent, with a greater risk reduction the longer oral contraceptives were used. The protective effect persists for many years after a woman stops using oral contraceptives. An analysis of women participating in the prospective National Institutes of Health (NIH)-American Association of Retired Persons (AARP) Diet and Health Study found that the risk reduction was especially pronounced in those long-time users of oral contraceptives who were smokers, obese, or exercised rarely.

- **Ovarian cancer:** Women who have ever used oral contraceptives have a 30–50 percent lower risk of ovarian cancer than women who have never used oral contraceptives. This protection has been found to increase with the length of time oral contraceptives are used and to continue for up to 30 years after a woman stops using oral contraceptives. A reduction in ovarian cancer risk with use of oral contraceptives is also seen among women who carry a harmful mutation in the *BRCA1* or *BRCA2* gene.

- **Colorectal cancer:** Oral contraceptive use is associated with 15–20 percent lower risks of colorectal cancer.

How Could Oral Contraceptives Influence Cancer Risk?

Naturally occurring estrogen and progesterone stimulate the development and growth of some cancers (e.g., cancers that express receptors for these hormones, such as breast cancer). Because birth control pills contain synthetic versions of these female hormones, they could potentially also increase cancer risk.

In addition, oral contraceptives might increase the risk of cervical cancer by changing the susceptibility of cervical cells to persistent infection with high-risk human papillomavirus (HPV) types (the cause of virtually all cervical cancers).

Researchers have proposed multiple ways that oral contraceptives may lower the risks of some cancers, including:

- Suppressing endometrial cell proliferation (endometrial cancer)

- Reducing the number of ovulations a woman experiences in her lifetime, thereby reducing exposure to naturally occurring female hormones (ovarian cancer)

- Lowering the levels of bile acids in the blood for women taking oral conjugated estrogens (colorectal cancer)

Section 6.2

Menopausal Hormone Therapy Use and Cancer

This section contains text excerpted from the following sources: Text beginning with the heading "What Is Menopause?" is excerpted from "Menopause and Hormones: Common Questions," U.S. Food and Drug Administration (FDA), February 16, 2018; Text beginning with the heading the heading "What Are the Health Risks of Menopausal Hormone Therapy (MHT)?" is excerpted from "Menopausal Hormone Therapy and Cancer," National Cancer Institute (NCI), December 5, 2011. Reviewed May 2018.

What Is Menopause?

Menopause is a normal change in a woman's life when her period stops. That's why some people call menopause "the change of life" or "the change." During menopause, a woman's body slowly produces less of the hormones estrogen and progesterone. This often happens between ages 45 and 55. A woman has reached menopause when she has not had a period for 12 months in a row.

What Are the Symptoms of Menopause?

Every woman's period will stop at menopause. Some women may not have any other symptoms at all. As you near menopause, you may have:

- Changes in your period—time between periods or flow may be different

- Hot flashes ("hot flushes")—getting warm in the face, neck and chest with and without sweating

- Night sweats, that may lead to problems sleeping and feeling tired, stressed, or tense

- Vaginal changes—the vagina may become dry and thin, and sex may be painful

- Thinning of your bones, which may lead to loss of height and bone breaks (osteoporosis)

Who Needs Treatment for Symptoms of Menopause?

- For some women, many of these changes will go away over time without treatment.
- Some women choose treatment for their symptoms and to prevent bone loss. If you choose hormone treatment, estrogen alone, or estrogen with progestin (for a woman who still has her uterus or womb) can be used.

What Is Hormone Therapy for Menopause?

Lower hormone levels in menopause may lead to hot flashes, vaginal dryness, and thin bones. To help with these problems, women are often given estrogen or estrogen with progestin (another hormone). Like all medicines, hormone therapy has risks and benefits. Talk to your doctor, nurse, or pharmacist about hormones. If you decide to use hormones, use them at the lowest dose that helps. Also, use them for the shortest time that you need them.

Who Should Not Take Hormone Therapy for Menopause?

Women who:

- Think they are pregnant
- Have problems with vaginal bleeding
- Have had certain kinds of cancers
- Have had a stroke or heart attack
- Have had blood clots
- Have liver disease

What Are the Benefits from Using Hormones for Menopause?

- Hormone therapy may help relieve hot flashes, night sweats, vaginal dryness, or dyspareunia (pain with sexual activity).

- Hormones may reduce your chances of getting thin, weak bones (osteoporosis) which break easily.

What Are the Health Risks of Menopausal Hormone Therapy (MHT)?

Before the Women's Health Initiative (WHI) studies began, it was known that MHT with estrogen alone increased the risk of endometrial cancer in women with an intact uterus. It was for this reason that, in the WHI trials, women randomly assigned to receive hormone therapy took estrogen plus progestin if they had a uterus and estrogen alone if they didn't have one.

Research from the WHI studies has shown that MHT is associated with the following harms:

- **Urinary incontinence.** Use of estrogen plus progestin increased the risk of urinary incontinence.

- **Dementia.** Use of estrogen plus progestin doubled the risk of developing dementia among postmenopausal women age 65 and older.

- **Stroke, blood clots, and heart attack.** Women who took either combined hormone therapy or estrogen alone had an increased risk of stroke, blood clots, and heart attack. For women in both groups, however, this risk returned to normal levels after they stopped taking the medication.

- **Breast cancer.** Women who took estrogen plus progestin were more likely to be diagnosed with breast cancer. The breast cancers in these women were larger and more likely to have spread to the lymph nodes by the time they were diagnosed. The number of breast cancers in this group of women increased with the length of time that they took the hormones and decreased after they stopped taking the hormones.

These studies also showed that both combination and estrogen-alone hormone use made mammography less effective for the early detection of breast cancer. Women taking hormones had more repeat mammograms to check on abnormalities found in a screening mammogram and more breast biopsies to determine whether abnormalities detected in mammograms were cancer.

The rate of death from breast cancer among those taking estrogen plus progestin was 2.6 per 10,000 women per year, compared with

1.3 per 10,000 women per year among those taking the placebo. The rate of death from any cause after a diagnosis of breast cancer was 5.3 per 10,000 women per year among women taking combined hormone therapy, compared with 3.4 per 10,000 women per year among those taking the placebo.

- **Lung cancer.** Women who took combined hormone therapy had the same risk of lung cancer as women who took the placebo. However, among those who were diagnosed with lung cancer, women who took estrogen plus progestin were more likely to die of the disease than those who took the placebo.

  There were no differences in the number of cases or the number of deaths from lung cancer among women who took estrogen alone compared with those among women who took the placebo.

- **Colorectal cancer.** In the initial study report, women taking combined hormone therapy had a lower risk of colorectal cancer than women who took the placebo. However, the colorectal tumors that arose in the combined hormone therapy group were more advanced at detection than those in the placebo group. There was no difference in either the risk of colorectal cancer or the stage of disease at diagnosis between women who took estrogen alone and those who took the placebo.

  However, a subsequent analysis of the WHI trials found no strong evidence that either estrogen alone or estrogen plus progestin had any effect on the risk of colorectal cancer, tumor stage at diagnosis, or death from colorectal cancer.

Do the Cancer Risks from MHT Change Over Time?

Women who have had a hysterectomy and who use estrogen-alone MHT have a reduced risk of breast cancer that continues for at least 5 years after they stop taking MHT.

Women who take combined hormone therapy have an increased risk of breast cancer that continues after they stop taking the medication. In the WHI study, where women took the combined hormone therapy for an average of 5.6 years, this increased risk persisted after an average follow-up period of 11 years. Breast cancers diagnosed in this group of women were larger and more likely to have spread to the lymph nodes (a sign of more advanced disease).

Studies have documented a decline in breast cancer diagnoses in the United States after the sharp reduction in the use of MHT that followed publication of the initial results of the Estrogen-plus-Progestin Study in July 2002. Additional factors, such as a reduction in the use of mammography, may also have contributed to this decline.

Is It Safe for Women Who Have Had a Cancer Diagnosis to Take MHT?

One of the roles of naturally occurring estrogen is to promote the normal growth of cells in the breast and uterus. For this reason, it is generally believed that MHT may promote further tumor growth in women who have already been diagnosed with breast cancer. However, studies of hormone use to treat menopausal symptoms in breast cancer survivors have produced conflicting results, with some showing an increased risk of breast cancer recurrence and others showing no increased risk of recurrence.

Section 6.3

Diethylstilbestrol Exposure and Cancer Risk

This section includes text excerpted from
"Diethylstilbestrol (DES) and Cancer," National Cancer
Institute (NCI), October 5, 2011. Reviewed May 2018.

What Is Diethylstilbestrol (DES)?

Diethylstilbestrol (DES) is a synthetic form of the female hormone estrogen. It was prescribed to pregnant women between 1940 and 1971 to prevent miscarriage, premature labor, and related complications of pregnancy. The use of DES declined after studies in the 1950s showed that it was not effective in preventing these problems.

In 1971, researchers linked prenatal (before birth) DES exposure to a type of cancer of the cervix and vagina called clear cell adenocarcinoma in a small group of women. Soon after, the U.S. Food and Drug

Administration (FDA) notified physicians throughout the country that DES should not be prescribed to pregnant women. The drug continued to be prescribed to pregnant women in Europe until 1978.

DES is now known to be an endocrine-disrupting chemical, one of a number of substances that interfere with the endocrine system to cause cancer, birth defects, and other developmental abnormalities. The effects of endocrine-disrupting chemicals are most severe when exposure occurs during fetal development.

What Is the Cancer Risk of Women Who Were Exposed to DES before Birth?

The daughters of women who used DES while pregnant—commonly called DES daughters—have about 40 times the risk of developing clear cell adenocarcinoma of the lower genital tract than unexposed women. However, this type of cancer is still rare; approximately 1 in 1,000 DES daughters develops it.

The first DES daughters who were diagnosed with clear cell adeno-carcinoma were very young at the time of their diagnoses. Subsequent research has shown that the risk of developing this disease remains elevated as women age into their 40s.

DES daughters have an increased risk of developing abnormal cells in the cervix and the vagina that are precursors of cancer (dysplasia, cervical intraepithelial neoplasia, and squamous intraepithelial lesions). These abnormal cells resemble cancer cells, but they do not invade nearby healthy tissue and are not cancer. They may develop into cancer, however, if left untreated. Scientists estimated that DES-exposed daughters were 2.2 times more likely to have these abnormal cell changes in the cervix than unexposed women. Approximately 4 percent of DES daughters developed these conditions because of their exposure. It has been recommended that DES daughters have a yearly Pap (Papanicolaou) test and pelvic exam to check for abnormal cells.

DES daughters may also have a slightly increased risk of breast cancer after age 40. A 2006 study from the United States suggested that, overall, breast cancer risk is not increased in DES daughters, but that, after age 40, DES daughters have approximately twice the risk of breast cancer as unexposed women of the same age and with similar risk factors. However, a 2010 study from Europe found no difference in breast cancer risk between DES daughters and unexposed women and no difference in overall cancer risk. A 2011 study found that about 2 percent of a large cohort of DES daughters has developed breast cancer due to their exposure.

DES daughters should be aware of these health risks, share their medical history with their doctors, and get regular physical examinations.

Do DES Daughters Have Problems with Fertility and Pregnancy?

Several studies have found increased risks of premature birth, miscarriage, and ectopic pregnancy associated with DES exposure. An analysis of updated data published in 2011 is outlined in the table 6.1 below.

Table 6.1. Fertility Problems in DES Daughters

Fertility Complication	Hazard Ratio	Percent Cumulative Risk* to Age 45, DES-Exposed Women	Percent Cumulative Risk* to Age 45, Unexposed Women
Premature delivery	4.68	53.3	17.8
Stillbirth	2.45	8.9	2.6
Neonatal death	8.12	7.8	0.6
Ectopic pregnancy	3.72	14.6	2.9
Miscarriage (second trimester)	3.77	16.4	1.7
Preeclampsia	1.42	26.4	13.7
Infertility	2.37	33.3	15.5

*The total risk (probability) that a certain problem will occur.

Some studies suggest that the increased risk of infertility is mainly due to uterine or fallopian tube problems.

What Other Health Problems Might DES Daughters Have?

Concerns have been raised that DES daughters may have problems with their immune system. However, research thus far suggests that DES daughters do not have an increased risk of auto-immune diseases. Researchers found no difference in the rates of lupus, rheumatoid arthritis (RA), optic neuritis (ON), and idiopathic thrombocytopenia purpura (ITP) between DES-exposed and unexposed women.

Studies examining the risk of depression among DES daughters have had conflicting results. One study found a 40 percent increase in risk of depression, whereas another found no increased risk for these women. A study published in 2003 found little support for the possibility that prenatal exposure to DES influences certain psychological and sexual characteristics of adult men and women, such as the likelihood of ever having been married, age at first sexual intercourse, number of sexual partners, and having had a same-sex sexual partner in adulthood.

DES daughters have more than twice the risk of early menopause (menopause that begins before age 45) as unexposed women. Scientists estimate that 3 percent of DES-exposed women have experienced early menopause due to their exposure to DES.

What Health Problems Might Women Who Took DES during Pregnancy Have?

Women who used DES may have a slight increase in the risk of developing and dying from breast cancer compared with women who did not use DES. No evidence exists to suggest that women who took DES are at higher risk for any other type of cancer.

What Health Problems Might DES-Exposed Grandchildren Have?

Researchers are also studying possible health effects among women and men who are the children of DES daughters. These groups are called DES granddaughters and DES grandsons, or the third generation. Researchers are studying these groups because studies in animal models suggest that DES may cause deoxyribonucleic acid (DNA) changes (i.e., altered patterns of methylation) in mice exposed to the chemical during early development. These changes can be heritable and have the potential to affect subsequent generations.

A comparison of the results of DES granddaughters' pelvic exams with those of their mothers' first pelvic exams found none of the changes that had been associated with prenatal DES exposure in their mothers. However, another analysis showed that DES granddaughters began their menstrual periods later and were more likely to have menstrual irregularities than other women of the same age. The data also suggested that infertility was greater among DES granddaughters, and that they tended to have fewer live births. However, this association is based on small numbers of events and was not statistically significant. Researchers will continue to follow these women to study the risk of infertility.

Recent studies have found that DES granddaughters and DES grandsons may have a slightly higher risk of cancer and birth defects, including hypospadias in DES grandsons. However, because each of these associations is based on small numbers of events, researchers will continue to study these groups to clarify the findings.

How Can People Find out If They Took DES during Pregnancy or Were Exposed to DES in Utero?

It is estimated that 5–10 million Americans—pregnant women and the children born to them—were exposed to DES between 1940 and 1971. DES was given widely to pregnant women between 1940 and 1971 to prevent complications during pregnancy. DES was provided under many different product names and also in various forms, such as pills, creams, and vaginal suppositories. The table 6.2 below includes examples of products that contained DES.

Table 6.2. DES Product Names

Nonsteroidal Estrogens		
Benzestrol	Gynben	Stil-Rol
Chlorotrianisene	Gyneben	Stilbal
Comestrol	Hexestrol	Stilbestrol
Cyren A	Hexoestrol	Stilbestronate
Cyren B.	Hi-Bestrol	Stilbetin
Delvinal	Menocrin	Stilbinol
DES	Meprane	Stilboestroform
Desplex	Mestilbol	Silboestrol
Dibestil	Microest	Stilboestrol DP
Diestryl	Methallenestril	Stilestrate
Dienestrol	Mikarol	Stilpalmitate
Dienoestrol	Mikarol forti	Stilphostrol
Diethylstilbestrol dipalmitate	Milestrol	Stilronate
Diethylstilbestrol diphosphate	Monomestrol	Stilrone
Diethylstilbestrol dipropionate	Neo-Oestranol I	Stils
Diethylstilbenediol	Neo-Oestranol II	Synestrin
Digestil	Nulabort	Synestrol

Table 6.2. Continued

Dienestrol	Oestrogenine	Synthosestrin
Domestrol	Oestromenin	Tace
Estilben	Oestromon	Vallestril
Estrobene	Orestol	Willestrol
Estrobene DP	Pabestrol D	
Estrosyn	Palestrol	
Fonatol	Restrol	
Nonsteroidal Estrogen-Androgen Combinations		
Amperone	Teserene	
Di-Erone	Tylandril	
Estan	Tylostereone	
Metystil		
Nonsteroidal Estrogen-Progesterone Combinations		
Progravidium		
Vaginal Cream Suppositories with Nonsteroidal Estrogens		
AVC Cream with Dienestrol		
Dienestrol Cream		

Women who think they used DES during pregnancy, or people who think that their mother used DES during pregnancy, can try contacting the physician or institution where they received their care to request a review of their medical records. If any pills were taken during pregnancy, obstetrical records could be checked to determine the name of the drug.

However, finding medical records after a long period of time can be difficult. If the doctor has retired or died, another doctor may have taken over the practice as well as the records. The county medical society or health department may know where the records have been stored. Some pharmacies keep records for a long time and can be contacted regarding prescription dispensing information. Military medical records are kept for 25 years. In most cases, however, it may be impossible to determine whether DES was used.

What Should DES-Exposed Daughters Do?

Women who know or believe they were exposed to DES before birth should be aware of the health effects of DES and inform their doctor about their possible exposure. It has been recommended that exposed women have an annual medical examination to check for the adverse health effects of DES. A thorough examination may include the following:

- Pelvic examination

- Pap test and colposcopy—A routine cervical Pap test is not adequate for DES daughters. The Pap test must gather cells from the cervix and the vagina. It is also good for a clinician to see the cervix and vaginal walls. They may use a colposcope to follow-up if there are any abnormal findings.

- Biopsy

- Breast examinations—It is recommended that DES daughters continue to rigorously follow the routine breast cancer screening recommendations for their age group.

What Should DES-Exposed Mothers Do?

A woman who took DES while pregnant or who suspects she may have taken it should inform her doctor. She should try to learn the dosage, when the medication was started, and how it was used. She also should inform her children who were exposed before birth so that this information can be included in their medical records.

It is recommended that DES-exposed mothers have regular breast cancer screenings and yearly medical checkups that include a pelvic examination and a Pap test.

What Should DES-Exposed Sons Do?

Men whose mothers took DES while pregnant should inform their physician of their exposure and be examined periodically. Although the risk of developing testicular cancer among DES-exposed sons is unclear, males with undescended or unusually small testicles have an increased risk of testicular cancer whether or not they were exposed to DES.

Is It Safe for DES Daughters to Use Hormone Replacement Therapy?

Each woman should discuss this question with her doctor. Studies have not shown that hormone replacement therapy is unsafe for DES daughters. However, some doctors believe that DES daughters should avoid these medications because they contain estrogen.

Section 6.4

Pregnancy and Cancer Risks

This section includes text excerpted from "Reproductive History and Cancer Risk," National Cancer Institute (NCI), November 9, 2016.

Is There a Relationship between Pregnancy and Breast Cancer Risk?

Studies have shown that a woman's risk of developing breast cancer is related to her exposure to hormones that are produced by her ovaries (endogenous estrogen and progesterone). Reproductive factors that increase the duration and/or levels of exposure to ovarian hormones, which stimulate cell growth, have been associated with an increase in breast cancer risk. These factors include early onset of menstruation, late onset of menopause, and factors that may allow breast tissue to be exposed to high levels of hormones for longer periods of time, such as later age at first pregnancy and never having given birth.

Conversely, pregnancy and breastfeeding, which both reduce a woman's lifetime number of menstrual cycles, and thus her cumulative exposure to endogenous hormones, are associated with a decrease in breast cancer risk. In addition, pregnancy and breastfeeding have direct effects on breast cells, causing them to differentiate, or mature, so they can produce milk. Some researchers hypothesize that these differentiated cells are more resistant to becoming transformed into cancer cells than cells that have not undergone differentiation.

Are Any Pregnancy-Related Factors Associated with a Lower Risk of Breast Cancer?

Some pregnancy-related factors have been associated with a reduced risk of developing breast cancer later in life. These factors include:

- **Early age at first full-term pregnancy.** Women who have their first full-term pregnancy at an early age have a decreased risk of developing breast cancer later in life. For example, in women who have a first full-term pregnancy before age 20, the risk of developing breast cancer is about half that of women whose first full-term pregnancy occurs after the age of 30. This risk reduction is limited to hormone receptor-positive breast cancer; age at first full-term pregnancy does not appear to affect the risk of hormone receptor-negative breast cancer.

- **Increasing number of births.** The risk of breast cancer declines with the number of children borne. Women who have given birth to five or more children have half the breast cancer risk of women who have not given birth. Some evidence indicates that the reduced risk associated with a higher number of births may be limited to hormone receptor-positive breast cancer.

- **History of preeclampsia.** Women who have had preeclampsia may have a decreased risk of developing breast cancer. Preeclampsia is a complication of pregnancy in which a woman develops high blood pressure and excess amounts of protein in her urine. Scientists are studying whether certain hormones and proteins associated with preeclampsia may affect breast cancer risk.

- **Longer duration of breastfeeding.** Breastfeeding for an extended period (at least a year) is associated with decreased risks of both hormone receptor-positive and hormone receptor-negative breast cancers.

Are Any Pregnancy-Related Factors Associated with an Increase in Breast Cancer Risk?

Some factors related to pregnancy may increase the risk of breast cancer. These factors include:

- **Older age at birth of first child.** The older a woman is when she has her first full-term pregnancy, the higher her risk of breast cancer. Women who are older than 30 when they give birth to their first child have a higher risk of breast cancer than women who have never given birth.

- **Recent childbirth.** Women who have recently given birth have a short-term increase in breast cancer risk that declines after about 10 years. The reason for this temporary increase is not known, but some researchers believe that it may be due to the effect of high levels of hormones on the development of cancers or to the rapid growth of breast cells during pregnancy.

- **Taking diethylstilbestrol (DES) during pregnancy.** DES is a synthetic form of estrogen that was used between the early 1940s and 1971 to prevent miscarriages and other pregnancy problems. Women who took DES during pregnancy may have a slightly higher risk of developing breast cancer than women who did not take DES during pregnancy. Some studies have shown that daughters of women who took DES during pregnancy may also have a slightly higher risk of developing breast cancer after age 40 than women who were not exposed to DES while in the womb, but the evidence is inconsistent.

Is Abortion Linked to Breast Cancer Risk?

A few retrospective (case-control) studies reported in the mid-1990s suggested that induced abortion (the deliberate ending of a pregnancy) was associated with an increased risk of breast cancer. However, these studies had important design limitations that could have affected the results. A key limitation was their reliance on self-reporting of medical history information by the study participants, which can introduce bias. Prospective studies, which are more rigorous in design and unaffected by such bias, have consistently shown no association between induced abortion and breast cancer risk. Moreover, in 2009, the Committee on Gynecologic Practice of the American College of Obstetricians and Gynecologists (ACOG) concluded that "more rigorous recent studies demonstrate no causal relationship between induced abortion and a subsequent increase in breast cancer risk." Major findings from these studies include:

- Women who have had an induced abortion have the same risk of breast cancer as other women

- Women who have had a spontaneous abortion (miscarriage) have the same risk of breast cancer as other women

- Cancers other than breast cancer also appear to be unrelated to a history of induced or spontaneous abortion

Does Pregnancy Affect the Risk of Other Cancers?

Research has shown the following with regard to pregnancy and the risk of other cancers:

- Women who have had a full-term pregnancy have reduced risks of ovarian and endometrial cancers. Furthermore, the risks of these cancers decline with each additional full-term pregnancy.

- Pregnancy also plays a role in an extremely rare type of tumor called a gestational trophoblastic tumor. In this type of tumor, which starts in the uterus, cancer cells grow in the tissues that are formed following conception.

- There is some evidence that pregnancy-related factors may affect the risk of other cancer types, but these relationships have not been as well studied as those for breast and gynecologic cancers. The associations require further study to clarify the exact relationships.

As in the development of breast cancer, exposures to hormones are thought to explain the role of pregnancy in the development of ovarian, endometrial, and other cancers. Changes in the levels of hormones during pregnancy may contribute to the variation in risk of these tumors after pregnancy.

Does Fertility Treatment Affect the Risk of Breast or Other Cancers?

Women who have difficulty becoming pregnant or carrying a pregnancy to term may receive fertility treatment. Such treatment can include surgery (to repair diseased, damaged, or blocked fallopian tubes or to remove uterine fibroids, patches of endometriosis, or adhesions); medications to stimulate ovulation; and assisted reproductive technology.

Ovarian stimulation and some assisted reproductive technologies involve treatments that temporarily change the levels of estrogen and progesterone in a woman's body. For example, women undergoing in vitro fertilization (IVF) receive multiple rounds of hormone treatment to first suppress ovulation until the developing eggs are ready, then stimulate development of multiple eggs, and finally promote maturation of the eggs. The use of hormones in some fertility treatments has raised concerns about possible increased risks of cancer, particularly cancers that are linked to elevated levels of these hormones.

Many studies have examined possible associations between use of fertility drugs or IVF and the risks of breast, ovarian, and endometrial cancers. The results of such studies can be hard to interpret because infertility itself is linked to increased risks of these cancers (that is, compared with fertile women, infertile women are at higher risk of these cancers even if they do not use fertility drugs). Also, these cancers are relatively rare and tend to develop years after treatment for infertility, which can make it difficult to link their occurrence to past use of fertility drugs.

- **Breast cancer:** The bulk of the evidence is consistent with no increased risk of breast cancer associated with the use of fertility drugs or IVF.

- **Ovarian cancer:** There is some uncertainty about whether treatment for infertility is a risk factor for ovarian cancer. A 2013 systematic review of 25 studies that included more than 180,000 women found, overall, no strong evidence of an increased risk of invasive ovarian cancer for women treated with fertility drugs. In one study, women who underwent IVF had an increase in risk of ovarian borderline malignant tumors.

- **Endometrial cancer:** Overall, the use of fertility drugs or IVF does not appear to increase the risk of endometrial cancer.

Chapter 7

Cancer-Causing Substances in the Environment

Cancer is caused by changes to certain genes that alter the way our cells function. Some of these genetic changes occur naturally when deoxyribonucleic acid (DNA) is replicated during the process of cell division. But others are the result of environmental exposures that damage DNA. These exposures may include substances, such as the chemicals in tobacco smoke, or radiation, such as ultraviolet rays from the sun.

People can avoid some cancer-causing exposures, such as tobacco smoke and the sun's rays. But others are harder to avoid, especially if they are in the air we breathe, the water we drink, the food we eat, or the materials we use to do our jobs. Scientists are studying which exposures may cause or contribute to the development of cancer. Understanding which exposures are harmful, and where they are found, may help people to avoid them.

The substances listed below are among the most likely carcinogens to affect human health. Simply because a substance has been designated as a carcinogen, however, does not mean that the substance will necessarily cause cancer. Many factors influence whether a person exposed to a carcinogen will develop cancer, including the amount and duration of the exposure and the individual's genetic background.

This chapter includes text excerpted from "Cancer-Causing Substances in the Environment," National Cancer Institute (NCI), March 18, 2015.

Aflatoxins

Aflatoxins are a family of toxins produced by certain fungi that are found on agricultural crops such as maize (corn), peanuts, cottonseed, and tree nuts.

Which Cancers Are Associated with Exposure to Aflatoxins?

Exposure to aflatoxins is associated with an increased risk of liver cancer.

How Can Aflatoxin Exposure Be Reduced?

You can reduce your aflatoxin exposure by buying only major commercial brands of nuts and nut butters and by discarding nuts that look moldy, discolored, or shriveled. To help minimize risk, the U.S. Food and Drug Administration (FDA) tests foods that may contain aflatoxins, such as peanuts and peanut butter. To date, no outbreak of human illness caused by aflatoxins has been reported in the United States, but such outbreaks have occurred in some developing countries.

Aristolochic Acids

Aristolochia clematitis, a plant that contains aristolochic acids.

Which Cancers Are Associated with Exposure to Aristolochic Acids?

Cancers of the upper urinary tract (renal pelvis and ureter) and bladder have been reported among individuals who had kidney damage caused by the consumption of herbal products containing aristolochic acids.

How Can Exposures Be Reduced?

To reduce your risk, do not use herbal products that contain aristolochic acids. The FDA provides a list of some products containing aristolochic acids.

Arsenic

Inorganic arsenic is naturally present at high levels in the groundwater of certain countries, including the United States.

Which Cancers Are Associated with Exposure to Arsenic?

Prolonged ingestion of arsenic-containing drinking water is associated with an increased risk of bladder cancer. In addition, cancers of the skin, lung, digestive tract, liver, kidney, and lymphatic and hematopoietic systems have been linked to arsenic exposure.

How Can Exposures Be Reduced?

Access to a safe water supply for drinking, food preparation, and irrigation of food crops is the most important way to prevent exposures to arsenic.

Asbestos

Asbestos is the name given to a group of naturally occurring fibrous minerals that are resistant to heat and corrosion.

Which Cancers Are Associated with Exposure to Asbestos?

Exposure to asbestos is associated with an increased risk of lung cancer and mesothelioma, which is a cancer of the thin membranes that line the chest and abdomen. Mesothelioma is the most common form of cancer associated with asbestos exposure, although the disease is relatively rare.

What Can Be Done to Reduce the Hazards of Asbestos?

The use of asbestos is now highly regulated in the United States. The Occupational Safety and Health Administration (OSHA) has issued standards for the construction industry, general industry, and shipyard employment sectors.

How Does Smoking Tobacco Affect the Risk of Asbestos-Associated Cancers?

Many studies have shown that the combination of tobacco smoking and asbestos exposure is particularly hazardous. However, there is also evidence that quitting smoking reduces the risk of lung cancer among asbestos-exposed workers.

Benzene

Outdoor air contains low levels of benzene from gasoline fumes, secondhand smoke, and other sources.

Which Cancers Are Associated with Exposure to Benzene?

Exposure to benzene may increase the risk of developing leukemia and other blood disorders.

How Can Exposure Be Reduced?

Don't smoke and avoid exposure to secondhand tobacco smoke. Try to limit exposure to gasoline fumes. For workers who may be exposed to benzene on the job, the United States Centers for Disease Control and Prevention (CDC) has information about how you can protect yourself and what to do if you are exposed.

Benzidine

Benzidine is a manufactured chemical that does not occur in nature. In the past, large amounts of benzidine were used to produce dyes for cloth, paper, and leather.

Which Cancers Are Associated with Exposure to Benzidine?

Occupational exposure to benzidine results in an increased risk of bladder cancer, according to studies of workers in different geographic locations.

Beryllium

Coal-fired power plants are a major source of beryllium-containing particles.

Which Cancers Are Associated with Exposure to Beryllium?

An increased risk of lung cancer has been observed in workers exposed to beryllium or beryllium compounds.

How Can Exposure Be Reduced?

The U.S. Occupational Safety and Health Administration (OSHA) has information about preventing adverse health effects from exposure to beryllium on the job.

Cadmium

Cadmium is a natural element found in the earth's crust, and has been used to make batteries and other products.

Which Cancers Are Associated with Exposure to Cadmium?

Occupational exposure to various cadmium compounds is associated with an increased risk of lung cancer.

How Can Exposures Be Reduced?

Dispose of nickel-cadmium batteries properly, and do not allow children to play with these batteries. Avoid tobacco smoke. If you work with cadmium, use all recommended safety precautions to avoid carrying cadmium-containing dust home from work on your clothing, skin, hair, or tools. The OSHA has more information about controlling exposures to cadmium.

Coal Tar and Coal-Tar Pitch

Coal-tar pitch is found in some types of asphalt and other coal-tar products.

Which Cancers Are Associated with Exposure to Coal Tar and Coal-Tar Pitch?

Occupational exposure to coal tar or coal-tar pitch is associated with an increased risk of skin cancer. Other types of cancer, including lung, bladder, kidney, and digestive tract cancer, have also been linked to occupational exposure to coal tar and coal-tar pitch.

How Can Exposures Be Reduced?

Exposures to coal tar and coal-tar pitch are regulated under the OSHA's Air Contaminants Standard for general industry, shipyard employment, and the construction industry. OSHA provides detailed safety and health information about coal-tar pitch to the public.

Coke Oven Emissions

Emissions from coking plants typically include carcinogens such as cadmium and arsenic.

85

Which Cancers Are Associated with Exposure to Coke Oven Emissions?

Exposure to coke oven emissions is associated with an increased risk of lung cancer.

How Can Exposures Be Reduced?

The OSHA provides information about exposure limits for coke oven emissions.

Crystalline Silica

Quartz is the most common form of crystalline silica.

Which Cancers Are Associated with Exposure to Crystalline Silica?

Exposure of workers to respirable crystalline silica is associated with elevated rates of lung cancer. The strongest link between human lung cancer and exposure to respirable crystalline silica has been seen in studies of quarry and granite workers and workers involved in ceramic, pottery, refractory brick, and certain earth industries.

How Can Exposures Be Reduced?

The Mine Safety and Health Administration (MSHA) and the U.S. Occupational Safety and Health Administration (OSHA) have regulations related to silica. For example, OSHA has a fact sheet on Controlling Silica Exposures in Construction While Operating Handheld Masonry Saws.

Erionite

Erionite is a fibrous mineral whose properties are similar to those of asbestos.

Which Cancers Are Associated with Exposure to Erionite?

Exposure to erionite is associated with increased risks of lung cancer and mesothelioma.

How Can Exposures Be Reduced?

There are no regulatory or consensus standards or occupational exposure limits for airborne erionite fibers. The OSHA's guidance for working with asbestos could serve as a model for limiting the generation and inhalation of dust known or thought to be contaminated with erionite.

Ethylene Oxide

Which Cancers Are Associated with Exposure to Ethylene Oxide?

Lymphoma and leukemia are the cancers most frequently reported to be associated with occupational exposure to ethylene oxide.

How Can Exposures Be Reduced?

The OSHA has information about limiting occupational exposure to ethylene oxide.

Formaldehyde

Formaldehyde is commonly used as a preservative.

Which Cancers Are Associated with Exposure to Formaldehyde?

Studies of workers exposed to high levels of formaldehyde, such as industrial workers and embalmers, have found that formaldehyde causes myeloid leukemia and rare cancers, including cancers of the paranasal sinuses, nasal cavity, and nasopharynx.

How Can Exposures Be Reduced?

The U.S. Environmental Protection Agency (EPA) recommends the use of "exterior-grade" pressed-wood products to limit formaldehyde exposure in the home. Formaldehyde levels in homes and work settings can also be reduced by ensuring adequate ventilation, moderate temperatures, and reduced humidity levels through the use of air conditioners and dehumidifiers.

Hexavalent Chromium Compounds

Hexavalent chromium compounds are used widely in metal finishing and chrome plating, stainless steel production, leather tanning, and wood preservatives.

Which Cancers Are Associated with Exposure to Hexavalent Chromium Compounds?

Occupational exposure to these compounds is associated with increased risks of lung cancer and cancer of the paranasal sinuses and nasal cavity.

How Can Exposures Be Reduced?

The OSHA has exposure limits and information about analytical methods used to evaluate hexavalent chromium exposure.

Indoor Emissions from the Household Combustion of Coal

Burning coal inside the home can release a number of harmful chemicals.

Which Cancers Are Associated with Exposure to Indoor Coal Combustion Emissions?

Lung cancer is associated with exposure to indoor coal combustion emissions.

How Can Exposures Be Reduced?

Installing indoor stoves with chimneys can reduce the level of indoor air pollution.

Nickel Compounds

Grinding, mining, welding, and other occupations expose workers to nickel compounds.

Which Cancers Are Associated with Exposure to Nickel and Nickel Compounds?

Exposure to various nickel compounds is associated with increased risks of lung cancer and nasal cancer.

How Can Exposures Be Reduced?

Exposures of the general population to nickel compounds are almost always too low to be of concern. To protect workers, the OSHA has issued exposure limits for nickel compounds.

1,3-Butadiene

1,3-Butadiene is used to produce synthetic rubber products, such as tires.

Which Cancers Are Associated with Exposure to 1,3-Butadiene?

Studies have consistently shown an association between occupational exposure to 1,3-butadiene and an increased incidence of leukemia.

How Can Exposures Be Reduced?

The OSHA has information on exposure limits for 1,3-butadiene. People can also reduce their exposure to 1,3-butadiene by avoiding tobacco smoke.

Radon

Radon is a radioactive gas that is released from the normal decay of the elements uranium, thorium, and radium in rocks and soil. The invisible, odorless gas seeps up through the ground and diffuses into the air. In a few areas, depending on local geology, radon dissolves into groundwater and can be released into the air when the water is used. Radon gas usually exists at very low levels outdoors, but the gas can accumulate in areas without adequate ventilation, such as underground mines.

Which Cancers Are Associated with Exposure to Radon?

Radon was identified as a health problem when scientists noted that underground uranium miners who were exposed to it died of lung cancer at high rates. Experimental studies in animals confirmed the results of the miner studies by showing higher rates of lung tumors among rodents exposed to high levels of radon. There has been a suggestion of an increased risk of leukemia associated with radon exposure in adults and children; the evidence, however, is not conclusive.

How Can Exposures Be Reduced?

Check the radon levels in your home regularly. The EPA has more information about residential radon exposure and what people can do about it in its Consumer's Guide to Radon Reduction.

Secondhand Tobacco Smoke (Environmental Tobacco Smoke)

At least 69 chemicals found in secondhand tobacco smoke are carcinogens.

Which Cancers Are Associated with Secondhand Smoke?

Inhaling secondhand smoke causes lung cancer in nonsmokers. Some research also suggests that secondhand smoke may increase the risk of some other cancers as well, though more research is needed on this subject.

How Can Exposures Be Reduced?

There is no safe level of exposure to secondhand smoke; even low levels of secondhand smoke can be harmful. In the United States, legislation has helped to reduce exposures. Federal law bans smoking on all domestic airline flights, nearly all flights between the United States and foreign destinations, interstate buses, and most trains. Smoking is also banned in most federally owned buildings. Many state and local governments have also passed laws prohibiting smoking in public facilities, such as schools, hospitals, and airports, as well as private workplaces, including restaurants and bars.

Internationally, a growing number of nations require all workplaces, including bars and restaurants, to be smoke free.

Strong Inorganic Acid Mists Containing Sulfuric Acid

Copper smelting and other manufacturing processes generate mists containing sulfuric acid.

Which Cancers Are Associated with Exposure to Strong Inorganic Acid Mists Containing Sulfuric Acid?

Occupational exposure to strong inorganic acid mists containing sulfuric acid is associated with increased risks of laryngeal and lung cancer.

The OSHA has information about exposure limits for sulfuric acid.

Thorium

Thorium is a naturally occurring radioactive metal found in soil, rock, and water.

Which Cancers Are Associated with Exposure to Thorium?

Studies of patients who received intravascular injections of Thorotrast found an increased risk of liver tumors among these individuals. And there is research evidence that inhaling thorium dust increases the risk of lung and pancreatic cancer. Individuals exposed to thorium also have an increased risk of bone cancer because thorium may be stored in bone.

How Can Exposures Be Reduced?

Occasionally, household items may be found to contain thorium, such as some older ceramic wares in which uranium was used in the glaze, or gas lantern mantles. Although these exposures generally do not pose serious health risks, such household items should be retired from use to avoid unnecessary exposures. A radiation counter is required to confirm if ceramics contain thorium.

Vinyl Chloride

Vinyl chloride is used primarily to make PVC, a substance used in products such as pipes.

Which Cancers Are Associated with Exposure to Vinyl Chloride?

Vinyl chloride exposure is associated with an increased risk of a rare form of liver cancer (hepatic angiosarcoma), as well as brain and lung cancers, lymphoma, and leukemia.

How Can Exposures Be Reduced?

The OSHA provides information about exposure limits to vinyl chloride.

Wood Dust

People who cut or shape wood for a living may inhale unhealthy amounts of wood dust.

Which Cancers Are Associated with Exposure to Wood Dust?

Strong and consistent associations with cancers of the paranasal sinuses and nasal cavity have been observed both in studies of people whose occupations were associated with wood-dust exposure and in studies that directly estimated wood-dust exposure.

How Can Exposures Be Reduced?

Exposures can be reduced through design and engineering modifications, such as installing an exhaust ventilation system with collectors placed at points where dust is produced. Personal protective equipment, such as respirators, is another short-term solution for reducing exposure. The OSHA provides information about exposure limits to wood dust.

Part Two

Breast Cancer

Chapter 8

Breast Cancer Statistics

Not counting some kinds of skin cancer, breast cancer in the United States is:

- The most common cancer in women, no matter your race or ethnicity

- The most common cause of death from cancer among Hispanic women

- The second most common cause of death from cancer among white, black, Asian/Pacific Islander, and American Indian/ Alaska native women

In 2014 (The most recent year numbers are available):

- 236,968 women and 2,141 men in the United States were diagnosed with breast cancer

- 41,211 women and 465 men in the United States died from breast cancer

Rates by Race and Ethnicity

The rate of women getting breast cancer or dying from breast cancer varies by race and ethnicity.

This chapter includes text excerpted from "Breast Cancer—Breast Cancer Statistics," Centers for Disease Control and Prevention (CDC), June 7, 2017.

Incidence Rates by Race/Ethnicity

"Incidence rate" means how many women out of a given number get the disease each year. In 2014, white women had the highest rate of getting breast cancer, followed by black, Hispanic, Asian/Pacific Islander (A/PI), and American Indian/Alaska Native (AI/AN) women.

Death Rates by Race/Ethnicity

From 1999–2014, the rate of women dying from breast cancer has varied, depending on their race and ethnicity. In 2014, black women were more likely to die of breast cancer than any other group, followed by white, Hispanic, Asian/Pacific Islander, and American Indian/Alaska Native women.

Breast Cancer Rates by State

The U.S. states are divided into groups based on the rates at which women developed or died from breast cancer in 2014, which is the most recent year for which incidence data are available. The rates are the numbers out of 100,000 women who developed or died from breast cancer each year. The number of people who get breast cancer is called breast cancer incidence. In the United States, the rate of getting breast cancer and the rate of dying from breast cancer vary from state to state.

Breast Cancer Trends

Incidence Trends

From 2003–2012 in the United States, the incidence rate of breast cancer:

- Remained level among women
- Remained level among white women
- Increased significantly by 0.8 percent per year among black women
- Remained level among Hispanic women
- Remained level among American Indian/Alaska Native women
- Increased significantly by 1.1 percent per year among Asian/Pacific Islander women

Mortality Trends

From 2003–2012 in the United States, the death rate from breast cancer:

- Decreased significantly by 1.9 percent per year among women

- Decreased significantly by 1.9 percent per year among white women

- Decreased significantly by 1.4 percent per year among black women

- Decreased significantly by 1.3 percent per year among Hispanic women

- Decreased significantly by 3.4 percent per year among American Indian/Alaska Native women

- Decreased significantly by 1.4 percent per year among Asian/ Pacific Islander women

Breast Cancer Risk by Age

The risk of getting breast cancer increases with age. The table below shows the percentage of women (how many out of 100) who will get breast cancer over different time periods. The time periods are based on the woman's current age.

For example, go to current age 60. The table 8.1 shows 3.46 percent of women who are 60 years old will get breast cancer sometime during the next 10 years. That is, 3 or 4 out of every 100 women who are 60 years old will get breast cancer by the age of 70.

Table 8.1. Percent of U.S. Women Who Develop Breast Cancer over 10-, 20-, and 30-Year Intervals According to Their Current Age, 2010–2012

Current Age	10 Years	20 Years	30 Years
30	0.44	1.87	4.05
40	1.44	3.65	6.8
50	2.28	5.53	8.75
60	3.46	6.89	8.89
70	3.89	6.16	N/A

Chapter 9

What You Need to Know about Breast Cancer

Breast cancer is a disease in which cells in the breast grow out of control. There are different kinds of breast cancer. The kind of breast cancer depends on which cells in the breast turn into cancer. Breast cancer can begin in different parts of the breast. A breast is made up of three main parts: lobules, ducts, and connective tissue. The lobules are the glands that produce milk. The ducts are tubes that carry milk to the nipple. The connective tissue (which consists of fibrous and fatty tissue) surrounds and holds everything together. Most breast cancers begin in the ducts or lobules. Breast cancer can spread outside the breast through blood vessels and lymph vessels. When breast cancer spreads to other parts of the body, it is said to have metastasized.

Kinds of Breast Cancer

The most common kinds of breast cancer are:

- **Invasive ductal carcinoma.** The cancer cells grow outside the ducts into other parts of the breast tissue. Invasive cancer cells can also spread, or metastasize, to other parts of the body.

This chapter includes text excerpted from "What Is Breast Cancer?" Centers for Disease Control and Prevention (CDC), July 25, 2017.

- **Invasive lobular carcinoma.** Cancer cells spread from the lobules to the breast tissues that are close by. These invasive cancer cells can also spread to other parts of the body.

There are several other less common kinds of breast cancer, such as Paget disease, medullary, mucinous, and inflammatory breast cancer. Ductal carcinoma in situ (DCIS) is a breast disease that may lead to breast cancer. The cancer cells are only in the lining of the ducts, and have not spread to other tissues in the breast.

What Are the Symptoms of Breast Cancer?

Different people have different symptoms of breast cancer. Some people do not have any signs or symptoms at all. A person may find out they have breast cancer after a routine mammogram.

Some warning signs of breast cancer are:

- New lump in the breast or underarm (armpit)
- Thickening or swelling of part of the breast
- Irritation or dimpling of breast skin
- Redness or flaky skin in the nipple area or the breast
- Pulling in of the nipple or pain in the nipple area
- Nipple discharge other than breast milk, including blood
- Any change in the size or the shape of the breast
- Pain in any area of the breast

Keep in mind that these symptoms can happen with other conditions that are not cancer. If you have any signs or symptoms that worry you, be sure to see your doctor right away.

What Is a Normal Breast?

No breast is typical. What is normal for you may not be normal for another woman. Most women say their breasts feel lumpy or uneven. The way your breasts look and feel can be affected by getting your period, having children, losing or gaining weight, and taking certain medications. Breasts also tend to change as you age.

What Do Lumps in My Breast Mean?

Many conditions can cause lumps in the breast, including cancer. But most breast lumps are caused by other medical conditions. The two most common causes of breast lumps are fibrocystic breast condition and cysts. Fibrocystic condition causes noncancerous changes in the breast that can make them lumpy, tender, and sore. Cysts are small fluid-filled sacs that can develop in the breast.

What Are the Risk Factors for Breast Cancer?

Studies have shown that your risk for breast cancer is due to a combination of factors. The main factors that influence your risk include being a woman and getting older. Most breast cancers are found in women who are 50 years old or older. Some women will get breast cancer even without any other risk factors that they know of. Having a risk factor does not mean you will get the disease, and not all risk factors have the same effect. Most women have some risk factors, but most women do not get breast cancer. If you have breast cancer risk factors, talk with your doctor about ways you can lower your risk and about screening for breast cancer.

How Is Breast Cancer Diagnosed?

Doctors often use additional tests to find or diagnose breast cancer. They may refer women to a breast specialist or a surgeon. This does not mean that she has cancer or that she needs surgery. These doctors are experts in diagnosing breast problems.

- **Breast ultrasound.** A machine that uses sound waves to make detailed pictures, called sonograms, of areas inside the breast.

- **Diagnostic mammogram.** If you have a problem in your breast, such as lumps, or if an area of the breast looks abnormal on a screening mammogram, doctors may have you get a diagnostic mammogram. This is a more detailed X-ray of the breast.

- **Magnetic resonance imaging (MRI).** A kind of body scan that uses a magnet linked to a computer. The MRI scan will make detailed pictures of areas inside the breast.

- **Biopsy.** This is a test that removes tissue or fluid from the breast to be looked at under a microscope and do more testing. There are different kinds of biopsies (for example, fine-needle aspiration, core biopsy, or open biopsy).

How Is Breast Cancer Treated?

Breast cancer is treated in several ways. It depends on the kind of breast cancer and how far it has spread. People with breast cancer often get more than one kind of treatment.

- **Surgery.** An operation where doctors cut out cancer tissue.

- **Chemotherapy.** Using special medicines to shrink or kill the cancer cells. The drugs can be pills you take or medicines given in your veins, or sometimes both.

- **Hormonal therapy.** Blocks cancer cells from getting the hormones they need to grow.

- **Biological therapy.** Works with your body's immune system to help it fight cancer cells or to control side effects from other cancer treatments.

- **Radiation therapy.** Using high-energy rays (similar to X-rays) to kill the cancer cells.

Doctors from different specialties often work together to treat breast cancer. Surgeons are doctors who perform operations. Medical oncologists are doctors who treat cancer with medicine. Radiation oncologists are doctors who treat cancer with radiation.

Chapter 10

Understanding the Risk of Breast Cancer

Chapter Contents

Section 10.1

Probability of Breast Cancer in American Women

This section includes text excerpted from "Breast Cancer Risk in American Women," National Cancer Institute (NCI), September 24, 2012. Reviewed May 2018.

What Is the Average American Woman's Risk of Developing Breast Cancer during Her Lifetime?

Based on current incidence rates, 12.4 percent of women born in the United States today will develop breast cancer at some time during their lives. This estimate, from the *Surveillance, Epidemiology, and End Results Program (SEER) Cancer Statistics Review* (a report published annually by the National Cancer Institute's (NCI) SEER Program), is based on breast cancer statistics for the years 2007 through 2009.

This estimate means that, if the current incidence rate stays the same, a woman born today has about a 1 in 8 chance of being diagnosed with breast cancer at some time during her life. On the other hand, the chance that she will never have breast cancer is 87.6 percent, or about 7 in 8.

In the 1970s, the lifetime risk of being diagnosed with breast cancer in the United States was just under 10 percent (or about 1 in 10).

The last five annual SEER reports show the following estimates of lifetime risk of breast cancer, all very close to a lifetime risk of 1 in 8:

- 12.7 percent for 2001 through 2003

- 12.3 percent for 2002 through 2004

- 12.0 percent for 2003 through 2005

- 12.1 percent for 2004 through 2006

- 12.4 percent for 2005 through 2007

SEER statisticians expect some variability from year to year. Slight changes, such as the ones observed over the last 5 years, may be explained by a variety of factors, including minor changes in risk factor levels in the population, slight changes in breast cancer screening rates, or just random variability inherent in the data.

What Is the Average American Woman's Risk of Being Diagnosed with Breast Cancer at Different Ages?

Many women are more interested in the risk of being diagnosed with breast cancer at specific ages or over specific time periods than in the risk of being diagnosed at some point during their lifetime. Estimates by decade of life are also less affected by changes in incidence and mortality rates than longer-term estimates. The SEER report estimates the risk of developing breast cancer in 10-year age intervals. According to the report, the risk that a woman will be diagnosed with breast cancer during the next 10 years, starting at the following ages, is as follows:

- Age 30—0.44 percent (or 1 in 227)

- Age 40—1.47 percent (or 1 in 68)

- Age 50—2.38 percent (or 1 in 42)

- Age 60—3.56 percent (or 1 in 28)

- Age 70—3.82 percent (or 1 in 26)

These probabilities are averages for the whole population. An individual woman's breast cancer risk may be higher or lower depending on a number of known factors and on factors that are not yet fully understood.

Section 10.2

Breast Cancer Risk and Protective Factors

This section includes text excerpted from "What Are
the Risk Factors for Breast Cancer?" Centers for
Disease Control and Prevention (CDC), July 25, 2017.

What Are the Risk Factors for Breast Cancer?

Studies have shown that your risk for breast cancer is due to a combination of factors. The main factors that influence your risk include being a woman and getting older. Most breast cancers are found in women who are 50 years old or older.

Some women will get breast cancer even without any other risk factors that they know of. Having a risk factor does not mean you will get the disease, and not all risk factors have the same effect. Most women have some risk factors, but most women do not get breast cancer. If you have breast cancer risk factors, talk with your doctor about ways you can lower your risk and about screening for breast cancer.

Risk factors include:

- **Getting older.** The risk for breast cancer increases with age; Most breast cancers are diagnosed after age 50.

- **Genetic mutations.** Inherited changes (mutations) to certain genes, such as *BRCA1* and *BRCA2*. Women who have inherited these genetic changes are at higher risk of breast and ovarian cancer.

- **Early menstrual period.** Women who start their periods before age 12 are exposed to hormones longer, raising the risk for breast cancer by a small amount.

- **Late or no pregnancy.** Having the first pregnancy after age 30 and never having a full-term pregnancy can raise breast cancer risk.

- **Starting menopause after age 55.** Like starting one's period early, being exposed to estrogen hormones for a longer time later in life also raises the risk of breast cancer.

- **Not being physically active.** Women who are not physically active have a higher risk of getting breast cancer.

- **Being overweight or obese after menopause.** Older women who are overweight or obese have a higher risk of getting breast cancer than those at a normal weight.

- **Having dense breasts.** Dense breasts have more connective tissue than fatty tissue, which can sometimes make it hard to see tumors on a mammogram. Women with dense breasts are more likely to get breast cancer.

- **Using combination hormone therapy.** Taking hormones to replace missing estrogen and progesterone in menopause for more than five years raises the risk for breast cancer. The hormones that have been shown to increase risk are estrogen and progestin when taken together.

- **Taking oral contraceptives (birth control pills).** Certain forms of oral contraceptive pills have been found to raise breast cancer risk.

- **Personal history of breast cancer.** Women who have had breast cancer are more likely to get breast cancer a second time.

- **Personal history of certain noncancerous breast diseases.** Some noncancerous breast diseases such as atypical hyperplasia or lobular carcinoma in situ are associated with a higher risk of getting breast cancer.

- **Family history of breast cancer.** A woman's risk for breast cancer is higher if she has a mother, sister, or daughter (first-degree relative) or multiple family members on either her mother's or father's side of the family who have had breast cancer. Having a first-degree male relative with breast cancer also raises a woman's risk.

- **Previous treatment using radiation therapy.** Women who had radiation therapy to the chest or breasts (like for treatment of Hodgkin lymphoma) before age 30 have a higher risk of getting breast cancer later in life.

- **Women who took the drug diethylstilbestrol (DES),** which was given to some pregnant women in the United States between 1940 and 1971 to prevent miscarriage, have a higher risk. Women whose mothers took DES while pregnant with them are also at risk.

- **Drinking alcohol.** Studies show that a woman's risk for breast cancer increases with the more alcohol she drinks.

What Can I Do to Reduce My Risk of Breast Cancer?

Many factors over the course of a lifetime can influence your breast cancer risk. You can't change some factors, such as getting older or your family history, but you can help lower your risk of breast cancer by taking care of your health in the following ways:

- Keep a healthy weight

- Exercise regularly (at least four hours a week)

- Research shows that lack of nighttime sleep can be a risk factor

- Don't drink alcohol, or limit alcoholic drinks to no more than one per day

- Avoid exposure to chemicals that can cause cancer (carcinogens) and chemicals that interfere with the normal function of the body

- Limit exposure to radiation from medical imaging tests like X-rays, computed tomography (CT) scans, and positron emission tomography (PET) scans if not medically necessary

- If you are taking, or have been told to take, hormone replacement therapy or oral contraceptives (birth control pills), ask your doctor about the risks and find out if it is right for you

- Breastfeed any children you may have, if possible

If you have a family history of breast cancer or inherited changes in your *BRCA1* and *BRCA2* genes, you may be at high risk for getting breast cancer. Talk to your doctor about more ways to lower your risk.

Staying healthy throughout your life will lower your risk of developing cancer, and improve your chances of surviving cancer if it occurs.

Who Is at High Risk for Breast Cancer?

If you have a family history of breast cancer or inherited changes in your *BRCA1* and *BRCA2* genes, you may have a high risk of getting breast cancer. You may also have a high risk for ovarian cancer. Talk to your doctor about these ways of reducing your risk, including any physical and emotional side effects from the surgeries:

- Antiestrogens or other medicines that block or decrease estrogen in your body.

- Surgery to reduce your risk of breast cancer:
  - Prophylactic (preventive) mastectomy (removal of breast tissue)
  - Prophylactic (preventive) salpingo-oophorectomy (removal of the ovaries and fallopian tubes)

It is important that you know your family history and talk to your doctor about how you can lower your risk.

Section 10.3

Alcohol and Breast Cancer Risk

This section includes text excerpted from "Women and Alcohol," National Institute on Alcohol Abuse and Alcoholism (NIAAA), June 2017.

Research shows that drinking, binge drinking, and extreme binge drinking by women are all increasing. While alcohol misuse by anyone presents serious public health concerns, women who drink have a higher risk of certain alcohol-related problems compared to men. Women should be aware of these health risks and make informed decisions about alcohol use.

Why Do Women Face Higher Risks?

Studies show that women start to have alcohol-related problems sooner and at lower drinking levels than men and for multiple reasons. On average, women weigh less than men. Also, alcohol resides predominantly in body water, and pound for pound, women have less water in their bodies than men. This means that after a woman and a man of the same weight drink the same amount of alcohol, the woman's blood alcohol concentration (BAC, the amount of alcohol in the blood) will tend to be higher, putting her at greater risk for harm. Other biological differences may contribute as well.

How Much Is Too Much?

In the United States, a standard drink is one that contains about 14 grams (0.6 fluid ounces) of "pure" alcohol, which is found in:

- 12 ounces of beer with about 5 percent alcohol content

- 5 ounces of wine with about 12 percent alcohol content

- 1.5 ounces of distilled spirits with about 40 percent alcohol content

The percent of pure alcohol varies within and across beverage types. Although the standard drink amounts are helpful for following health guidelines, they may not reflect customary serving sizes. A large cup of beer, an overpoured glass of wine, or a single mixed drink could contain much more alcohol than a standard drink.

According to the *Dietary Guidelines for Americans* (DGA), which are intended to help individuals improve and maintain overall health and reduce the risk of many chronic diseases, moderate alcohol consumption is up to one drink per day for women and up to two drinks per day for men.

At-Risk Drinking

The National Institute on Alcohol Abuse and Alcoholism (NIAAA) defines how much drinking can put a person at risk for developing alcohol use disorder (AUD). Low-risk drinking limits for developing AUD are:

- **Women:** No more than 3 drinks on any single day and no more than 7 drinks per week

- **Men:** No more than 4 drinks on any single day and no more than 14 drinks per week

Drinking more than the single day or weekly low-risk limits shown here is considered at-risk drinking. People who regularly exceed the low-risk drinking limits include those who engage in binge drinking and heavy alcohol use. NIAAA defines binge drinking as a pattern of drinking that brings BAC levels to 0.08 g/dL (0.08%) or higher. This typically occurs after 4 drinks for women and 5 drinks for men—in about 2 hours. Binge drinking and heavy alcohol use (binge drinking five or more times a month) increase the likelihood of developing AUD, as well as experiencing alcohol-related injuries and other harms.

What Are the Long-Term Health Risks?

Alcohol Use Disorder (AUD)

AUD is a chronic relapsing brain disease characterized by an impaired ability to stop or control alcohol use despite adverse social, occupational, or health consequences. AUD can range from mild to severe, and recovery is possible regardless of severity.

Table 10.1. Snapshot: Alcohol Use by Women In the United States

Alcohol Use by Women	Women	Men
Drank alcohol in the past month	51.10%	61.30%
Engaged in binge drinking in the past month	22.00%	32.10%
Engaged in heavy alcohol use in the past month	4.50%	9.80%
Had alcohol use disorder in the past year	4.20%	8.40%
Had AUD and received any treatment in the past year	5.40%	7.40%
Pregnant and used alcohol in the past month	9.30%	

Percentages represent U.S. adults aged 18 years and older who used alcohol or had AUD, with the exception of "pregnant and used alcohol in the past month," which represents females aged 15–44.

Breast Cancer

There is an association between drinking alcohol and developing breast cancer. Studies demonstrate that women who consume about one drink per day have a 5–9 percent higher chance of developing breast cancer than women who do not drink at all. That risk increases for every additional drink they have per day.

Pregnancy

Any drinking during pregnancy can be harmful. A woman who drinks during pregnancy puts her fetus at risk for physical, cognitive,

111

or behavioral problems. Drinking during pregnancy can also increase the risk for preterm labor.

Some women should avoid alcohol entirely, including:

- Anyone who is pregnant or trying to conceive
- Anyone younger than age 21
- Anyone who takes medications that can interact negatively with alcohol

Liver Damage

Women who regularly misuse alcohol are more likely to develop alcoholic hepatitis, a serious acute illness, than men who drink the same amount of alcohol. This pattern of drinking can also lead to cirrhosis (liver scarring and shrinkage).

Heart Disease

Long-term alcohol misuse is a leading cause of heart disease. Women are more susceptible to alcohol-related heart disease than men, even though they may consume less alcohol over their lifetime than men.

Brain Damage

Research suggests that alcohol misuse produces brain damage more quickly in women than in men. In addition, because alcohol can disrupt the development of the brain during the adolescent years, teen girls who drink may be more vulnerable to brain damage than teen boys who drink. Women also may be more susceptible than men to alcohol-related blackouts, defined as periods of memory loss of events during intoxication without loss of consciousness.

Chapter 11

Genes Associated with Breast Cancer

What Are BRCA1 *and* BRCA2*?*

BRCA1 and *BRCA2* are human genes that produce tumor suppressor proteins. These proteins help repair damaged deoxyribonucleic acid (DNA) and, therefore, play a role in ensuring the stability of each cell's genetic material. When either of these genes is mutated, or altered, such that its protein product is not made or does not function correctly, DNA damage may not be repaired properly. As a result, cells are more likely to develop additional genetic alterations that can lead to cancer.

Specific inherited mutations in *BRCA1* and *BRCA2* most notably increase the risk of female breast and ovarian cancers, but they have also been associated with increased risks of several additional types of cancer. People who have inherited mutations in *BRCA1* and *BRCA2* tend to develop breast and ovarian cancers at younger ages than people who do not have these mutations.

A harmful *BRCA1* or *BRCA2* mutation can be inherited from a person's mother or father. Each child of a parent who carries a mutation in one of these genes has a 50 percent chance (or 1 chance in 2) of inheriting the mutation. The effects of mutations in *BRCA1* and *BRCA2* are seen even when a person's second copy of the gene is normal.

This chapter includes text excerpted from "BRCA Mutations: Cancer Risk and Genetic Testing," National Cancer Institute (NCI), January 30, 2018.

How Much Does Having a BRCA1 or BRCA2 Gene Mutation Increase a Woman's Risk of Breast and Ovarian Cancer?

A woman's lifetime risk of developing breast and/or ovarian cancer is greatly increased if she inherits a harmful mutation in *BRCA1* or *BRCA2*.

Breast cancer: About 12 percent of women in the general population will develop breast cancer sometime during their lives. By contrast, a recent large study estimated that about 72 percent of women who inherit a harmful *BRCA1* mutation and about 69 percent of women who inherit a harmful *BRCA2* mutation will develop breast cancer by the age of 80.

Like women from the general population, those with harmful *BRCA1* or *BRCA2* mutations also have a high risk of developing a new primary cancer in the opposite (contralateral) breast in the years following a breast cancer diagnosis. It has been estimated that, by 20 years after a first breast cancer diagnosis, about 40 percent of women who inherit a harmful *BRCA1* mutation and about 26 percent of women who inherit a harmful *BRCA2* mutation will develop cancer in their other breast.

Ovarian cancer: About 1.3 percent of women in the general population will develop ovarian cancer sometime during their lives. By contrast, it is estimated that about 44 percent of women who inherit a harmful *BRCA1* mutation and about 17 percent of women who inherit a harmful *BRCA2* mutation will develop ovarian cancer by the age of 80.

What Other Cancers Have Been Linked to Mutations in BRCA1 and BRCA2?

Harmful mutations in *BRCA1* and *BRCA2* increase the risk of several cancers in addition to breast and ovarian cancer. These include fallopian tube cancer and peritoneal cancer. Both men and women with harmful *BRCA1* or *BRCA2* mutations are at increased risk of pancreatic cancer.

Certain mutations in *BRCA2* (also known as *FANCD1*), if they are inherited from both parents, can cause a rare form of Fanconi anemia (subtype FA-D1), a syndrome that is associated with childhood solid tumors and development of acute myeloid leukemia. Likewise, certain mutations in *BRCA1* (also known as *FANCS*), if they are inherited from both parents, can cause another Fanconi anemia subtype.

Are Mutations in BRCA1 *and* BRCA2 *More Common in Certain Racial/Ethnic Populations than Others?*

Yes. For example, people of Ashkenazi Jewish descent have a higher prevalence of harmful *BRCA1* and *BRCA2* mutations than people in the general U.S. population. Other ethnic and geographic populations around the world, such as the Norwegian, Dutch, and Icelandic peoples, also have a higher prevalence of specific harmful *BRCA1* and *BRCA2* mutations.

In addition, the prevalence of specific harmful *BRCA1* and *BRCA2* mutations may vary among individual racial and ethnic groups in the United States, including African Americans, Hispanics, Asian Americans, and non-Hispanic whites. This question is under intensive study, since identifying population-specific mutations in these genes can greatly simplify the genetic testing for *BRCA1* and *BRCA2* mutations.

Are Genetic Tests Available to Detect BRCA1 *and* BRCA2 *Mutations?*

Yes, several different tests are available. Some tests look for a specific harmful *BRCA1* or *BRCA2* gene mutation that has already been identified in another family member. Other tests check for all of the known harmful mutations in both genes. Multigene (panel) testing uses next-generation sequencing to look for harmful mutations in many genes that are associated with an increased risk of breast and ovarian cancer, including *BRCA1* and *BRCA2*, at the same time. Deoxyribonucleic acid (usually from a blood or saliva sample) is needed for all of these tests. The sample is sent to a laboratory for analysis. It usually takes about a month to get the test results.

Who Should Consider Genetic Testing for BRCA1 *and* BRCA2 *Mutations?*

Because harmful *BRCA1* and *BRCA2* gene mutations are relatively rare in the general population, most experts agree that mutation testing of individuals who do not have cancer should be performed only when the person's individual or family history suggests the possible presence of a harmful mutation in *BRCA1* or *BRCA2*.

The U.S. Preventive Services Task Force (USPSTF) recommends that women who have family members with breast, ovarian, fallopian tube, or peritoneal cancer be evaluated to see if they have a family history that is associated with an increased risk of a harmful mutation in one of these genes.

Several screening tools are available to help healthcare providers with this evaluation. These tools assess personal or family history factors that are associated with an increased likelihood of having a harmful mutation in *BRCA1* or *BRCA2*, such as:

- Breast cancer diagnosed before age 50 years

- Cancer in both breasts in the same woman

- Both breast and ovarian cancers in either the same woman or the same family

- Multiple breast cancers in the family

- Two or more primary types of *BRCA1*- or *BRCA2*-related cancers in a single family member

- Cases of male breast cancer

- Ashkenazi Jewish ethnicity

When an individual has a family history that is suggestive of the presence of a *BRCA1* or *BRCA2* mutation, it may be most informative to first test a family member who has cancer, if that person is still alive and willing to be tested. If that person has a harmful *BRCA1* or *BRCA2* mutation, then other family members may want to consider genetic counseling to learn more about their potential risks and whether genetic testing for mutations in *BRCA1* and *BRCA2* might be appropriate for them.

If it can't be determined whether the family member with cancer has a harmful *BRCA1* or *BRCA2* mutation, members of a family whose history is suggestive of the presence of a *BRCA1* or *BRCA2* gene mutation may still want to consider genetic counseling for possible testing.

Some individuals—for example, those who were adopted at birth— may not know their family history. If a woman with an unknown family history has an early-onset breast cancer or ovarian cancer or a man with an unknown family history is diagnosed with breast cancer, that individual may want to consider genetic counseling and testing for a *BRCA1* or *BRCA2* mutation.

Professional societies do not recommend that children under age 18, even those with a family history suggestive of a harmful *BRCA1* or

BRCA2 mutation, undergo genetic testing for *BRCA1* or *BRCA2*. This is because there are no risk-reduction strategies that are specifically meant for children, and children's risks of developing a cancer type associated with a *BRCA1* or *BRCA2* mutation are extremely low.

Should People Considering Genetic Testing for BRCA1 and BRCA2 Mutations Talk with a Genetic Counselor?

Genetic counseling is generally recommended before and after any genetic test for an inherited cancer syndrome. This counseling should be performed by a healthcare professional who is experienced in cancer genetics. Genetic counseling usually covers many aspects of the testing process, including:

- A hereditary cancer risk assessment based on an individual's personal and family medical history
- Discussion of:
  - The appropriateness of genetic testing
  - The medical implications of a positive or a negative test result
  - The possibility that a test result might not be informative (that is, it might find an alteration whose effect on cancer risk is not known)
  - The psychological risks and benefits of genetic test results
  - The risk of passing a mutation to children
- Explanation of the specific test(s) that might be used and the technical accuracy of the test(s)

Does Health Insurance Cover the Cost of BRCA1 and BRCA2 Mutation Testing?

People considering *BRCA1* and *BRCA2* mutation testing may want to confirm their insurance coverage for genetic counseling and testing. The Affordable Care Act (ACA) considers genetic counseling and *BRCA1* and *BRCA2* mutation testing a covered preventive service for women who have not already been diagnosed with a cancer related to a mutation in *BRCA1* or *BRCA2* and who meet the USPSTF recommendations for testing.

117

Medicare covers *BRCA1* and *BRCA2* mutation testing for women who have signs and symptoms of breast, ovarian, or other cancers that are related to mutations in *BRCA1* and *BRCA2* but not for unaffected women. Some of the genetic testing companies that offer testing for *BRCA1* and *BRCA2* mutations may offer testing at no charge to patients who lack insurance and meet specific financial and medical criteria.

What Do BRCA1 *or* BRCA2 *Genetic Test Results Mean?*

BRCA1 and *BRCA2* gene mutation testing can give several possible results: a positive result, a negative result, or an ambiguous or uncertain result.

Positive result. A positive test result indicates that a person has inherited a known harmful mutation in *BRCA1* or *BRCA2* and, therefore, has an increased risk of developing certain cancers. However, a positive test result cannot tell whether or when an individual will actually develop cancer. Some women who inherit a harmful *BRCA1* or *BRCA2* mutation never develop breast or ovarian cancer.

A positive test result may also have important implications for family members, including future generations.

- Both men and women who inherit a harmful *BRCA1* or *BRCA2* mutation, whether or not they develop cancer themselves, may pass the mutation on to their sons and daughters. Each child has a 50 percent chance of inheriting a parent's mutation.

- If a person learns that he or she has inherited a harmful *BRCA1* or *BRCA2* mutation, this will mean that each of his or her full siblings has a 50 percent chance of having inherited the mutation as well.

Negative result. A negative test result can be more difficult to understand than a positive result because what the result means depends in part on an individual's family history of cancer and whether a *BRCA1* or *BRCA2* mutation has been identified in a blood relative.

If a close (first- or second-degree) relative of the tested person is known to carry a harmful *BRCA1* or *BRCA2* mutation, a negative test result is clear: it means that person does not carry the harmful mutation that is responsible for their family's cancer risk, and thus cannot pass it on to their children. Such a test result is called a true negative. A person with such a test result is currently thought to have the same risk of cancer as someone in the general population.

If the tested person has a family history that suggests the possibility of having a harmful mutation in *BRCA1* or *BRCA2* but complete gene testing identifies no such mutation in the family, a negative result is less clear. The likelihood that genetic testing will miss a known harmful *BRCA1* or *BRCA2* mutation is very low, but it could happen. Moreover, scientists continue to discover new *BRCA1* and *BRCA2* mutations and have not yet identified all potentially harmful ones. Therefore, it is possible that a person in this scenario with a "negative" test result may actually have a harmful *BRCA1* or *BRCA2* mutation that has not previously been identified.

It is also possible for people to have a mutation in a gene other than *BRCA1* or *BRCA2* that increases their cancer risk but is not detectable by the test used. It is important that people considering genetic testing for *BRCA1* and *BRCA2* mutations discuss these potential uncertainties with a genetic counselor before undergoing testing.

Ambiguous or uncertain result. Sometimes, a genetic test finds a change in *BRCA1* or *BRCA2* that has not been previously associated with cancer. This type of test result may be described as "ambiguous" (often referred to as "a genetic variant of uncertain significance") because it isn't known whether this specific genetic change is harmful. One study found that 10 percent of women who underwent *BRCA1* and *BRCA2* mutation testing had this type of ambiguous result.

As more research is conducted and more people are tested for *BRCA1* and *BRCA2* mutations, scientists will learn more about these changes and cancer risk. Genetic counseling can help a person understand what an ambiguous change in *BRCA1* or *BRCA2* may mean in terms of cancer risk. Over time, additional studies of variants of uncertain significance may result in a specific mutation being reclassified as either clearly harmful or clearly not harmful.

How Can a Person Who Has a Harmful BRCA1 or BRCA2 Gene Mutation Manage Their Risk of Cancer?

Several options are available for managing cancer risk in individuals who have a known harmful *BRCA1* or *BRCA2* mutation. These include enhanced screening, prophylactic (risk-reducing) surgery, and chemoprevention.

Enhanced screening. Some women who test positive for *BRCA1* and *BRCA2* mutations may choose to start breast cancer screening at younger ages, and/or have more frequent screening, than women at average risk of breast cancer. For example, some experts recommend that women who carry a harmful *BRCA1* or *BRCA2* mutation undergo clinical breast examinations beginning at age 25–35 years. And some expert groups recommend that women who carry such a mutation have a mammogram every year, beginning at age 25–35 years.

Enhanced screening may increase the chance of detecting breast cancer at an early stage, when it may have a better chance of being treated successfully. Studies have shown that magnetic resonance imaging (MRI) may be better able than mammography to find tumors, particularly in younger women at high risk of breast cancer. However, mammography can also identify some breast cancers that are not identified by MRI. Also, MRI may be less specific (that is, lead to more false-positive results) than mammography.

Several organizations, such as the American Cancer Society (ACS) and the National Comprehensive Cancer Network (NCCN), now recommend annual screening with both mammography and MRI for women who have a high risk of breast cancer. Women who test positive for a *BRCA1* or *BRCA2* mutation should ask their healthcare provider about the possible harms of diagnostic tests that involve radiation (mammograms or X-rays).

No effective ovarian cancer screening methods currently exist. Some groups recommend transvaginal ultrasound, blood tests for the antigen CA-125, and clinical examinations for ovarian cancer screening in women with harmful *BRCA1* or *BRCA2* mutations, but none of these methods appears to detect ovarian tumors at an early enough stage to reduce the risk of dying from ovarian cancer. For a screening method to be considered effective, it must have demonstrated reduced mortality from the disease of interest. This standard has not yet been met for ovarian cancer screening.

Prophylactic (risk-reducing) surgery. Prophylactic surgery involves removing as much of the "at-risk" tissue as possible. Women may choose to have both breasts removed (bilateral prophylactic mastectomy) to reduce their risk of breast cancer. Surgery to remove a woman's ovaries and fallopian tubes (bilateral prophylactic salpingo-oophorectomy) can help reduce her risk of ovarian cancer. (Ovarian cancers often originate in the fallopian tubes, so it is essential that they be removed along with the ovaries.) Removing the ovaries may also reduce the risk of breast cancer in premenopausal women by eliminating a source of hormones that can fuel the growth of some types of breast cancer.

Whether bilateral prophylactic mastectomy reduces breast cancer risk in men with a harmful *BRCA1* or *BRCA2* mutation or a family history of breast cancer isn't known. Therefore, bilateral prophylactic mastectomy for men at high risk of breast cancer is considered an experimental procedure, and insurance companies will not normally cover it.

Prophylactic surgery does not guarantee that cancer will not develop because not all at-risk tissue can be removed by these procedures. That is why these surgical procedures are often described as "risk-reducing" rather than "preventive." Some women have developed breast cancer, ovarian cancer, or primary peritoneal carcinomatosis (a type of cancer similar to ovarian cancer) even after risk-reducing surgery. Nevertheless, these surgical procedures confer substantial benefits. For example, research demonstrates that women who underwent bilateral prophylactic salpingo-oophorectomy had a nearly 80 percent reduction in risk of dying from ovarian cancer, a 56 percent reduction in risk of dying from breast cancer, and a 77 percent reduction in risk of dying from any cause during the studies' follow-up periods.

The reduction in breast and ovarian cancer risk from removal of the ovaries and fallopian tubes appears to be similar for carriers of *BRCA1* and *BRCA2* mutations.

Chemoprevention. Chemoprevention is the use of medicines to try to reduce the risk of cancer. Although two chemopreventive drugs (tamoxifen and raloxifene) have been approved by the U.S. Food and Drug Administration (FDA) to reduce the risk of breast cancer in women at increased risk, the role of these drugs in women with harmful *BRCA1* or *BRCA2* mutations is not yet clear. However, these medications may be an option for women who don't choose, or can't undergo, surgery.

Data from three studies suggest that tamoxifen may be able to help lower the risk of breast cancer in women who carry harmful mutations in *BRCA2*, as well as the risk of cancer in the opposite breast among *BRCA1* and *BRCA2* mutation carriers previously diagnosed with breast cancer. Studies have not examined the effectiveness of raloxifene in *BRCA1* and *BRCA2* mutation carriers specifically.

Oral contraceptives (birth control pills) are thought to reduce the risk of ovarian cancer by about 50 percent both in the general population and in women with harmful *BRCA1* or *BRCA2* mutations.

What Are Some of the Benefits of Genetic Testing for Breast and Ovarian Cancer Risk?

There can be benefits to genetic testing, regardless of whether a person receives a positive or a negative result. The potential benefits of a true negative result include a sense of relief regarding the future risk of cancer, learning that one's children are not at risk of inheriting the family's cancer susceptibility, and the possibility that special checkups, tests, or preventive surgeries may not be needed.

A positive test result may bring relief by resolving uncertainty regarding future cancer risk and may allow people to make informed decisions about their future healthcare, including taking steps to reduce their cancer risk. In addition, people who have a positive test result may choose to participate in medical research that could, in the long run, help reduce deaths from hereditary breast and ovarian cancer.

What Are Some of the Possible Harms of Genetic Testing for BRCA Gene Mutations?

The direct medical harms of genetic testing are minimal, but knowledge of test results may have harmful effects on a person's emotions, social relationships, finances, and medical choices.

People who receive a positive test result may feel anxious, depressed, or angry, particularly immediately after they learn the result. People who learn that they carry a *BRCA* mutation may have difficulty making choices about whether to have preventive surgery or about which surgery to have.

People who receive a negative test result may experience "survivor guilt," caused by the knowledge that they likely do not have an increased risk of developing a disease that affects one or more loved ones.

Because genetic testing can reveal information about more than one family member, the emotions caused by test results can create tension within families. Test results can also affect personal life choices, such as decisions about career, marriage, and childbearing.

Violations of privacy and of the confidentiality of genetic test results are additional potential risks. However, the federal Health Insurance Portability and Accountability Act (HIPAA) and various state laws protect the privacy of a person's genetic information. Moreover, the federal Genetic Information Nondiscrimination Act (GINA), along with many state laws, prohibits discrimination based on genetic information in relation to health insurance and employment, although it does not cover life insurance, disability insurance, or long-term care insurance.

Finally, there is a small chance that test results may not be accurate, leading people to make medical decisions based on incorrect information. Although it is rare that results are inaccurate, people with these concerns should address them during genetic counseling.

What Are the Implications of Having a Harmful BRCA1 *or* BRCA2 *Mutation for Breast and Ovarian Cancer Prognosis and Treatment?*

Some studies have investigated whether there are clinical differences between breast and ovarian cancers that are associated with harmful *BRCA1* or *BRCA2* mutations and cancers that are not associated with these mutations.

- There is evidence that, over the long term, women who carry these mutations are more likely to develop a second cancer in either the same (ipsilateral) breast or the opposite (contralateral) breast than women who do not carry these mutations. Thus, some women with a harmful *BRCA1* or *BRCA2* mutation who develop breast cancer in one breast opt for a bilateral mastectomy, even if they would otherwise be candidates for breast-conserving surgery. Because of the increased risk of a second breast cancer among *BRCA1* and *BRCA2* mutation carriers, some doctors recommend that women with early onset breast cancer and those whose family history is consistent with a mutation in one of these genes have genetic testing when breast cancer is diagnosed.

- Breast cancers in women with a harmful *BRCA1* mutation tend to be "triple-negative cancers" (that is, the breast cancer cells do not have estrogen receptors, progesterone receptors, or large amounts of HER2/neu protein), which generally have poorer prognosis than other breast cancers.

- Because the *BRCA1* and *BRCA2* genes are involved in DNA repair, some investigators have suggested that cancer cells with a harmful mutation in either of these genes may be more sensitive to anticancer agents that act by damaging DNA, such as cisplatin. A class of drugs called PARP inhibitors, which block the repair of DNA damage, have been found to arrest the growth of cancer cells that have *BRCA1* or *BRCA2* mutations. Several

PARP inhibitors, including olaparib (Lynparza™) and rucaparib (Rubraca®), have been approved by the U.S. Food and Drug Administration (FDA) for the treatment of advanced ovarian cancers in women with a *BRCA1* or *BRCA2* mutation. Olaparib is also approved for the treatment of HER2-negative metastatic breast cancers in women with a *BRCA1* or *BRCA2* mutation.

Do Inherited Mutations in Other Genes Increase the Risk of Breast and/or Ovarian Tumors?

Yes. Although harmful mutations in *BRCA1* and *BRCA2* are responsible for the disease in nearly half of families with multiple cases of breast cancer and up to 90 percent of families with both breast and ovarian cancer, mutations in a number of other genes have been associated with increased risks of breast and/or ovarian cancers. These other genes include several that are associated with the inherited disorders Cowden syndrome (CS), Peutz-Jeghers syndrome (PJS), Li-Fraumeni syndrome (LFS), and Fanconi anemia (FA), which increase the risk of many cancer types.

Most mutations in these other genes do not increase breast cancer risk to the same extent as mutations in *BRCA1* and *BRCA2*. However, researchers have reported that inherited mutations in the *PALB2* gene are associated with a risk of breast cancer nearly as high as that associated with inherited *BRCA1* and *BRCA2* mutations. They estimated that 33 percent of women who inherit a harmful mutation in *PALB2* will develop breast cancer by age 70 years.

Recently, mutations in other genes that increase breast and ovarian cancer risk have been identified. These include mutations in the genes *TP53*, *CDH1*, and *CHEK2*, which increase the risk of breast cancer, and in *RAD51C*, *RAD51D*, and *STK11*, which increase the risk of ovarian cancer. Genetic testing for these other mutations is available as part of multigene (panel) testing. However, expert groups have not yet developed specific guidelines for who should be tested, or for the management of breast or ovarian cancer risk in people with these other high-risk mutations.

Chapter 12

Breast Cancer Screening

Breast cancer screening means checking a woman's breasts for cancer before there are signs or symptoms of the disease. All women need to be informed by their healthcare provider about the best screening options for them. When you are told about the benefits and risks and decide with your healthcare provider what screening test, if any, is right for you, this is called informed and shared decision-making. Although breast cancer screening cannot prevent breast cancer, it can help find breast cancer early, when it is easier to treat. Talk to your doctor about which breast cancer screening tests are right for you, and when you should have them.

Breast Cancer Screening Recommendations

The U.S. Preventive Services Task Force (USPSTF) Is an organization made up of doctors and disease experts who look at research on the best way to prevent diseases and make recommendations on how doctors can help patients avoid diseases or find them early.

The USPSTF recommends that women who are 50–74 years old and are at average risk for breast cancer get a mammogram every two

This chapter contains text excerpted from the following sources: Text in this chapter begins with excerpts from "What Is Breast Cancer Screening?" Centers for Disease Control and Prevention (CDC), July 25, 2017; Text under the heading "Risks for Breast Cancer Screening" is excerpted from "Breast Cancer Screening (PDQ®)—Patient Version," National Cancer Institute (NCI), August 11, 2017.

years. Women who are 40–49 years old should talk to their doctor or other healthcare professional about when to start and how often to get a mammogram. Women should weigh the benefits and risks of screening tests when deciding whether to begin getting mammograms at age 40.

Breast Cancer Screening Tests

Mammogram

A mammogram is an X-ray of the breast. Mammograms are the best way to find breast cancer early, when it is easier to treat and before it is big enough to feel or cause symptoms. Having regular mammograms can lower the risk of dying from breast cancer.

Breast Magnetic Resonance Imaging (MRI)

A breast MRI uses magnets and radio waves to take pictures of the breast. MRI is used along with mammograms to screen women who are at high risk for getting breast cancer. Because breast MRIs may appear abnormal even when there is no cancer, it is not used for women at average risk.

Where Can I Go to Get Screened?

You can get screened for breast cancer at a clinic, hospital, or doctor's office. If you want to be screened for breast cancer, call your doctor's office. They can help you schedule an appointment. Most health insurance plans are required to cover mammograms every 1–2 years for women beginning at age 40 with no out-of-pocket cost (Like a copay, deductible, or coinsurance).

Other Exams

The best way to find breast cancer is with a mammogram.

Clinical Breast Exam

A clinical breast exam is an examination by a doctor or nurse, who uses his or her hands to feel for lumps or other changes.

Breast Self-Awareness

Being familiar with how your breasts look and feel can help you notice symptoms such as lumps, pain, or changes in size that may be of concern. These could include changes found during a breast self-exam. You should report any changes that you notice to your doctor or healthcare provider. Having a clinical breast exam or doing a breast self-exam has not been found to lower the risk of dying from breast cancer.

Risks for Breast Cancer Screening

Screening tests have risks. Decisions about screening tests can be difficult. Not all screening tests are helpful and most have risks. Before having any screening test, you may want to discuss the test with your doctor. It is important to know the risks of the test and whether it has been proven to reduce the risk of dying from cancer.

The risks of breast cancer screening tests include the following:

- **False-positive test results can occur.**

  Screening test results may appear to be abnormal even though no cancer is present. A false-positive test result (one that shows there is cancer when there really isn't) is usually followed by more tests (such as biopsy), which also have risks.

  When a breast biopsy result is abnormal, getting a second opinion from a different pathologist may improve the accuracy of a breast cancer diagnosis.

  Most abnormal test results turn out not to be cancer. False-positive results are more common in the following:

  - Younger women

  - Women who have had previous breast biopsies

  - Women with a family history of breast cancer

  - Women who take hormones, such as estrogen and progestin

  False-positive results are more likely the first time a screening mammogram is done than with later screenings. Being able to compare a current mammogram with a past mammogram lowers the risk of a false-positive result.

  The skill of the radiologist also can affect the chance of a false-positive result.

- **False-negative test results can occur.**

  Screening test results may appear to be normal even though breast cancer is present. A woman who receives a false-negative test result (one that shows there is no cancer when there really is) may delay seeking medical care even if she has symptoms.

One in 5 cancers may be missed by mammography. False-negative results occur more often in younger women than in older women because the breast tissue of younger women is more dense. The chance of a false-negative result is also affected by the following:

- The size of the tumor

- The rate of tumor growth

- The level of hormones, such as estrogen and progesterone, in the woman's body

- The skill of the radiologist

- **Finding breast cancer may not improve health or help a woman live longer.**

Screening may not help you if you have fast-growing breast cancer or if it has already spread to other places in your body. Also, some breast cancers found on a screening mammogram may never cause symptoms or become life-threatening. Finding these cancers is called overdiagnosis. When such cancers are found, treatment would not help you live longer and may instead cause serious side effects.

- **There may be pain or discomfort during a mammogram.**

During a mammogram, the breast is placed between 2 plates that are pressed together. Pressing the breast helps to get a better X-ray of the breast. Some women have pain or discomfort during a mammogram. Some women have more pain than others. The amount of pain depends on the following:

- The phase of the woman's menstrual cycle

- The woman's anxiety level

- How much pain the woman expected

- **Mammograms expose the breast to radiation.**

Being exposed to radiation is a risk factor for breast cancer. The risk of breast cancer from radiation exposure is higher in women who received radiation before age 30 and at high doses. For women older than 40 years, the benefits of an annual screening mammogram may be greater than the risks from radiation exposure.

- **Anxiety from additional testing may result from false positive results.**

  Studies have shown that false-positive results from screening mammograms are usually followed by more testing that can lead to anxiety. In one study, women who had a false-positive screening mammogram followed by more testing reported feeling anxiety 3 months later, even though cancer was not diagnosed. Another study found that women who had a false-positive screening mammogram had anxiety right after screening, but it went away within a few months. A third study found that some women had anxiety several years after having a false-positive screening mammogram. However, several studies show that women who feel anxiety after false-positive test results are more likely to schedule regular breast screening exams in the future.

- **The risks and benefits of screening for breast cancer may be different in different age groups.**

  The benefits of breast cancer screening may vary among age groups:

  - In women who are expected to live 5 years or fewer, finding and treating early-stage breast cancer may reduce their quality of life without helping them live longer.

  - As with other women, in women older than 65 years, the results of a screening test may lead to more diagnostic tests and anxiety while waiting for the test results. Also, the breast cancers found are usually not life-threatening.

  - It has not been shown that women with an average risk of developing breast cancer benefit from starting screening mammography before age 40.

  Women who have had radiation treatment to the chest, especially at a young age, are advised to have routine breast cancer screening. Yearly MRI screening may begin 8 years after treatment or by age 25 years, whichever is later. The benefits and risks of mammograms and MRIs for these women have not been studied.

  There is no information on the benefits or risks of breast cancer screening in men.

  No matter how old you are, if you have risk factors for breast cancer you should ask for medical advice about when to begin having breast cancer screening tests and how often to have them.

- **Talk to your doctor about your risk of breast cancer and your need for screening tests.**

  Talk to your doctor or other healthcare provider about your risk of breast cancer, whether a screening test is right for you, and the benefits and harms of the screening test. You should take part in the decision about whether you want to have a screening test, based on what is best for you.

Chapter 13

Staging and Treating Breast Cancer

Staging

After breast cancer has been diagnosed, tests are done to find out if cancer cells have spread within the breast or to other parts of the body. The process used to find out whether the cancer has spread within the breast or to other parts of the body is called staging. The information gathered from the staging process determines the stage of the disease. It is important to know the stage in order to plan treatment. The results of some of the tests used to diagnose breast cancer are also used to stage the disease.

The following tests and procedures also may be used in the staging process:

- **Sentinel lymph node biopsy.** The removal of the sentinel lymph node during surgery. The sentinel lymph node is the first lymph node to receive lymphatic drainage from a tumor. It is the first lymph node the cancer is likely to spread to from the tumor. A radioactive substance and/or blue dye is injected near the tumor. The substance or dye flows through the lymph ducts to the lymph nodes. The first lymph node to receive the substance

---

This chapter includes text excerpted from "Breast Cancer Treatment (PDQ®)— Patient Version," National Cancer Institute (NCI), April 12, 2018.

or dye is removed. A pathologist views the tissue under a microscope to look for cancer cells. If cancer cells are not found, it may not be necessary to remove more lymph nodes.

- **Chest X-ray.** An X-ray of the organs and bones inside the chest. An X-ray is a type of energy beam that can go through the body and onto film, making a picture of areas inside the body.

- **Computerized axial tomography (CAT) scan.** A procedure that makes a series of detailed pictures of areas inside the body, taken from different angles. The pictures are made by a computer linked to an X-ray machine. A dye may be injected into a vein or swallowed to help the organs or tissues show up more clearly. This procedure is also called computed tomography, computerized tomography, or computerized axial tomography.

- **Bone scan.** A procedure to check if there are rapidly dividing cells, such as cancer cells, in the bone. A very small amount of radioactive material is injected into a vein and travels through the bloodstream. The radioactive material collects in the bones with cancer and is detected by a scanner.

- **Positron emission tomography (PET) scan.** A procedure to find malignant tumor cells in the body. A small amount of radioactive glucose (sugar) is injected into a vein. The PET scanner rotates around the body and makes a picture of where glucose is being used in the body. Malignant tumor cells show up brighter in the picture because they are more active and take up more glucose than normal cells do.

Stages of Breast Cancer

The breast cancer stage is based on the results of tests that are done on the tumor and lymph nodes removed during surgery and on other tests.

Stage 0 (Carcinoma in Situ)

There are 3 types of breast carcinoma in situ:

- Ductal carcinoma in situ (DCIS) is a noninvasive condition in which abnormal cells are found in the lining of a breast duct. The abnormal cells have not spread outside the duct to other tissues in the breast. In some cases, DCIS may become invasive cancer and spread to other tissues. At this time, there is no way to know which lesions could become invasive.

- Lobular carcinoma in situ (LCIS) is a condition in which abnormal cells are found in the lobules of the breast. This condition seldom becomes invasive cancer.

- Paget disease of the nipple is a condition in which abnormal cells are found in the nipple only.

Stage I

In stage I, cancer has formed. Stage I is divided into stages IA and IB.

- In stage IA, the tumor is 2 centimeters or smaller. Cancer has not spread outside the breast.

- In stage IB, small clusters of breast cancer cells (larger than 0.2 millimeter but not larger than 2 millimeters) are found in the lymph nodes and either:

  - no tumor is found in the breast; or

  - the tumor is 2 centimeters or smaller.

Stage II

Stage II is divided into stages IIA and IIB.
In stage IIA:

- no tumor is found in the breast or the tumor is 2 centimeters or smaller. Cancer (larger than 2 millimeters) is found in 1–3 axillary lymph nodes or in the lymph nodes near the breastbone (found during a sentinel lymph node biopsy); or

- the tumor is larger than 2 centimeters but not larger than 5 centimeters. Cancer has not spread to the lymph nodes.

In stage IIB, the tumor is:

- larger than 2 centimeters but not larger than 5 centimeters. Small clusters of breast cancer cells (larger than 0.2 millimeter but not larger than 2 millimeters) are found in the lymph nodes; or

- larger than 2 centimeters but not larger than 5 centimeters. Cancer has spread to 1–3 axillary lymph nodes or to the lymph nodes near the breastbone (found during a sentinel lymph node biopsy); or

- larger than 5 centimeters. Cancer has not spread to the lymph nodes.

Stage III

In stage IIIA,

- no tumor is found in the breast or the tumor may be any size. Cancer is found in 4–9 axillary lymph nodes or in the lymph nodes near the breastbone (found during imaging tests or a physical exam); or

- the tumor is larger than 5 centimeters. Small clusters of breast cancer cells (larger than 0.2 millimeter but not larger than 2 millimeters) are found in the lymph nodes; or

- the tumor is larger than 5 centimeters. Cancer has spread to 1–3 axillary lymph nodes or to the lymph nodes near the breastbone (found during a sentinel lymph node biopsy).

In stage IIIB, the tumor may be any size and cancer has spread to the chest wall and/or to the skin of the breast and caused swelling or an ulcer. Also, cancer may have spread to:

- up to 9 axillary lymph nodes; or

- the lymph nodes near the breastbone.

Cancer that has spread to the skin of the breast may also be inflammatory breast cancer.

In stage IIIC, no tumor is found in the breast or the tumor may be any size. Cancer may have spread to the skin of the breast and caused swelling or an ulcer and/or has spread to the chest wall. Also, cancer has spread to:

- Ten or more axillary lymph nodes; or

- lymph nodes above or below the collarbone; or

- axillary lymph nodes and lymph nodes near the breastbone.

Cancer that has spread to the skin of the breast may also be inflammatory breast cancer.

Stage IV

In stage IV, cancer has spread to other organs of the body, most often the bones, lungs, liver, or brain.

Treatment Option Overview

Different types of treatment are available for patients with breast cancer. Some treatments are standard (the currently used treatment), and some are being tested in clinical trials. A treatment clinical trial is a research study meant to help improve current treatments or obtain information on new treatments for patients with cancer. When clinical trials show that a new treatment is better than the standard treatment, the new treatment may become the standard treatment. Patients may want to think about taking part in a clinical trial. Some clinical trials are open only to patients who have not started treatment.

Surgery

Most patients with breast cancer have surgery to remove the cancer. Sentinel lymph node biopsy is the removal of the sentinel lymph node during surgery. The sentinel lymph node is the first lymph node to receive lymphatic drainage from a tumor. It is the first lymph node where the cancer is likely to spread. A radioactive substance and/or blue dye is injected near the tumor. The substance or dye flows through the lymph ducts to the lymph nodes. The first lymph node to receive the substance or dye is removed. A pathologist views the tissue under a microscope to look for cancer cells. After the sentinel lymph node biopsy, the surgeon removes the tumor using breast-conserving surgery or mastectomy. If cancer cells were not found in the sentinel lymph node, it may not be necessary to remove more lymph nodes. If cancer cells were found, more lymph nodes will be removed through a separate incision. This is called a lymph node dissection.

Types of surgery include the following:

- **Breast-conserving surgery:** An operation to remove the cancer and some normal tissue around it, but not the breast itself. Part of the chest wall lining may also be removed if the cancer is near it. This type of surgery may also be called lumpectomy, partial mastectomy, segmental mastectomy, quadrantectomy, or breast-sparing surgery.

- **Total mastectomy:** Surgery to remove the whole breast that has cancer. This procedure is also called a simple mastectomy. Some of the lymph nodes under the arm may be removed and checked for cancer. This may be done at the same time as the breast surgery or after. This is done through a separate incision.

- **Modified radical mastectomy:** Surgery to remove the whole breast that has cancer, many of the lymph nodes under the arm, the lining over the chest muscles, and sometimes, part of the chest wall muscles.

Chemotherapy may be given before surgery to remove the tumor. When given before surgery, chemotherapy will shrink the tumor and reduce the amount of tissue that needs to be removed during surgery. Treatment given before surgery is called preoperative therapy or neo-adjuvant therapy.

After the doctor removes all the cancer that can be seen at the time of the surgery, some patients may be given radiation therapy, chemotherapy, targeted therapy, or hormone therapy after surgery, to kill any cancer cells that are left. Treatment given after the surgery, to lower the risk that the cancer will come back, is called postoperative therapy or adjuvant therapy.

Breast Reconstruction

If a patient is going to have a mastectomy, breast reconstruction (surgery to rebuild a breast's shape after a mastectomy) may be considered. Breast reconstruction may be done at the time of the mastectomy or at some time after. The reconstructed breast may be made with the patient's own (nonbreast) tissue or by using implants filled with saline or silicone gel. Before the decision to get an implant is made, patients can call the U.S. Food and Drug Administration's (FDA) Center for Devices and Radiological Health (CDRH) at 888-INFO-FDA (888-463-6332) or visit the FDA website for more information on breast implants.

Radiation Therapy

Radiation therapy is a cancer treatment that uses high-energy X-rays or other types of radiation to kill cancer cells or keep them from growing. There are two types of radiation therapy:

- External radiation therapy uses a machine outside the body to send radiation toward the cancer.

- Internal radiation therapy uses a radioactive substance sealed in needles, seeds, wires, or catheters that are placed directly into or near the cancer.

The way the radiation therapy is given depends on the type and stage of the cancer being treated. External radiation therapy is used to treat breast cancer. Internal radiation therapy with strontium-89 (a radionuclide) is used to relieve bone pain caused by breast cancer that has spread to the bones. Strontium-89 is injected into a vein and travels to the surface of the bones. Radiation is released and kills cancer cells in the bones.

Chemotherapy

Chemotherapy is a cancer treatment that uses drugs to stop the growth of cancer cells, either by killing the cells or by stopping them from dividing. When chemotherapy is taken by mouth or injected into a vein or muscle, the drugs enter the bloodstream and can reach cancer cells throughout the body (systemic chemotherapy). When chemotherapy is placed directly into the cerebrospinal fluid, an organ, or a body cavity such as the abdomen, the drugs mainly affect cancer cells in those areas (regional chemotherapy). The way the chemotherapy is given depends on the type and stage of the cancer being treated. Systemic chemotherapy is used in the treatment of breast cancer.

Hormone Therapy

Hormone therapy is a cancer treatment that removes hormones or blocks their action and stops cancer cells from growing. Hormones are substances made by glands in the body and circulated in the bloodstream. Some hormones can cause certain cancers to grow. If tests show that the cancer cells have places where hormones can attach (receptors), drugs, surgery, or radiation therapy is used to reduce the production of hormones or block them from working. The hormone estrogen, which makes some breast cancers grow, is made mainly by the ovaries. Treatment to stop the ovaries from making estrogen is called ovarian ablation.

Hormone therapy with tamoxifen is often given to patients with early localized breast cancer that can be removed by surgery and those with metastatic breast cancer (cancer that has spread to other parts of the body). Hormone therapy with tamoxifen or estrogens can act on cells all over the body and may increase the chance of developing endometrial cancer. Women taking tamoxifen should have a pelvic exam every year to look for any signs of cancer. Any vaginal bleeding, other than menstrual bleeding, should be reported to a doctor as soon as possible.

Hormone therapy with a luteinizing hormone-releasing hormone (LHRH) agonist is given to some premenopausal women who have just been diagnosed with hormone receptor-positive breast cancer. LHRH agonists decrease the body's estrogen and progesterone.

Hormone therapy with an aromatase inhibitor is given to some postmenopausal women who have hormone receptor-positive breast cancer. Aromatase inhibitors decrease the body's estrogen by blocking an enzyme called aromatase from turning androgen into estrogen. Anastrozole, letrozole, and exemestane are types of aromatase inhibitors.

For the treatment of early localized breast cancer that can be removed by surgery, certain aromatase inhibitors may be used as adjuvant therapy instead of tamoxifen or after 2–3 years of tamoxifen use. For the treatment of metastatic breast cancer, aromatase inhibitors are being tested in clinical trials to compare them to hormone therapy with tamoxifen. Other types of hormone therapy include megestrol acetate or anti-estrogen therapy such as fulvestrant.

Targeted Therapy

Targeted therapy is a type of treatment that uses drugs or other substances to identify and attack specific cancer cells without harming normal cells. Monoclonal antibodies (mAbs), tyrosine kinase inhibitors (TKIs), cyclin-dependent kinase inhibitors (CDKIs), mammalian target of rapamycin (mTOR) inhibitors, and poly (ADP-ribose polymerase (PARP) inhibitors are types of targeted therapies used in the treatment of breast cancer.

Monoclonal antibody therapy is a cancer treatment that uses antibodies made in the laboratory, from a single type of immune system cell. These antibodies can identify substances on cancer cells or normal substances that may help cancer cells grow. The antibodies attach to the substances and kill the cancer cells, block their growth, or keep them from spreading. Monoclonal antibodies are given by infusion. They may be used alone or to carry drugs, toxins, or radioactive material directly to cancer cells. Monoclonal antibodies may be used in combination with chemotherapy as adjuvant therapy.

Types of monoclonal antibody therapy include the following:

- Trastuzumab is a monoclonal antibody that blocks the effects of the growth factor protein HER2 (human epidermal growth factor receptor 2), which sends growth signals to breast cancer cells. It may be used with other therapies to treat HER2 positive breast cancer.

- Pertuzumab is a monoclonal antibody that may be combined with trastuzumab and chemotherapy to treat breast cancer. It may be used to treat certain patients with HER2 positive breast cancer that has metastasized (spread to other parts of the body). It may also be used as neoadjuvant therapy in certain patients with early-stage HER2 positive breast cancer.

- Ado-trastuzumab emtansine is a monoclonal antibody linked to an anticancer drug. This is called an antibody-drug conjugate. It is used to treat HER2 positive breast cancer that has spread to other parts of the body or recurred (comeback).

Tyrosine kinase inhibitors are targeted therapy drugs that block signals needed for tumors to grow. Tyrosine kinase inhibitors may be used with other anticancer drugs as adjuvant therapy. Tyrosine kinase inhibitors include the following:

- Lapatinib is a tyrosine kinase inhibitor that blocks the effects of the HER2 protein and other proteins inside tumor cells. It may be used with other drugs to treat patients with HER2 positive breast cancer that has progressed after treatment with trastuzumab.

- Neratinib is a tyrosine kinase inhibitor that blocks the effects of the HER2 protein and other proteins inside tumor cells. It may be used to treat patients with early stage HER2 positive breast cancer after treatment with trastuzumab.

Cyclin-dependent kinase inhibitors (CDI) are targeted therapy drugs that block proteins called cyclin-dependent kinases, which cause the growth of cancer cells. Cyclin-dependent kinase inhibitors include the following:

- Palbociclib is a cyclin-dependent kinase inhibitor used with the drug letrozole to treat breast cancer that is estrogen receptor positive and HER2 negative and has spread to other parts of the body. It is used in postmenopausal women whose cancer has not been treated with hormone therapy. Palbociclib may also be used with fulvestrant in women whose disease has gotten worse after treatment with hormone therapy.

- Ribociclib is a cyclin-dependent kinase inhibitor used with letrozole to treat breast cancer that is hormone receptor positive and HER2 negative and has come back or spread to other parts of the body. It is used in postmenopausal women whose cancer has not been treated with hormone therapy.

- Abemaciclib is a cyclin-dependent kinase inhibitor used to treat hormone receptor positive and HER2 negative breast cancer that is advanced or has spread to other parts of the body. It may be used alone or with other drugs to treat breast cancer that has gotten worse after other treatment.

Mammalian target of rapamycin (mTOR) inhibitors block a protein called mTOR, which may keep cancer cells from growing and prevent the growth of new blood vessels that tumors need to grow. mTOR inhibitors include the following:

- Everolimus is an mTOR inhibitor used in postmenopausal women with advanced hormone receptor-positive breast cancer that is also HER2 negative and has not gotten better with other treatment.

PARP inhibitors are a type of targeted therapy that block deoxyribonucleic acid (DNA) repair and may cause cancer cells to die. PARP inhibitor therapy is being studied for the treatment of patients with triple-negative breast cancer or tumors with *BRCA1* or *BRCA2* mutations.

Side Effects of Breast Cancer Treatment

Some treatments for breast cancer may cause side effects that continue or appear months or years after treatment has ended. These are called late effects.

Late effects of radiation therapy are not common, but may include:

- Inflammation of the lung after radiation therapy to the breast, especially when chemotherapy is given at the same time

- Arm lymphedema, especially when radiation therapy is given after lymph node dissection

- In women younger than 45 years who receive radiation therapy to the chest wall after mastectomy, there may be a higher risk of developing breast cancer in the other breast

Late effects of chemotherapy depend on the drugs used, but may include:

- Heart failure
- Blood clots
- Premature menopause
- Second cancer, such as leukemia

Late effects of targeted therapy with trastuzumab, lapatinib, or pertuzumab may include:

- Heart problems such as heart failure

Chapter 14

Breast Cancer Treatment and Pregnancy

Breast cancer occurs about once in every 3,000 pregnancies. It occurs most often in women aged 32–38 years. Because many women are choosing to delay having children, it is likely that the number of new cases of breast cancer during pregnancy will increase. Signs of breast cancer include a lump or change in the breast.

These and other signs may be caused by breast cancer or by other conditions. Check with your doctor if you have any of the following:

- A lump or thickening in or near the breast or in the underarm area

- A change in the size or shape of the breast

- A dimple or puckering in the skin of the breast

- A nipple turned inward into the breast

- Fluid, other than breast milk, from the nipple, especially if it's bloody

- Scaly, red, or swollen skin on the breast, nipple, or areola (the dark area of skin around the nipple)

This chapter includes text excerpted from "Breast Cancer Treatment during Pregnancy (PDQ®)—Patient Version," National Cancer Institute (NCI), April 9, 2018.

- Dimples in the breast that look like the skin of an orange, called peau d'orange

It may be difficult to detect (find) breast cancer early in pregnant or nursing women. The breasts usually get larger, tender, or lumpy in women who are pregnant, nursing, or have just given birth. This occurs because of normal hormone changes that take place during pregnancy. These changes can make small lumps difficult to detect. The breasts may also become denser. It is more difficult to detect breast cancer in women with dense breasts using mammography. Because these breast changes can delay diagnosis, breast cancer is often found at a later stage in these women.

Breast exams should be part of prenatal and postnatal care. To detect breast cancer, pregnant and nursing women should examine their breasts themselves. Women should also receive clinical breast exams during their regular prenatal and postnatal check-ups. Talk to your doctor if you notice any changes in your breasts that you do not expect or that worry you. Tests that examine the breasts are used to detect (find) and diagnose breast cancer.

The following tests and procedures may be used:

- **Physical exam and history:** An exam of the body to check general signs of health, including checking for signs of disease, such as lumps or anything else that seems unusual. A history of the patient's health habits and past illnesses and treatments will also be taken.

- **Clinical breast exam (CBE):** An exam of the breast by a doctor or other health professional. The doctor will carefully feel the breasts and under the arms for lumps or anything else that seems unusual.

- **Ultrasound exam:** A procedure in which high-energy sound waves (ultrasound) are bounced off internal tissues or organs and make echoes. The echoes form a picture of body tissues called a sonogram. The picture can be printed to look at later.

- **Mammogram:** An X-ray of the breast. A mammogram can be done with little risk to the unborn baby. Mammograms in pregnant women may appear negative even though cancer is present.

- **Biopsy:** The removal of cells or tissues so they can be viewed under a microscope by a pathologist to check for signs of cancer. If a lump in the breast is found, a biopsy may be done.

There are four types of breast biopsies:

- **Excisional biopsy:** The removal of an entire lump of tissue.

- **Core biopsy:** The removal of tissue using a wide needle.

- **Fine-needle aspiration (FNA) biopsy:** The removal of tissue or fluid, using a thin needle.

If cancer is found, tests are done to study the cancer cells. Decisions about the best treatment are based on the results of these tests and the age of the unborn baby. The tests give information about:

- How quickly the cancer may grow

- How likely it is that the cancer will spread to other parts of the body

- How well certain treatments might work

- How likely the cancer is to recur (come back)

Tests may include the following:

- **Estrogen and progesterone receptor test:** A test to measure the amount of estrogen and progesterone (hormones) receptors in cancer tissue. If there are more estrogen or progesterone receptors than normal, the cancer is called estrogen receptor positive or progesterone receptor positive. This type of breast cancer may grow more quickly. The test results show whether treatment to block estrogen and progesterone given after the baby is born may stop the cancer from growing.

- **Human epidermal growth factor type 2 receptor (HER2/neu) test:** A laboratory test to measure how many *HER2/neu* genes there are and how much HER2/neu protein is made in a sample of tissue. If there are more *HER2/neu* genes or higher levels of HER2/neu protein than normal, the cancer is called HER2/neu positive. This type of breast cancer may grow more quickly and is more likely to spread to other parts of the body. The cancer may be treated with drugs that target the HER2/neu protein, such as trastuzumab and pertuzumab, after the baby is born.

- **Multigene tests:** Tests in which samples of tissue are studied to look at the activity of many genes at the same time. These tests may help predict whether cancer will spread to other parts of the body or recur (come back).

145

- **Oncotype DX:** This test helps predict whether stage I or stage II breast cancer that is estrogen receptor positive (ER+) and node-negative will spread to other parts of the body. If the risk of the cancer spreading is high, chemotherapy may be given to lower the risk.

- **MammaPrint:** This test helps predict whether stage I or stage II breast cancer that is node-negative will spread to other parts of the body. If the risk of the cancer spreading is high, chemotherapy may be given to lower the risk.

Stages of Breast Cancer

After breast cancer has been diagnosed, tests are done to find out if cancer cells have spread within the breast or to other parts of the body. The process used to find out if the cancer has spread within the breast or to other parts of the body is called staging. The information gathered from the staging process determines the stage of the disease. It is important to know the stage in order to plan treatment.

Some procedures may expose the unborn baby to harmful radiation or dyes. These procedures are done only if absolutely necessary. Certain actions can be taken to expose the unborn baby to as little radiation as possible, such as the use of a lead-lined shield to cover the abdomen.

The following tests and procedures may be used to stage breast cancer during pregnancy:

- **Chest X-ray:** An X-ray of the organs and bones inside the chest. An X-ray is a type of energy beam that can go through the body and onto film, making a picture of areas inside the body.

- **Bone scan:** A procedure to check if there are rapidly dividing cells, such as cancer cells, in the bone. A very small amount of radioactive material is injected into a vein and travels through the bloodstream. The radioactive material collects in bones with cancer and is detected by a scanner.

- **Ultrasound exam:** A procedure in which high-energy sound waves (ultrasound) are bounced off internal tissues or organs, such as the liver, and make echoes. The echoes form a picture of body tissues called a sonogram. The picture can be printed to be looked at later.

- **Magnetic resonance imaging (MRI):** A procedure that uses a magnet, radio waves, and a computer to make a series of detailed pictures of areas inside the body, such as the brain. This procedure is also called nuclear magnetic resonance imaging (NMRI).

There are three ways that cancer spreads in the body. Cancer can spread through tissue, the lymph system, and the blood:

- **Tissue.** The cancer spreads from where it began by growing into nearby areas.

- **Lymph system.** The cancer spreads from where it began by getting into the lymph system. The cancer travels through the lymph vessels to other parts of the body.

- **Blood.** The cancer spreads from where it began by getting into the blood. The cancer travels through the blood vessels to other parts of the body.

Cancer may spread from where it began to other parts of the body. When cancer spreads to another part of the body, it is called metastasis. Cancer cells break away from where they began (the primary tumor) and travel through the lymph system or blood.

- **Lymph system.** The cancer gets into the lymph system, travels through the lymph vessels, and forms a tumor (metastatic tumor) in another part of the body.

- **Blood.** The cancer gets into the blood, travels through the blood vessels, and forms a tumor (metastatic tumor) in another part of the body.

The metastatic tumor is the same type of cancer as the primary tumor. For example, if breast cancer spreads to the bone, the cancer cells in the bone are actually breast cancer cells. The disease is metastatic breast cancer, not bone cancer.

The following stages are used for breast cancer:

This section describes the stages of breast cancer. The breast cancer stage is based on the results of testing that is done on the tumor and lymph nodes removed during surgery and other tests.

Stage 0 (Carcinoma in Situ (CIS))

There are 3 types of breast carcinoma in situ:

- Ductal carcinoma in situ (DCIS) is a noninvasive condition in which abnormal cells are found in the lining of a breast duct.

The abnormal cells have not spread outside the duct to other tissues in the breast. In some cases, DCIS may become invasive cancer and spread to other tissues. At this time, there is no way to know which lesions could become invasive.

- Lobular carcinoma in situ (LCIS) is a condition in which abnormal cells are found in the lobules of the breast. This condition seldom becomes invasive cancer. However, having LCIS in one breast increases the risk of developing breast cancer in either breast.

- Paget disease of the nipple is a condition in which abnormal cells are found in the nipple only.

Stage I

In stage I, cancer has formed. Stage I is divided into stages IA and IB.

- In stage IA, the tumor is 2 centimeters or smaller. Cancer has not spread outside the breast.

- In stage IB, small clusters of breast cancer cells (larger than 0.2 millimeter but not larger than 2 millimeters) are found in the lymph nodes and either:

  - no tumor is found in the breast; or

  - the tumor is 2 centimeters or smaller

Stage II

Stage II is divided into stages IIA and IIB.
In stage IIA:

- no tumor is found in the breast or the tumor is 2 centimeters or smaller. Cancer (larger than 2 millimeters) is found in 1–3 axillary lymph nodes or in the lymph nodes near the breastbone (found during a sentinel lymph node biopsy); or

- the tumor is larger than 2 centimeters but not larger than 5 centimeters. Cancer has not spread to lymph nodes.

In stage IIB, the tumor is:

- larger than 2 centimeters but not larger than 5 centimeters. Small clusters of breast cancer cells (larger than 0.2 millimeter but not larger than 2 millimeters) are found in the lymph nodes; or

- larger than 2 centimeters but not larger than 5 centimeters. Cancer has spread to 1–3 axillary lymph nodes or to the lymph nodes near the breastbone (found during a sentinel lymph node biopsy); or

- larger than 5 centimeters. Cancer has not spread to lymph nodes.

Stage III

In stage IIIA:

- no tumor is found in the breast or the tumor may be any size. Cancer is found in 4–9 axillary lymph nodes or in lymph nodes near the breastbone (found during imaging tests or a physical exam); or

- the tumor is larger than 5 centimeters. Small clusters of breast cancer cells (larger than 0.2 millimeter but not larger than 2 millimeters) are found in the lymph nodes; or

- the tumor is larger than 5 centimeters. Cancer has spread to 1–3 axillary lymph nodes or to lymph nodes near the breastbone (found during a sentinel lymph node biopsy).

In stage IIIB, the tumor may be any size and cancer has spread to the chest wall and/or to the skin of the breast and caused swelling or an ulcer. Also, cancer may have spread to:

- up to 9 axillary lymph nodes; or

- the lymph nodes near the breastbone

Cancer that has spread to the skin of the breast may also be inflammatory breast cancer.

In stage IIIC, no tumor is found in the breast or the tumor may be any size. Cancer may have spread to the skin of the breast and caused swelling or an ulcer and/or has spread to the chest wall. Also, cancer has spread to:

- 10 or more axillary lymph nodes; or

- lymph nodes above or below the collarbone; or

- axillary lymph nodes and lymph nodes near the breastbone.

Cancer that has spread to the skin of the breast may also be inflammatory breast cancer.

For treatment, stage IIIC breast cancer is divided into operable and inoperable cancer.

Stage IV

In stage IV, cancer has spread to other organs of the body, most often the bones, lungs, liver, or brain.

Treatment Option Overview

Treatment options for pregnant women depend on the stage of the disease and the age of the unborn baby.

Three types of standard treatment are used:

Surgery

Most pregnant women with breast cancer have surgery to remove the breast. Some of the lymph nodes under the arm may be removed so they can be checked under a microscope by a pathologist for signs of cancer.

Types of surgery to remove the cancer include:

- **Modified radical mastectomy:** Surgery to remove the whole breast that has cancer, many of the lymph nodes under the arm, the lining over the chest muscles, and sometimes, part of the chest wall muscles. This type of surgery is most common in pregnant women.

- **Breast-conserving surgery (BCS):** Surgery to remove the cancer and some normal tissue around it, but not the breast itself. Part of the chest wall lining may also be removed if the cancer is near it. This type of surgery may also be called lumpectomy, partial mastectomy, segmental mastectomy, quadrantectomy, or breast-sparing surgery.

After the doctor removes all of the cancer that can be seen at the time of surgery, some patients may be given chemotherapy or radiation therapy after surgery to kill any cancer cells that are left. For pregnant women with early-stage breast cancer, radiation therapy and hormone therapy are given after the baby is born. Treatment given after surgery, to lower the risk that the cancer will come back, is called adjuvant therapy.

Radiation Therapy

Radiation therapy is a cancer treatment that uses high-energy X-rays or other types of radiation to kill cancer cells or keep them from growing. There are two types of radiation therapy:

- External radiation therapy uses a machine outside the body to send radiation toward the cancer.

- Internal radiation therapy uses a radioactive substance sealed in needles, seeds, wires, or catheters that are placed directly into or near the cancer.

The way the radiation therapy is given depends on the type and stage of the cancer being treated.

External radiation therapy may be given to pregnant women with early-stage (stage I or II) breast cancer after the baby is born. Women with late-stage (stage III or IV) breast cancer may be given external radiation therapy after the first 3 months of pregnancy or, if possible, radiation therapy is delayed until after the baby is born.

Chemotherapy

Chemotherapy is a cancer treatment that uses drugs to stop the growth of cancer cells, either by killing the cells or by stopping the cells from dividing. When chemotherapy is taken by mouth or injected into a vein or muscle, the drugs enter the bloodstream and can reach cancer cells throughout the body (systemic chemotherapy). When chemotherapy is placed directly into the cerebrospinal fluid, an organ, or a body cavity such as the abdomen, the drugs mainly affect cancer cells in those areas (regional chemotherapy).

The way the chemotherapy is given depends on the type and stage of the cancer being treated. Systemic chemotherapy is used to treat breast cancer during pregnancy.

Chemotherapy is usually not given during the first 3 months of pregnancy. Chemotherapy given after this time does not usually harm the unborn baby but may cause early labor or low birth weight. Ending the pregnancy does not seem to improve the mother's chance of survival. Because ending the pregnancy is not likely to improve the mother's chance of survival, it is not usually a treatment option. Treatment for breast cancer may cause side effects.

Treatment Options for Breast Cancer during Pregnancy

Early-Stage Breast Cancer

Pregnant women with early-stage breast cancer (stage I and stage II) are usually treated in the same way as patients who are not pregnant, with some changes to protect the unborn baby. Treatment may include the following:

- Modified radical mastectomy, if the breast cancer was diagnosed early in pregnancy

- Breast-conserving surgery (BCS), if the breast cancer is diagnosed later in pregnancy. Radiation therapy may be given after the baby is born.

- Modified radical mastectomy or BCS during pregnancy. After the first 3 months of pregnancy, certain types of chemotherapy may be given before or after surgery.

Hormone therapy and trastuzumab should not be given during pregnancy.

Late-Stage Breast Cancer

There is no standard treatment for patients with late-stage breast cancer (stage III or stage IV) during pregnancy. Treatment may include the following:

- Radiation therapy

- Chemotherapy

Radiation therapy and chemotherapy should not be given during the first 3 months of pregnancy.

Special Issues about Breast Cancer during Pregnancy

Lactation (breast milk production) and breastfeeding should be stopped if surgery or chemotherapy is planned. If surgery is planned, breastfeeding should be stopped to reduce blood flow in the breasts and make them smaller. Many chemotherapy drugs, especially cyclophosphamide and methotrexate, may occur in high levels in breast milk and may harm the nursing baby. Women receiving chemotherapy should not breastfeed.

Stopping lactation does not improve the mother's prognosis. Breast cancer does not appear to harm the unborn baby. Breast cancer cells do not seem to pass from the mother to the unborn baby. Pregnancy does not seem to affect the survival of women who have had breast cancer in the past. For women who have had breast cancer, pregnancy does not seem to affect their survival. However, some doctors recommend that a woman wait 2 years after treatment for breast cancer before trying to have a baby, so that any early return of the cancer would be detected. This may affect a woman's decision to become pregnant. The unborn baby does not seem to be affected if the mother has had breast cancer.

Chapter 15

Surgery to Reduce the Risk of Breast Cancer

What Kinds of Surgery Can Reduce the Risk of Breast Cancer?

Two kinds of surgery can be performed to reduce the risk of breast cancer in a woman who has never been diagnosed with breast cancer but is known to be at very high risk of the disease.

A woman can be at very high risk of developing breast cancer if she has a strong family history of breast and/or ovarian cancer, a deleterious (disease-causing) mutation in the *BRCA1* gene or the *BRCA2* gene, or a high-penetrance mutation in one of several other genes associated with breast cancer risk, such as *TP53* or *PTEN*.

The most common risk-reducing surgery is bilateral prophylactic mastectomy (also called bilateral risk-reducing mastectomy). Bilateral prophylactic mastectomy may involve complete removal of both breasts, including the nipples (total mastectomy), or it may involve removal of as much breast tissue as possible while leaving the nipples intact (subcutaneous or nipple-sparing mastectomy). Subcutaneous mastectomies preserve the nipple and allow for more natural-looking breasts if a woman chooses to have breast reconstruction surgery

---

This chapter includes text excerpted from "Surgery to Reduce the Risk of Breast Cancer," National Cancer Institute (NCI), August 12, 2013. Reviewed May 2018.

afterward. However, total mastectomy provides the greatest breast cancer risk reduction because more breast tissue is removed in this procedure than in a subcutaneous mastectomy.

Even with total mastectomy, not all breast tissue that may be at risk of becoming cancerous in the future can be removed. The chest wall, which is not typically removed during a mastectomy, may contain some breast tissue, and breast tissue can sometimes be found in the armpit, above the collarbone, and as far down as the abdomen—and it is impossible for a surgeon to remove all of this tissue.

The other kind of risk-reducing surgery is bilateral prophylactic salpingo-oophorectomy, which is sometimes called prophylactic oophorectomy. This surgery involves removal of the ovaries and fallopian tubes and may be done alone or along with bilateral prophylactic mastectomy in premenopausal women who are at very high risk of breast cancer. Removing the ovaries in premenopausal women reduces the amount of estrogen that is produced by the body. Because estrogen promotes the growth of some breast cancers, reducing the amount of this hormone in the body by removing the ovaries may slow the growth of those breast cancers.

How Effective Are Risk-Reducing Surgeries?

Bilateral prophylactic mastectomy has been shown to reduce the risk of breast cancer by at least 95 percent in women who have a deleterious (disease-causing) mutation in the *BRCA1* gene or the *BRCA2* gene and by up to 90 percent in women who have a strong family history of breast cancer.

Bilateral prophylactic salpingo-oophorectomy has been shown to reduce the risk of ovarian cancer by approximately 90 percent and the risk of breast cancer by approximately 50 percent in women at very high risk of developing these diseases.

Which Women Might Consider Having Surgery to Reduce Their Risk of Breast Cancer?

Women who inherit a deleterious mutation in the *BRCA1* gene or the *BRCA2* gene or mutations in certain other genes that greatly increase the risk of developing breast cancer may consider having bilateral prophylactic mastectomy and/or bilateral prophylactic salpingo-oophorectomy to reduce this risk.

In two studies, the estimated risks of developing breast cancer by age 70 years were 55–65 percent for women who carry a deleterious mutation in the *BRCA1* gene and 45–47 percent for women who carry a deleterious mutation in the *BRCA2* gene. Estimates of the lifetime risk of breast cancer for women with Cowden syndrome, which is caused by certain mutations in the PTEN gene, range from 25–50 percent or higher, and for women with Li-Fraumeni syndrome, which is caused by certain mutations in the *TP53* gene, from 49–60 percent. (By contrast, the lifetime risk of breast cancer for the average American woman is about 12%.)

Other women who are at very high risk of breast cancer may also consider bilateral prophylactic mastectomy, including:

- those with a strong family history of breast cancer (such as having a mother, sister, and/or daughter who was diagnosed with bilateral breast cancer or with breast cancer before age 50 years or having multiple family members with breast or ovarian cancer)

- those with lobular carcinoma in situ (LCIS) plus a family history of breast cancer (LCIS is a condition in which abnormal cells are found in the lobules of the breast. It is not cancer, but women with LCIS have an increased risk of developing invasive breast cancer in either breast. Many breast surgeons consider prophylactic mastectomy to be an overly aggressive approach for women with LCIS who do not have a strong family history or other risk factors.)

- those who have had radiation therapy to the chest (including the breasts) before the age of 30 years—for example, if they were treated with radiation therapy for Hodgkin lymphoma (Such women are at high risk of developing breast cancer throughout their lives.)

Can a Woman Have Risk-Reducing Surgery If She Has Already Been Diagnosed with Breast Cancer?

Yes. Some women who have been diagnosed with cancer in one breast, particularly those who are known to be at very high risk, may consider having the other breast (called the contralateral breast) removed as well, even if there is no sign of cancer in that breast. Prophylactic surgery to remove a contralateral breast during breast cancer surgery (known as contralateral prophylactic mastectomy) reduces the risk of breast cancer in that breast, although it is not yet known whether this risk reduction translates into longer survival for the patient.

157

However, doctors often discourage contralateral prophylactic mastectomy for women with cancer in one breast who do not meet the criteria of being at very high risk of developing a contralateral breast cancer. For such women, the risk of developing another breast cancer, either in the same or the contralateral breast, is very small, especially if they receive adjuvant chemotherapy or hormone therapy as part of their cancer treatment.

Given that most women with breast cancer have a low risk of developing the disease in their contralateral breast, women who are not known to be at very high risk but who remain concerned about cancer development in their other breast may want to consider options other than surgery to further reduce their risk of a contralateral breast cancer.

What Are the Potential Harms of Risk-Reducing Surgeries?

As with any other major surgery, bilateral prophylactic mastectomy and bilateral prophylactic salpingo-oophorectomy (BPSO) have potential complications or harms, such as bleeding or infection. Also, both surgeries are irreversible.

Bilateral prophylactic mastectomy can also affect a woman's psychological well-being due to a change in body image and the loss of normal breast functions. Although most women who choose to have this surgery are satisfied with their decision, they can still experience anxiety and concerns about body image. The most common psychological side effects include difficulties with body appearance, with feelings of femininity, and with sexual relationships. Women who undergo total mastectomies lose nipple sensation, which may hinder sexual arousal.

Bilateral prophylactic salpingo-oophorectomy causes a sudden drop in estrogen production, which will induce early menopause in a premenopausal woman (this is also called surgical menopause). Surgical menopause can cause an abrupt onset of menopausal symptoms, including hot flashes, insomnia, anxiety, and depression, and some of these symptoms can be severe. The long-term effects of surgical menopause include decreased sex drive, vaginal dryness, and decreased bone density.

Women who have severe menopausal symptoms after undergoing bilateral prophylactic salpingo-oophorectomy may consider using short-term menopausal hormone therapy (MHT) after surgery to alleviate these symptoms. (The increase in breast cancer risk associated with certain types of menopausal hormone therapy is much less than the decrease in breast cancer risk associated with bilateral prophylactic salpingo-oophorectomy.)

What Are the Cancer Risk Reduction Options for Women Who Are at Increased Risk of Breast Cancer but Not at the Highest Risk?

Risk-reducing surgery is not considered an appropriate cancer prevention option for women who are not at the highest risk of breast cancer (that is, for those who do not carry a high-penetrance gene mutation that is associated with breast cancer or who do not have a clinical or medical history that puts them at very high risk). However, some women who are not at very high risk of breast cancer but are, nonetheless, considered as being at increased risk of the disease may choose to use drugs to reduce their risk.

Healthcare providers use several types of tools, called risk assessment models, to estimate the risk of breast cancer for women who do not have a deleterious mutation in *BRCA1*, *BRCA2*, or another gene associated with breast cancer risk. One widely used tool is the Breast Cancer Risk Assessment Tool (BRCAT), a computer model that takes a number of factors into account in estimating the risks of breast cancer over the next 5 years and up to age 90 years (lifetime risk). Women who have an estimated 5-year risk of 1.67 percent or higher are classified as "high-risk," which means that they have a higher than average risk of developing breast cancer. This high-risk cutoff (that is, an estimated 5-year risk of 1.67% or higher) is widely used in research studies and in clinical counseling.

Two drugs, tamoxifen and raloxifene, are approved by the U.S. Food and Drug Administration (FDA) to reduce the risk of breast cancer in women who have a 5-year risk of developing breast cancer of 1.67 percent or more. Tamoxifen is approved for risk reduction in both premenopausal and postmenopausal women, and raloxifene is approved for risk reduction in postmenopausal women only. In large randomized clinical trials, tamoxifen, taken for 5 years, reduced the risk of invasive breast cancer by about 50 percent in high-risk postmenopausal women; raloxifene, taken for 5 years, reduced breast cancer risk by about 38 percent in high-risk postmenopausal women. Both drugs block the activity of estrogen, thereby inhibiting the growth of some breast cancers. The U.S. Preventive Services Task Force (USPSTF) recommends that women at increased risk of breast cancer talk with their healthcare professional about the potential benefits and harms of taking tamoxifen or raloxifene to reduce their risk.

Another drug, exemestane, was recently shown to reduce the incidence of breast cancer in postmenopausal women who are at increased risk of the disease by 65 percent. Exemestane belongs to a class of drugs called aromatase inhibitors (AIs), which block the production of estrogen by the body. It is not known, however, whether any of these drugs reduces the very high risk of breast cancer for women who carry a known mutation that is strongly associated with an increased risk of breast cancer, such as deleterious mutations in *BRCA1* and *BRCA2*.

Some women who have undergone breast cancer surgery, regardless of their risk of recurrence, may be given drugs to reduce the likelihood that their breast cancer will recur. (This additional treatment is called adjuvant therapy.) Such treatment also reduces the already low risks of contralateral and second primary breast cancers. Drugs that are used as adjuvant therapy to reduce the risk of breast cancer after breast cancer surgery include tamoxifen, aromatase inhibitors, traditional chemotherapy agents, and trastuzumab.

What Can Women at Very High Risk Do If They Do Not Want to Undergo Risk-Reducing Surgery?

Some women who are at very high risk of breast cancer (or of contralateral breast cancer) may undergo more frequent breast cancer screening (also called enhanced screening). For example, they may have yearly mammograms and yearly magnetic resonance imaging (MRI) screening—with these tests staggered so that the breasts are imaged every 6 months—as well as clinical breast examinations performed regularly by a healthcare professional. Enhanced screening may increase the chance of detecting breast cancer at an early stage, when it may have a better chance of being treated successfully.

Women who carry mutations in some genes that increase their risk of breast cancer may be more likely to develop radiation-associated breast cancer than the general population because those genes are involved in the repair of deoxyribonucleic acid (DNA) breaks, which can be caused by exposure to radiation. Women who are at high risk of breast cancer should ask their healthcare provider about the risks of diagnostic tests that involve radiation (mammograms or X-rays). Ongoing clinical trials are examining various aspects of enhanced screening for women who are at high risk of breast cancer.

Chemoprevention (the use of drugs or other agents to reduce cancer risk or delay its development) may be an option for some women who wish to avoid surgery. Tamoxifen and raloxifene have both been approved by the FDA to reduce the risk of breast cancer in women at increased risk. Whether these drugs can be used to prevent breast cancer in women at much higher risk, such as women with harmful mutations in *BRCA1* or *BRCA2* or other breast cancer susceptibility genes, is not yet clear, although tamoxifen may be able to help lower the risk of contralateral breast cancer among *BRCA1* and *BRCA2* mutation carriers previously diagnosed with breast cancer.

Does Health Insurance Cover the Cost of Risk-Reducing Surgeries?

Many health insurance companies have official policies about whether and under what conditions they will pay for prophylactic mastectomy (bilateral or contralateral) and bilateral prophylactic salpingo-oophorectomy for breast and ovarian cancer risk reduction. However, the criteria used for considering these procedures as medically necessary may vary among insurance companies. Some insurance companies may require a second opinion or a letter of medical necessity from the healthcare provider before they will approve coverage of any surgical procedure. A woman who is considering prophylactic surgery to reduce her risk of breast and/or ovarian cancer should discuss insurance coverage issues with her doctor and insurance company before choosing to have the surgery.

The Women's Health and Cancer Rights Act (WHCRA), enacted in 1999, requires most health plans that offer mastectomy coverage to also pay for breast reconstruction surgery after mastectomy.

Who Should a Woman Talk to When Considering Surgery to Reduce Her Risk of Breast Cancer?

The decision to have any surgery to reduce the risk of breast cancer is a major one. A woman who is at high risk of breast cancer may wish to get a second opinion on risk-reducing surgery as well as on alternatives to surgery.

A woman who is considering prophylactic mastectomy may also want to talk with a surgeon who specializes in breast reconstruction. Other healthcare professionals, including a breast health specialist, medical social worker, or cancer clinical psychologist or psychiatrist, can also help a woman consider her options for reducing her risk of breast cancer.

Many factors beyond the risk of disease itself may influence a woman's decision about whether to undergo risk-reducing surgery. For example, for women who have been diagnosed with cancer in one breast, these factors can include distress about the possibility of having to go through cancer treatment a second time and the worry and inconvenience associated with long-term breast surveillance. For this reason, women who are considering risk-reducing surgery may want to talk with other women who have considered or had the procedure. Support groups can help connect women with others who have had similar cancer experiences. The searchable National Cancer Institute (NCI) database National Organizations That Offer Cancer-Related Services has listings for many support groups.

Finally, if a woman has a strong family history of breast cancer, ovarian cancer, or both, she and other members of her family may want to obtain genetic counseling services. A genetic counselor or other healthcare provider trained in genetics can review the family's risks of disease and help family members obtain genetic testing for mutations in cancer-predisposing genes, if appropriate.

Part Three

Gynecologic Cancers

Chapter 16

Cervical Cancer

Chapter Contents

Section 16.1

Understanding Cervical Cancer

This section includes text excerpted from "Cervical Cancer," Office on Women's Health (OWH), U.S. Department of Health and Human Services (HHS), January 2, 2018.

What Is Cervical Cancer?

Cervical cancer is cancer that starts in the cervix, the lower, narrow part of the uterus (womb). Most cervical cancers are caused by the human papillomavirus (HPV). Cervical cancer is the easiest gynecological cancer to prevent with regular screening tests and vaccination. It is also very curable when found and treated early. It happens when the body's cervical cells divide very fast and grow out of control. These extra cells form a tumor.

Who Gets Cervical Cancer?

Each year, about 12,000 women in the United States get cervical cancer. Cervical cancer happens most often in women 30 years or older, but all women are at risk.

What Causes Cervical Cancer?

Most cases of cervical cancer are caused by a high-risk type of HPV. HPV is a virus that is passed from person to person through genital contact, such as vaginal, anal, or oral sex. If the HPV infection does not go away on its own, it may cause cervical cancer over time.

Other things may increase the risk of developing cancer following a high-risk HPV infection. These other things include:

- Smoking

- Having human immunodeficiency virus (HIV) or reduced immunity

- Taking birth control pills for a long time (more than 5 years)

- Having given birth to three or more children

What Are the Symptoms of Cervical Cancer?

You may not notice any signs or symptoms of cervical cancer. Signs of advanced cervical cancer may include bleeding or discharge from the vagina. These symptoms may not be caused by cervical cancer, but the only way to be sure is to see your doctor.

How Do I Find out If I Have Cervical Cancer?

Women should start getting screened at age 21. You can get a Pap (Papanicolaou) test to look for changes in cervical cells that could become cancerous if not treated. If the Pap test finds major changes in the cells of the cervix, your doctor may suggest more tests to look for cancer. Women between the ages of 30 and 65 can also get an HPV test with your Pap test to see if you have HPV.

What Is the Difference between a Pap Test and an HPV Test?

The Pap test and the HPV test look for different things. A Pap test checks the cervix for abnormal cell changes that, if not found and treated, can lead to cervical cancer. Your doctor takes cells from your cervix to examine under a microscope. How often you need a Pap test depends on your age and health history. Talk with your doctor about what is best for you. An HPV test looks for HPV on a woman's cervix. Certain types of HPV can lead to cervical cancer. Your doctor will swab the cervix for cells. An HPV test is not the same as the HPV vaccine. According to the U.S. Preventive Services Task Force (USPSTF), women ages 30–65 can combine the HPV test with a Pap test every 5 years. The USPSTF does not recommend the HPV test for women under age 30.

How Often Do I Need to Be Screened for Cervical Cancer?

How often you need to be screened depends on your age and health history. Talk with your doctor about what is best for you. Most women can follow these guidelines:

- If you are between ages 21–29, you should get a Pap test every 3 years

- If you are between ages 30–64, you should get a Pap test and HPV test together every 5 years or a Pap test alone every 3 years

- If you are 65 or older, ask your doctor if you can stop having Pap tests

If you had a hysterectomy, you should follow these guidelines:

- If you no longer have a cervix because you had a hysterectomy for reasons other than cancer, you do not need Pap tests

- If you had a hysterectomy because of abnormal cervical cells or cervical cancer, you should have a yearly Pap test until you have three normal tests

- If you had your uterus removed but you still have a cervix (this type of hysterectomy is not common), you need regular Pap tests until you are 65 and have had three normal Pap tests in a row with no abnormal results in the last 10 years

What Can I Do to Prevent Cervical Cancer?

You can lower your risk of getting cervical cancer with the following steps. The steps work best when used together. No single step can protect you from cervical cancer. The best ways to prevent cervical cancer include:

- **Get an HPV vaccine (if you are 26 or younger).** The HPV vaccine is recommended for girls who are 11–12 years old. But any girl or woman can get the HPV vaccine between 9 and 26 years. HPV vaccines are licensed, safe, and effective.

- **Get regular Pap tests.** Regular Pap tests help your doctor find and treat any changing cells before they turn into cancer. Women who have had the HPV vaccine still need to have regular Pap tests.

- **Be monogamous.** Being monogamous means that you only have sex with one partner and no one else. The best way to prevent any sexually transmitted infection (STI), including HPV, is to not have vaginal, oral, or anal sex. But having sex with just one partner can lower your risk. That means that you only have sex with each other and no one else.

- **Use condoms.** Research shows that condoms can lower your risk of getting cervical cancer when used correctly and every time you have vaginal, anal, or oral sex. Protect yourself with a condom every time you have vaginal, anal, or oral sex.

Who Should Get the HPV Vaccine?

HPV vaccines are approved for girls and young women from ages 9 to 26. Experts recommend that all girls get an HPV vaccine before any sexual activity, by the time they are 11 or 12. The Gardasil 9 HPV vaccine gives the most protection against cervical cancer for girls and women. Some girls younger than 15 may be able to get just two doses of the HPV vaccine, but others may need three doses of the HPV vaccine. The HPV vaccine is not recommended for pregnant women. Talk to your doctor to find out how many doses are best for you.

Can I Still Benefit from the HPV Vaccine If I Have Already Had Sexual Contact?

Yes. You can still benefit from the HPV vaccine if you have already had sexual contact before getting all three doses. This only applies if you have not been infected with the HPV types included in the vaccine.

Section 16.2

Staging and Treating Cervical Cancer

This section includes text excerpted from "Cervical Cancer Treatment (PDQ®)—Patient Version," National Cancer Institute (NCI), March 28, 2018.

Stages of Cervical Cancer

After cervical cancer has been diagnosed, tests are done to find out if cancer cells have spread within the cervix or to other parts of the body.

The process used to find out if cancer has spread within the cervix or to other parts of the body is called staging. The information gathered from the staging process determines the stage of the disease. It is important to know the stage in order to plan treatment.

The following tests and procedures may be used in the staging process:

- **Computerized axial tomography (CAT) or computed tomography (CT) scan:** A procedure that makes a series of detailed pictures of areas inside the body, taken from different angles. The pictures are made by a computer linked to an X-ray machine. A dye may be injected into a vein or swallowed to help the organs or tissues show up more clearly. This procedure is also called computed tomography, computerized tomography, or computerized axial tomography.

- **Positron emission tomography (PET) scan:** A procedure to find malignant tumor cells in the body. A small amount of radioactive glucose (sugar) is injected into a vein. The PET scanner rotates around the body and makes a picture of where glucose is being used in the body. Malignant tumor cells show up brighter in the picture because they are more active and take up more glucose than normal cells do.

- **Magnetic resonance imaging (MRI):** A procedure that uses a magnet, radio waves, and a computer to make a series of detailed pictures of areas inside the body. This procedure is also called nuclear magnetic resonance imaging (NMRI).

- **Ultrasound exam:** A procedure in which high-energy sound waves (ultrasound) are bounced off internal tissues or organs and make echoes. The echoes form a picture of body tissues called a sonogram. This picture can be printed to be looked at later.

- **Chest X-ray:** An X-ray of the organs and bones inside the chest. An X-ray is a type of energy beam that can go through the body and onto film, making a picture of areas inside the body.

- **Cystoscopy:** A procedure to look inside the bladder and urethra to check for abnormal areas. A cystoscope is inserted through the urethra into the bladder. A cystoscope is a thin, tube-like instrument with a light and a lens for viewing. It may also have a tool to remove tissue samples, which are checked under a microscope for signs of cancer.

- **Laparoscopy:** A surgical procedure to look at the organs inside the abdomen to check for signs of disease. Small incisions (cuts) are made in the wall of the abdomen and a laparoscope (a thin, lighted tube) is inserted into one of the incisions. Other instruments may be inserted through the same or other incisions to perform procedures such as removing organs or taking tissue samples to be checked under a microscope for signs of disease.

- **Pretreatment surgical staging:** Surgery (an operation) is done to find out if the cancer has spread within the cervix or to other parts of the body. In some cases, the cervical cancer can be removed at the same time. Pretreatment surgical staging is usually done only as part of a clinical trial.

The results of these tests are viewed together with the results of the original tumor biopsy to determine the cervical cancer stage. There are three ways that cancer spreads in the body.

Cancer can spread through tissue, the lymph system, and the blood:

- **Tissue.** The cancer spreads from where it began by growing into nearby areas.

- **Lymph system.** The cancer spreads from where it began by getting into the lymph system. The cancer travels through the lymph vessels to other parts of the body.

- **Blood.** The cancer spreads from where it began by getting into the blood. The cancer travels through the blood vessels to other parts of the body.

Cancer may spread from where it began to other parts of the body. When cancer spreads to another part of the body, it is called metastasis. Cancer cells break away from where they began (the primary tumor) and travel through the lymph system or blood.

- **Lymph system.** The cancer gets into the lymph system, travels through the lymph vessels, and forms a tumor (metastatic tumor) in another part of the body.

- **Blood.** The cancer gets into the blood, travels through the blood vessels, and forms a tumor (metastatic tumor) in another part of the body.

The metastatic tumor is the same type of cancer as the primary tumor. For example, if cervical cancer spreads to the lung, the cancer cells in the lung are actually cervical cancer cells. The disease is metastatic cervical cancer, not lung cancer.

The following stages are used for cervical cancer:

Stage 0 (Carcinoma in Situ (CIS))

In carcinoma in situ (stage 0), abnormal cells are found in the inner-most lining of the cervix. These abnormal cells may become cancer and spread into nearby normal tissue.

Stage I

In stage I, cancer is found in the cervix only.

Stage I is divided into stages IA and IB, based on the amount of cancer that is found.

- **Stage IA:**

  A very small amount of cancer that can only be seen with a microscope is found in the tissues of the cervix.

  Stage IA is divided into stages IA1 and IA2, based on the size of the tumor.

  - In stage IA1, the cancer is not more than 3 millimeters deep and not more than 7 millimeters wide.

  - In stage IA2, the cancer is more than 3 but not more than 5 millimeters deep, and not more than 7 millimeters wide.

- **Stage IB:**

  Stage IB is divided into stages IB1 and IB2, based on the size of the tumor.

  In stage IB1:

  - the cancer can only be seen with a microscope and is more than 5 millimeters deep and more than 7 millimeters wide; or

  - the cancer can be seen without a microscope and is not more than 4 centimeters.

In stage IB2, the cancer can be seen without a microscope and is more than 4 centimeters.

Stage II

In stage II, cancer has spread beyond the uterus but not onto the pelvic wall (the tissues that line the part of the body between the hips) or to the lower third of the vagina.

Stage II is divided into stages IIA and IIB, based on how far the cancer has spread.

- **Stage IIA:** Cancer has spread beyond the cervix to the upper two-thirds of the vagina but not to tissues around the uterus. Stage IIA is divided into stages IIA1 and IIA2, based on the size of the tumor.

  - In stage IIA1, the tumor can be seen without a microscope and is not more than 4 centimeters.

  - In stage IIA2, the tumor can be seen without a microscope and is more than 4 centimeters.

- **Stage IIB:** Cancer has spread beyond the cervix to the tissues around the uterus but not onto the pelvic wall.

Stage III

In stage III, cancer has spread to the lower third of the vagina, and/or onto the pelvic wall, and/or has caused kidney problems.

Stage III is divided into stages IIIA and IIIB, based on how far the cancer has spread.

In stage IIIA:

- Cancer has spread to the lower third of the vagina but not onto the pelvic wall.

In stage IIIB:

- Cancer has spread onto the pelvic wall; or

- the tumor has become large enough to block one or both ureters (tubes that connect the kidneys to the bladder) and has caused one or both kidneys to get bigger or stop working.

Stage IV

In stage IV, cancer has spread beyond the pelvis, or can be seen in the lining of the bladder and/or rectum, or has spread to other parts of the body.

Stage IV is divided into stages IVA and IVB, based on where the cancer has spread.

In stage IVA:

- Cancer has spread to nearby organs, such as the bladder or rectum.

In stage IVB:

- Cancer has spread to other parts of the body, such as the liver, lungs, bones, or distant lymph nodes.

Treatment Option Overview

Different types of treatment are available for patients with cervical cancer. Some treatments are standard (the currently used treatment), and some are being tested in clinical trials. A treatment clinical trial is a research study meant to help improve current treatments or obtain information on new treatments for patients with cancer. When clinical trials show that a new treatment is better than the standard treatment, the new treatment may become the standard treatment. Patients may want to think about taking part in a clinical trial. Some clinical trials are open only to patients who have not started treatment.

Four types of standard treatment are used:

Surgery

Surgery (removing the cancer in an operation) is sometimes used to treat cervical cancer. The following surgical procedures may be used:

- **Conization:** A procedure to remove a cone-shaped piece of tissue from the cervix and cervical canal. A pathologist views the tissue under a microscope to look for cancer cells. Conization may be used to diagnose or treat a cervical condition. This procedure is also called a cone biopsy.

  Conization may be done using one of the following procedures:

  - **Cold-knife conization:** A surgical procedure that uses a scalpel (sharp knife) to remove abnormal tissue or cancer.

  - **Loop electrosurgical excision procedure (LEEP):** A surgical procedure that uses electrical current passed through a thin wire loop as a knife to remove abnormal tissue or cancer.

  - **Laser surgery:** A surgical procedure that uses a laser beam (a narrow beam of intense light) as a knife to make bloodless cuts in tissue or to remove a surface lesion such as a tumor.

  The type of conization procedure used depends on where the cancer cells are in the cervix and the type of cervical cancer.

- **Total hysterectomy:** Surgery to remove the uterus, including the cervix. If the uterus and cervix are taken out through the vagina, the operation is called a vaginal hysterectomy. If the uterus and cervix are taken out through a large incision (cut) in the abdomen, the operation is called a total abdominal hysterectomy. If the uterus and cervix are taken out through a small incision in the abdomen using a laparoscope, the operation is called a total laparoscopic hysterectomy.

- **Radical hysterectomy:** Surgery to remove the uterus, cervix, part of the vagina, and a wide area of ligaments and tissues around these organs. The ovaries, fallopian tubes, or nearby lymph nodes may also be removed.

- **Modified radical hysterectomy:** Surgery to remove the uterus, cervix, upper part of the vagina, and ligaments and tissues that closely surround these organs. Nearby lymph nodes may also be removed. In this type of surgery, not as many tissues and/or organs are removed as in a radical hysterectomy.

- **Radical trachelectomy:** Surgery to remove the cervix, nearby tissue and lymph nodes, and the upper part of the vagina. The uterus and ovaries are not removed.

- **Bilateral salpingo-oophorectomy (BSO):** Surgery to remove both ovaries and both fallopian tubes.

- **Pelvic exenteration:** Surgery to remove the lower colon, rectum, and bladder. The cervix, vagina, ovaries, and nearby lymph nodes are also removed. Artificial openings (stoma) are made for urine and stool to flow from the body to a collection bag. Plastic surgery may be needed to make an artificial vagina after this operation.

Radiation Therapy

Radiation therapy is a cancer treatment that uses high-energy X-rays or other types of radiation to kill cancer cells or keep them from growing. There are two types of radiation therapy:

- External radiation therapy uses a machine outside the body to send radiation toward the cancer. Certain ways of giving radiation therapy can help keep radiation from damaging nearby healthy tissue. This type of radiation therapy includes the following:

- Intensity-modulated radiation therapy (IMRT): IMRT is a type of 3-dimensional (3D) radiation therapy that uses a computer to make pictures of the size and shape of the tumor. Thin beams of radiation of different intensities (strengths) are aimed at the tumor from many angles.

- Internal radiation therapy uses a radioactive substance sealed in needles, seeds, wires, or catheters that are placed directly into or near the cancer.

The way the radiation therapy is given depends on the type and stage of the cancer being treated. External and internal radiation therapy are used to treat cervical cancer, and may also be used as palliative therapy to relieve symptoms and improve quality of life.

Chemotherapy

Chemotherapy is a cancer treatment that uses drugs to stop the growth of cancer cells, either by killing the cells or by stopping them from dividing. When chemotherapy is taken by mouth or injected into a vein or muscle, the drugs enter the bloodstream and can reach cancer cells throughout the body (systemic chemotherapy). When chemotherapy is placed directly into the cerebrospinal fluid, an organ, or a body cavity such as the abdomen, the drugs mainly affect cancer cells in those areas (regional chemotherapy). The way the chemotherapy is given depends on the type and stage of the cancer being treated.

Targeted Therapy

Targeted therapy is a type of treatment that uses drugs or other substances to identify and attack specific cancer cells without harming normal cells.

Monoclonal antibody therapy is a type of targeted therapy that uses antibodies made in the laboratory from a single type of immune system cell. These antibodies can identify substances on cancer cells or normal substances that may help cancer cells grow. The antibodies attach to the substances and kill the cancer cells, block their growth, or keep them from spreading. Monoclonal antibodies are given by infusion. They may be used alone or to carry drugs, toxins, or radioactive material directly to cancer cells.

Bevacizumab is a monoclonal antibody that binds to a protein called vascular endothelial growth factor (VEGF) and may prevent the growth of new blood vessels that tumors need to grow. Bevacizumab is used to treat cervical cancer that has metastasized (spread to other parts of the body) and recurrent cervical cancer.

Chapter 17

Endometrial Cancer

Endometrial cancer is a disease in which malignant (cancer) cells form in the tissues of the endometrium. The endometrium is the lining of the uterus, a hollow, muscular organ in a woman's pelvis. The uterus is where a fetus grows. In most nonpregnant women, the uterus is about 3 inches long. The lower, narrow end of the uterus is the cervix, which leads to the vagina. Cancer of the endometrium is different from cancer of the muscle of the uterus, which is called sarcoma of the uterus.

Obesity and having metabolic syndrome may increase the risk of endometrial cancer. Anything that increases your chance of getting a disease is called a risk factor. Having a risk factor does not mean that you will get cancer; not having risk factors doesn't mean that you will not get cancer. Talk to your doctor if you think you may be at risk for endometrial cancer.

Risk Factors of Endometrial Cancer

Risk factors for endometrial cancer include the following:

- Taking estrogen-only hormone replacement therapy (HRT) after menopause

- Taking tamoxifen to prevent or treat breast cancer

This chapter includes text excerpted from "Endometrial Cancer Treatment (PDQ®)—Patient Version," National Cancer Institute (NCI), March 30, 2018.

- Obesity

- Having metabolic syndrome

- Having type 2 diabetes

- Exposure of endometrial tissue to estrogen made by the body. This may be caused by:

  - Never giving birth

  - Menstruating at an early age

  - Starting menopause at a later age

- Having polycystic ovarian syndrome (PCOS)

- Having a family history of endometrial cancer in a first-degree relative (mother, sister, or daughter)

- Having certain genetic conditions, such as Lynch syndrome

- Having endometrial hyperplasia

Older age is the main risk factor for most cancers. The chance of getting cancer increases as you get older. Taking tamoxifen for breast cancer or taking estrogen alone (without progesterone) can increase the risk of endometrial cancer. Endometrial cancer may develop in breast cancer patients who have been treated with tamoxifen. A patient who takes this drug and has abnormal vaginal bleeding should have a follow-up exam and a biopsy of the endometrial lining if needed. Women taking estrogen (a hormone that can affect the growth of some cancers) alone also have an increased risk of endometrial cancer. Taking estrogen combined with progesterone (another hormone) does not increase a woman's risk of endometrial cancer.

Signs and Symptoms of Endometrial Cancer

Signs and symptoms of endometrial cancer include unusual vaginal bleeding or pain in the pelvis. These and other signs and symptoms may be caused by endometrial cancer or by other conditions. Check with your doctor if you have any of the following:

- Vaginal bleeding or discharge not related to menstruation (periods)

- Vaginal bleeding after menopause

- Difficult or painful urination

- Pain during sexual intercourse

- Pain in the pelvic area

Diagnosis of Endometrial Cancer

Tests that examine the endometrium are used to detect (find) and diagnose endometrial cancer. Because endometrial cancer begins inside the uterus, it does not usually show up in the results of a Pap (Papanicolaou) test. For this reason, a sample of endometrial tissue must be removed and checked under a microscope to look for cancer cells. One of the following procedures may be used:

- **Endometrial biopsy:** The removal of tissue from the endometrium (inner lining of the uterus) by inserting a thin, flexible tube through the cervix and into the uterus. The tube is used to gently scrape a small amount of tissue from the endometrium and then remove the tissue samples. A pathologist views the tissue under a microscope to look for cancer cells.

- **Dilatation and curettage (D&C):** A procedure to remove samples of tissue from the inner lining of the uterus. The cervix is dilated and a curette (spoon-shaped instrument) is inserted into the uterus to remove tissue. The tissue samples are checked under a microscope for signs of disease. This procedure is also called a D&C.

- **Hysteroscopy:** A procedure to look inside the uterus for abnormal areas. A hysteroscope is inserted through the vagina and cervix into the uterus. A hysteroscope is a thin, tube-like instrument with a light and a lens for viewing. It may also have a tool to remove tissue samples, which are checked under a microscope for signs of cancer.

Other tests and procedures used to diagnose endometrial cancer include the following:

- **Physical exam and history:** An exam of the body to check general signs of health, including checking for signs of disease, such as lumps or anything else that seems unusual. A history of the patient's health habits and past illnesses and treatments will also be taken.

- **Transvaginal ultrasound exam:** A procedure used to examine the vagina, uterus, fallopian tubes, and bladder. An ultrasound transducer (probe) is inserted into the vagina and used to bounce high-energy sound waves (ultrasound) off internal tissues or organs and make echoes. The echoes form a picture of body tissues called a sonogram. The doctor can identify tumors by looking at the sonogram.

Stages of Endometrial Cancer

After endometrial cancer has been diagnosed, tests are done to find out if cancer cells have spread within the uterus or to other parts of the body. The process used to find out whether the cancer has spread within the uterus or to other parts of the body is called staging. The information gathered from the staging process determines the stage of the disease. It is important to know the stage in order to plan treatment. Certain tests and procedures are used in the staging process. A hysterectomy (an operation in which the uterus is removed) will usually be done to treat endometrial cancer. Tissue samples are taken from the area around the uterus and checked under a microscope for signs of cancer to help find out whether the cancer has spread.

The following procedures may be used in the staging process:

- **Pelvic exam:** An exam of the vagina, cervix, uterus, fallopian tubes, ovaries, and rectum. A speculum is inserted into the vagina and the doctor or nurse looks at the vagina and cervix for signs of disease. A Pap test of the cervix is usually done. The doctor or nurse also inserts one or two lubricated, gloved fingers of one hand into the vagina and places the other hand over the lower abdomen to feel the size, shape, and position of the uterus and ovaries. The doctor or nurse also inserts a lubricated, gloved finger into the rectum to feel for lumps or abnormal areas.

- **Chest X-ray:** An X-ray of the organs and bones inside the chest. An X-ray is a type of energy beam that can go through the body and onto film, making a picture of areas inside the body.

- **Computerized axial tomography (CAT) or computed tomography (CT) scan:** A procedure that makes a series of detailed pictures of areas inside the body, taken from different angles. The pictures are made by a computer linked to an X-ray machine. A dye may be injected into a vein or swallowed to help the organs or tissues show up more clearly. This procedure is also called computed tomography, computerized tomography, or computerized axial tomography.

- **Magnetic resonance imaging (MRI):** A procedure that uses a magnet, radio waves, and a computer to make a series of detailed pictures of areas inside the body. This procedure is also called nuclear magnetic resonance imaging (NMRI).

- **Positron emission tomography (PET) scan:** A procedure to find malignant tumor cells in the body. A small amount of radioactive glucose (sugar) is injected into a vein. The PET scanner rotates around the body and makes a picture of where glucose is being used in the body. Malignant tumor cells show up brighter in the picture because they are more active and take up more glucose than normal cells do.

- **Lymph node dissection:** A surgical procedure in which the lymph nodes are removed from the pelvic area and a sample of tissue is checked under a microscope for signs of cancer. This procedure is also called lymphadenectomy.

The following stages are used for endometrial cancer:

Stage I

In stage I, cancer is found in the uterus only. Stage I is divided into stages IA and IB, based on how far the cancer has spread.

- **Stage IA:** Cancer is in the endometrium only or less than halfway through the myometrium (muscle layer of the uterus).

- **Stage IB:** Cancer has spread halfway or more into the myometrium.

Stage II

In stage II, cancer has spread into connective tissue of the cervix, but has not spread outside the uterus.

Stage III

In stage III, cancer has spread beyond the uterus and cervix, but has not spread beyond the pelvis. Stage III is divided into stages IIIA, IIIB, and IIIC, based on how far the cancer has spread within the pelvis.

- **Stage IIIA:** Cancer has spread to the outer layer of the uterus and/or to the fallopian tubes, ovaries, and ligaments of the uterus.

- **Stage IIIB:** Cancer has spread to the vagina and/or to the parametrium (connective tissue and fat around the uterus).

- **Stage IIIC:** Cancer has spread to lymph nodes in the pelvis and/ or around the aorta (largest artery in the body, which carries blood away from the heart).

Stage IV

In stage IV, cancer has spread beyond the pelvis. Stage IV is divided into stages IVA and IVB, based on how far the cancer has spread.

- **Stage IVA:** Cancer has spread to the bladder and/or bowel wall.

- **Stage IVB:** Cancer has spread to other parts of the body beyond the pelvis, including the abdomen and/or lymph nodes in the groin.

Endometrial cancer may be grouped for treatment as follows:

Low-Risk Endometrial Cancer

Grades 1 and 2 tumors are usually considered low-risk. They usually do not spread to other parts of the body.

High-Risk Endometrial Cancer

Grade 3 tumors are considered high-risk. They often spread to other parts of the body. Uterine papillary serous, clear cell, and carcinosarcoma are three subtypes of endometrial cancer that are considered grade 3.

Treatment Option Overview

There are different types of treatment for patients with endometrial cancer. Different types of treatment are available for patients with endometrial cancer. Some treatments are standard (the currently used treatment), and some are being tested in clinical trials. A treatment clinical trial is a research study meant to help improve current treatments or obtain information on new treatments for patients with cancer. When clinical trials show that a new treatment is better than the standard treatment, the new treatment may become the standard treatment. Patients may want to think about taking part in a clinical trial. Some clinical trials are open only to patients who have not started treatment.

Five types of standard treatment are used:

Surgery

Surgery (removing the cancer in an operation) is the most common treatment for endometrial cancer. The following surgical procedures may be used:

- **Total hysterectomy:** Surgery to remove the uterus, including the cervix. If the uterus and cervix are taken out through the vagina, the operation is called a vaginal hysterectomy. If the uterus and cervix are taken out through a large incision (cut) in the abdomen, the operation is called a total abdominal hysterectomy. If the uterus and cervix are taken out through a small incision (cut) in the abdomen using a laparoscope, the operation is called a total laparoscopic hysterectomy.

- **Bilateral salpingo-oophorectomy (BSO):** Surgery to remove both ovaries and both fallopian tubes.

- **Radical hysterectomy:** Surgery to remove the uterus, cervix, and part of the vagina. The ovaries, fallopian tubes, or nearby lymph nodes may also be removed.

- **Lymph node dissection:** A surgical procedure in which the lymph nodes are removed from the pelvic area and a sample of tissue is checked under a microscope for signs of cancer. This procedure is also called lymphadenectomy.

Even if the doctor removes all the cancer that can be seen at the time of the surgery, some patients may be given radiation therapy or hormone treatment after surgery to kill any cancer cells that are left. Treatment given after the surgery, to lower the risk that the cancer will come back, is called adjuvant therapy.

Radiation Therapy

Radiation therapy is a cancer treatment that uses high-energy X-rays or other types of radiation to kill cancer cells or keep them from growing. There are two types of radiation therapy:

- External radiation therapy uses a machine outside the body to send radiation toward the cancer.

- Internal radiation therapy uses a radioactive substance sealed in needles, seeds, wires, or catheters that are placed directly into or near the cancer.

The way the radiation therapy is given depends on the type and stage of the cancer being treated. External and internal radiation therapy are used to treat endometrial cancer, and may also be used as palliative therapy to relieve symptoms and improve quality of life.

Chemotherapy

Chemotherapy is a cancer treatment that uses drugs to stop the growth of cancer cells, either by killing the cells or by stopping the cells from dividing. When chemotherapy is taken by mouth or injected into a vein or muscle, the drugs enter the bloodstream and can reach cancer cells throughout the body (systemic chemotherapy). When chemotherapy is placed directly into the cerebrospinal fluid, an organ, or a body cavity such as the abdomen, the drugs mainly affect cancer cells in those areas (regional chemotherapy).

The way the chemotherapy is given depends on the type and stage of the cancer being treated.

Hormone Therapy

Hormone therapy is a cancer treatment that removes hormones or blocks their action and stops cancer cells from growing. Hormones are substances made by glands in the body and circulated in the bloodstream. Some hormones can cause certain cancers to grow. If tests show that the cancer cells have places where hormones can attach (receptors), drugs, surgery, or radiation therapy is used to reduce the production of hormones or block them from working.

Targeted Therapy

Targeted therapy is a type of treatment that uses drugs or other substances to identify and attack specific cancer cells without harming normal cells. Monoclonal antibodies (mAb), mechanistic target of rapamycin (mTOR) inhibitors, and signal transduction inhibitors are three types of targeted therapy used to treat endometrial cancer.

- Monoclonal antibody (mAb) therapy is a cancer treatment that uses antibodies made in the laboratory from a single type of immune system cell. These antibodies can identify substances on cancer cells or normal substances that may help cancer cells grow. The antibodies attach to the substances and kill the cancer cells, block their growth, or keep them from spreading. Monoclonal antibodies (mAb) are given by infusion. They may be used alone or to carry drugs, toxins, or radioactive material directly to cancer cells. Bevacizumab is used to treat stage III, stage IV, and recurrent endometrial cancer.

- mTOR inhibitors block a protein called mTOR, which helps control cell division. mTOR inhibitors may keep cancer cells from growing and prevent the growth of new blood vessels that tumors need to grow. Everolimus and ridaforolimus are used to treat stage III, stage IV, and recurrent endometrial cancer.

- Signal transduction inhibitors block signals that are passed from one molecule to another inside a cell. Blocking these signals may kill cancer cells. Metformin is being studied to treat stage III, stage IV, and recurrent endometrial cancer.

Chapter 18

Gestational Trophoblastic Tumors

Gestational trophoblastic disease (GTD) is a tumor that develops inside the uterus from tissue that forms after conception (the joining of sperm and egg). This tissue is made of trophoblast cells and normally surrounds the fertilized egg in the uterus. Trophoblast cells help connect the fertilized egg to the wall of the uterus and form part of the placenta (the organ that passes nutrients from the mother to the fetus).

Sometimes there is a problem with the fertilized egg and trophoblast cells. Instead of a healthy fetus developing, a tumor forms. Until there are signs or symptoms of the tumor, the pregnancy will seem like a normal pregnancy.

Most GTD is benign (not cancer) and does not spread, but some types become malignant (cancer) and spread to nearby tissues or distant parts of the body.

GTD is a general term that includes different types of disease:

- Hydatidiform moles (HM)

  - Complete HM

  - Partial HM

- Gestational trophoblastic neoplasia (GTN)

This chapter includes text excerpted from "Gestational Trophoblastic Disease Treatment (PDQ®)—Patient Version," National Cancer Institute (NCI), October 13, 2017.

- Invasive moles
- Choriocarcinomas
- Placental site trophoblastic tumors (PSTT; very rare)
- Epithelioid trophoblastic tumors (ETT; even more rare)

Risks of Gestational Trophoblastic Disease

Age and a previous molar pregnancy affect the risk of GTD. Anything that increases your risk of getting a disease is called a risk factor. Having a risk factor does not mean that you will get cancer; not having risk factors doesn't mean that you will not get cancer. Talk to your doctor if you think you may be at risk. Risk factors for GTD include the following:

- Being pregnant when you are younger than 20 or older than 35 years of age
- Having a personal history of hydatidiform mole

Signs and Symptoms of Gestational Trophoblastic Disease

Signs of GTD include abnormal vaginal bleeding and a uterus that is larger than normal. These and other signs and symptoms may be caused by GTD or by other conditions. Check with your doctor if you have any of the following:

- Vaginal bleeding not related to menstruation
- A uterus that is larger than expected during pregnancy
- Pain or pressure in the pelvis
- Severe nausea and vomiting during pregnancy
- High blood pressure with headache and swelling of feet and hands early in the pregnancy
- Vaginal bleeding that continues for longer than normal after delivery
- Fatigue, shortness of breath, dizziness, and a fast or irregular heartbeat caused by anemia

GTD sometimes causes an overactive thyroid. Signs and symptoms of an overactive thyroid include the following:

- Fast or irregular heartbeat
- Shakiness
- Sweating
- Frequent bowel movements
- Trouble sleeping
- Feeling anxious or irritable
- Weight loss

Diagnostic Tests for Gestational Trophoblastic Disease

Tests that examine the uterus are used to detect (find) and diagnose GTD. The following tests and procedures may be used:

Physical exam and history: An exam of the body to check general signs of health, including checking for signs of disease, such as lumps or anything else that seems unusual. A history of the patient's health habits and past illnesses and treatments will also be taken.

Pelvic exam: An exam of the vagina, cervix, uterus, fallopian tubes, ovaries, and rectum. A speculum is inserted into the vagina and the doctor or nurse looks at the vagina and cervix for signs of disease. A Pap (Papanicolaou) test of the cervix is usually done. The doctor or nurse also inserts one or two lubricated, gloved fingers of one hand into the vagina and places the other hand over the lower abdomen to feel the size, shape, and position of the uterus and ovaries. The doctor or nurse also inserts a lubricated, gloved finger into the rectum to feel for lumps or abnormal areas.

Ultrasound exam of the pelvis: A procedure in which high-energy sound waves (ultrasound) are bounced off internal tissues or organs in the pelvis and make echoes. The echoes form a picture of body tissues called a sonogram. Sometimes a transvaginal ultrasound (TVUS) will be done. For TVUS, an ultrasound transducer (probe) is inserted into the vagina to make the sonogram.

Blood chemistry studies: A procedure in which a blood sample is checked to measure the amounts of certain substances released into the blood by organs and tissues in the body. An unusual (higher or lower than normal) amount of a substance can be a sign of disease. Blood is also tested to check the liver, kidney, and bone marrow.

Serum tumor marker test: A procedure in which a sample of blood is checked to measure the amounts of certain substances made by organs, tissues, or tumor cells in the body. Certain substances are linked to specific types of cancer when found in increased levels in the body. These are called tumor markers. For GTD, the blood is checked for the level of beta-human chorionic gonadotropin (β-hCG), a hormone that is made by the body during pregnancy. β-hCG in the blood of a woman who is not pregnant may be a sign of GTD.

Urinalysis: A test to check the color of urine and its contents, such as sugar, protein, blood, bacteria, and the level of β-hCG.

Stages of Gestational Trophoblastic Disease

After GTN has been diagnosed, tests are done to find out if cancer has spread from where it started to other parts of the body. The process used to find out the extent or spread of cancer is called staging, The information gathered from the staging process helps determine the stage of the disease. For GTN, stage is one of the factors used to plan treatment. The following tests and procedures may be done to help find out the stage of the disease:

- **Chest X-ray:** An X-ray of the organs and bones inside the chest. An X-ray is a type of energy beam that can go through the body onto film, making pictures of areas inside the body.

- **Computerized axial tomography (CAT) or computed tomography (CT) scan:** A procedure that makes a series of detailed pictures of areas inside the body, taken from different angles. The pictures are made by a computer linked to an X-ray machine. A dye may be injected into a vein or swallowed to help the organs or tissues show up more clearly. This procedure is also called computed tomography, computerized tomography, or computerized axial tomography.

- **Magnetic resonance imaging (MRI) with gadolinium:** A procedure that uses a magnet, radio waves, and a computer to make a series of detailed pictures of areas inside the body, such as brain and spinal cord. A substance called gadolinium is injected into a vein. The gadolinium collects around the cancer cells so they show up brighter in the picture. This procedure is also called nuclear magnetic resonance imaging (NMRI).

- **Lumbar puncture:** A procedure used to collect cerebrospinal fluid (CSF) from the spinal column. This is done by placing a needle between two bones in the spine and into the CSF around the spinal cord and removing a sample of the fluid. The sample of CSF is checked under a microscope for signs that the cancer has spread to the brain and spinal cord. This procedure is also called an LP or spinal tap.

There is no staging system for hydatidiform moles (HM). HM are found in the uterus only and do not spread to other parts of the body. The following stages are used for GTN:

Stage I

In stage I, the tumor is in the uterus only.

Stage II

In stage II, cancer has spread outside of the uterus to the ovary, fallopian tube, vagina, and/or the ligaments that support the uterus.

Stage III

In stage III, cancer has spread to the lung.

Stage IV

In stage IV, cancer has spread to distant parts of the body other than the lungs.

The treatment of GTN is based on the type of disease, stage, or risk group. Invasive moles and choriocarcinomas are treated based on risk groups. The stage of the invasive mole or choriocarcinoma is one factor used to determine risk group. Other factors include the following:

- The age of the patient when the diagnosis is made

- Whether the GTN occurred after a molar pregnancy, miscarriage, or normal pregnancy

- How soon the tumor was diagnosed after the pregnancy began

- The level of beta-human chorionic gonadotropin (β-hCG) in the blood

- The size of the largest tumor

- Where the tumor has spread to and the number of tumors in the body

- How many chemotherapy drugs the tumor has been treated with (for recurrent or resistant tumors)

There are two risk groups for invasive moles and choriocarcinomas: low risk and high risk. Patients with low-risk disease usually receive less aggressive treatment than patients with high-risk disease. Placental-site trophoblastic tumor (PSTT) and epithelioid trophoblastic tumor (ETT) treatments depend on the stage of disease.

Treatment Option Overview

There are different types of treatment for patients with GTD. Different types of treatment are available for patients with GTD. Some treatments are standard (the currently used treatment), and some are being tested in clinical trials. Before starting treatment, patients may want to think about taking part in a clinical trial. A treatment clinical trial is a research study meant to help improve current treatments or obtain information on new treatments for patients with cancer. When clinical trials show that a new treatment is better than the standard treatment, the new treatment may become the standard treatment.

Three types of standard treatment are used:

Surgery

The doctor may remove the cancer using one of the following operations:

- **Dilatation and curettage (D&C) with suction evacuation:** A surgical procedure to remove abnormal tissue and parts of the inner lining of the uterus. The cervix is dilated and the material inside the uterus is removed with a small vacuum-like device. The walls of the uterus are then gently scraped with a curette (spoon-shaped instrument) to remove any material that may remain in the uterus. This procedure may be used for molar pregnancies.

- **Hysterectomy:** Surgery to remove the uterus, and sometimes the cervix. If the uterus and cervix are taken out through the vagina, the operation is called a vaginal hysterectomy. If the uterus and cervix are taken out through a large incision (cut) in the abdomen, the operation is called a total abdominal hysterectomy. If the uterus and cervix are taken out through a small incision (cut) in the abdomen using a laparoscope, the operation is called a total laparoscopic hysterectomy.

Chemotherapy

Chemotherapy is a cancer treatment that uses drugs to stop the growth of cancer cells, either by killing the cells or by stopping them from dividing. When chemotherapy is taken by mouth or injected into a vein or muscle, the drugs enter the bloodstream and can reach cancer cells throughout the body (systemic chemotherapy). When chemotherapy is placed directly into the cerebrospinal fluid, an organ, or a body cavity such as the abdomen, the drugs mainly affect cancer cells in those areas (regional chemotherapy). The way the chemotherapy is given depends on the type and stage of the cancer being treated, or whether the tumor is low-risk or high-risk.

Combination chemotherapy is treatment using more than one anti-cancer drug. Even if the doctor removes all the cancer that can be seen at the time of the surgery, some patients may be given chemotherapy after surgery to kill any tumor cells that are left. Treatment given after the surgery, to lower the risk that the cancer will come back, is called adjuvant therapy.

Radiation Therapy

Radiation therapy is a cancer treatment that uses high-energy X-rays or other types of radiation to kill cancer cells or keep them from growing. There are two types of radiation therapy:

- External radiation therapy uses a machine outside the body to send radiation toward the cancer.

- Internal radiation therapy uses a radioactive substance sealed in needles, seeds, wires, or catheters that are placed directly into or near the cancer.

The way the radiation therapy is given depends on the type of GTD being treated. External radiation therapy is used to treat GTD.

Chapter 19

Ovarian Cancer

Chapter Contents

Section 19.1

What You Need to Know about Ovarian Cancer

This section includes text excerpted from "Gynecologic Cancers—Ovarian Cancer," Centers for Disease Control and Prevention (CDC), September 13, 2017.

Cancer is a disease in which abnormal cells in the body grow out of control. Cancer is always named for the part of the body where it starts, even if it spreads to other body parts later. Ovarian cancer is a group of diseases that originates in the ovaries, or in the related areas of the fallopian tubes and the peritoneum. Women have two ovaries that are located in the pelvis, one on each side of the uterus. The ovaries make female hormones and produce eggs. Women have two fallopian tubes that are a pair of long, slender tubes on each side of the uterus. Eggs pass from the ovaries through the fallopian tubes to the uterus. The peritoneum is the tissue lining that covers organs in the abdomen.

Ovarian cancer causes more deaths than any other cancer of the female reproductive system. But when ovarian cancer is found in its early stages, treatment works best. Ovarian cancer often causes signs and symptoms, so it is important to pay attention to your body and know what is normal for you. Symptoms may be caused by something other than cancer, but the only way to know is to see your doctor, nurse, or other healthcare professional. Some mutations (changes in genes) can raise your risk for ovarian cancer. Mutations in the breast cancer susceptibility genes 1 and 2 (*BRCA1* and *BRCA2*), and those associated with Lynch syndrome, raise ovarian cancer risk.

What Are the Risk Factors for Ovarian Cancer?

There is no way to know for sure if you will get ovarian cancer. Most women get it without being at high risk. However, several factors may increase a woman's risk for ovarian cancer, including if you:

- Are middle-aged or older

198

- Have close family members (such as your mother, sister, aunt, or grandmother) on either your mother's or your father's side, who have had ovarian cancer

- Have a genetic mutation (abnormality) called *BRCA1* or *BRCA2*, or one associated with Lynch syndrome

- Have had breast, uterine, or colorectal (colon), cancer

- Have an Eastern European or Ashkenazi Jewish background

- Have endometriosis (a condition where tissue from the lining of the uterus grows elsewhere in the body)

- Have never given birth or have had trouble getting pregnant

In addition, some studies suggest that women who take estrogen by itself (without progesterone) for 10 or more years may have an increased risk of ovarian cancer.

If one or more of these factors is true for you, it does not mean you will get ovarian cancer. But you should speak with your doctor about your risk. If you or your family have a history of ovarian cancer, speak to your doctor about genetic counseling.

What Can I Do to Reduce My Risk of Ovarian Cancer?

There is no known way to prevent ovarian cancer, but these things are associated with a lower chance of getting ovarian cancer:

- Having used birth control pills for five or more years

- Having had a tubal ligation (getting your tubes tied), both ovaries removed, or a hysterectomy (an operation in which the uterus, and sometimes the cervix, is removed)

- Having given birth

- Breastfeeding. Some studies suggest that women who breastfeed for a year or more may have a modestly reduced risk of ovarian cancer.

While these things may help reduce the chance of getting ovarian cancer, they are not recommended for everybody, and risks and benefits are associated with each. Avoiding risk factors may lower your risk, but it does not mean that you will not get cancer. Talk to your doctor about ways to reduce your risk.

What Are the Symptoms of Ovarian Cancer?

Ovarian cancer may cause the following signs and symptoms:

- Vaginal bleeding (particularly if you are past menopause), or discharge from your vagina that is not normal for you

- Pain or pressure in the pelvic area

- Abdominal or back pain

- Bloating

- Feeling full too quickly, or difficulty eating

- A change in your bathroom habits, such as more frequent or urgent need to urinate and/or constipation

Pay attention to your body, and know what is normal for you. If you have unusual vaginal bleeding, see a doctor right away. If you have any of the other signs for two weeks or longer and they are not normal for you, see a doctor. They may be caused by something other than cancer, but the only way to know is to see a doctor.

What Should I Know about Screening?

There is no simple and reliable way to screen for ovarian cancer in women who do not have any signs or symptoms. Screening is when a test is used to look for a disease before there are any symptoms. Cancer screening tests work when they can find the disease early, when treatment works best. Diagnostic tests are used when a person has symptoms. The purpose of diagnostic tests is to find out, or diagnose, what is causing the symptoms. Diagnostic tests also may be used to check a person who is considered at high risk for cancer.

The Pap (Papanicolaou) test does not check for ovarian cancer. The only cancer the Pap test screens for is cervical cancer. Since there is no simple and reliable way to screen for any gynecologic cancer except for cervical cancer, it is especially important to recognize warning signs, and learn what you can do to reduce your risk.

Here is what you can do:

- Pay attention to your body, and know what is normal for you.

- If you notice any changes in your body that are not normal for you and could be a sign of ovarian cancer, talk to your doctor about them.

Ask your doctor if you should have a diagnostic test, like a rectovaginal pelvic exam, a transvaginal ultrasound, or a CA-125 (cancer antigen 125) blood test if you have any unexplained signs or symptoms of ovarian cancer. These tests sometimes help find or rule out ovarian cancer.

How Is Ovarian Cancer Treated?

If your doctor says that you have ovarian, fallopian tube, or primary peritoneal cancers, ask to be referred to a gynecologic oncologist—a doctor who was trained to treat cancers of a woman's reproductive system. Gynecologic oncologists can perform surgery on and give chemotherapy (medicine) to women with ovarian cancer. Your doctor can work with you to create a treatment plan.

Types of Treatment

Treatment for ovarian cancer usually involves a combination of surgery and chemotherapy.

- **Surgery:** Doctors remove cancer tissue in an operation.

- **Chemotherapy:** Using special medicines to shrink or kill the cancer. The drugs can be pills you take or medicines given in your veins, or sometimes both.

Different treatments may be provided by different doctors on your medical team.

- Gynecologic oncologists are doctors who have been trained to treat cancers of a woman's reproductive system. They perform surgery and give chemotherapy (medicine).

- Surgeons are doctors who perform operations.

- Medical oncologists are doctors who treat cancer with medicine (chemotherapy).

Which Treatment Is Right for Me?

Choosing the treatment that is right for you may be hard. Talk to your cancer doctor about the treatment options available for your type and stage of cancer. Your doctor can explain the risks and benefits of each treatment and their side effects. Side effects are how your body reacts to drugs or other treatments.

Sometimes people get an opinion from more than one cancer doctor. This is called a "second opinion." Getting a second opinion may help you choose the treatment that is right for you.

Section 19.2

Ovarian Germ Cell Tumors

This section includes text excerpted from "Ovarian Germ Cell Tumors Treatment (PDQ®)—Patient Version," National Cancer Institute (NCI), October 13, 2017.

Ovarian germ cell tumor (OGCT) is a disease in which malignant (cancer) cells form in the germ (egg) cells of the ovary. Germ cell tumors begin in the reproductive cells (egg or sperm) of the body. OGCTs usually occur in teenage girls or young women and most often affect just one ovary. The ovaries are a pair of organs in the female reproductive system. They are in the pelvis, one on each side of the uterus (the hollow, pear-shaped organ where a fetus grows). Each ovary is about the size and shape of an almond. The ovaries make eggs and female hormones. OGCT is a general name that is used to describe several different types of cancer. The most common OGCT is called dysgerminoma.

Signs of Ovarian Germ Cell Tumor

Signs of OGCT are swelling of the abdomen or vaginal bleeding after menopause. OGCTs can be hard to diagnose (find) early. Often there are no symptoms in the early stages, but tumors may be found during regular gynecologic exams (checkups). Check with your doctor if you have either of the following:

- Swollen abdomen without weight gain in other parts of the body

- Bleeding from the vagina after menopause (when you are no longer having menstrual periods)

Diagnosing Ovarian Germ Cell Tumor

Tests that examine the ovaries, pelvic area, blood, and ovarian tissue are used to detect (find) and diagnose OGCT.

The following tests and procedures may be used:

- **Physical exam and history:** An exam of the body to check general signs of health, including checking for signs of disease, such as lumps or anything else that seems unusual. A history of the patient's health habits and past illnesses and treatments will also be taken.

- **Pelvic exam:** An exam of the vagina, cervix, uterus, fallopian tubes, ovaries, and rectum. A speculum is inserted into the vagina and the doctor or nurse looks at the vagina and cervix for signs of disease. A Pap test of the cervix is usually done. The doctor or nurse also inserts one or two lubricated, gloved fingers of one hand into the vagina and places the other hand over the lower abdomen to feel the size, shape, and position of the uterus and ovaries. The doctor or nurse also inserts a lubricated, gloved finger into the rectum to feel for lumps or abnormal areas.

- **Laparotomy:** A surgical procedure in which an incision (cut) is made in the wall of the abdomen to check the inside of the abdomen for signs of disease. The size of the incision depends on the reason the laparotomy is being done. Sometimes organs are removed or tissue samples are taken and checked under a microscope for signs of disease.

- **Computerized axial tomography (CAT) or computed tomography (CT) scan:** A procedure that makes a series of detailed pictures of areas inside the body, taken from different angles. The pictures are made by a computer linked to an X-ray machine. A dye may be injected into a vein or swallowed to help the organs or tissues show up more clearly. This procedure is also called computed tomography, computerized tomography, or computerized axial tomography.

- **Serum tumor marker test:** A procedure in which a sample of blood is checked to measure the amounts of certain substances released into the blood by organs, tissues, or tumor cells in the body. Certain substances are linked to specific types of cancer when found in increased levels in the blood. These are called tumor markers. An increased level of alpha-fetoprotein (AFP) or human chorionic gonadotropin (HCG) in the blood may be a sign of OGCT.

Stages of Ovarian Germ Cell Tumors

Many of the tests used to diagnose OGCT are also used for staging. The following tests and procedures may also be used for staging:

- **Positron emission tomography (PET) scan:** A procedure to find malignant tumor cells in the body. A small amount of radioactive glucose (sugar) is injected into a vein. The PET scanner rotates around the body and makes a picture of where glucose is being used in the body. Malignant tumor cells show up brighter in the picture because they are more active and take up more glucose than normal cells do.

- **Magnetic resonance imaging (MRI):** A procedure that uses a magnet, radio waves, and a computer to make a series of detailed pictures of areas inside the body. This procedure is also called nuclear magnetic resonance imaging (NMRI).

- **Transvaginal ultrasound exam:** A procedure used to examine the vagina, uterus, fallopian tubes, and bladder. An ultrasound transducer (probe) is inserted into the vagina and used to bounce high-energy sound waves (ultrasound) off internal tissues or organs and make echoes. The echoes form a picture of body tissues called a sonogram. The doctor can identify tumors by looking at the sonogram.

The following stages are used for OGCTs:

Stage I

In stage I, cancer is found in one or both ovaries. Stage I is divided into stage IA, stage IB, and stage IC.

- **Stage IA:** Cancer is found inside a single ovary.
- **Stage IB:** Cancer is found inside both ovaries.
- **Stage IC:** Cancer is found inside one or both ovaries and one of the following is true:
  - Cancer is also found on the outside surface of one or both ovaries.
  - The capsule (outer covering) of the ovary has ruptured (broken open).
  - Cancer cells are found in the fluid of the peritoneal cavity (the body cavity that contains most of the organs in the abdomen) or in washings of the peritoneum (tissue lining the peritoneal cavity).

Stage II

In stage II, cancer is found in one or both ovaries and has spread into other areas of the pelvis. Stage II is divided into stage IIA, stage IIB, and stage IIC.

- **Stage IIA:** Cancer has spread to the uterus and/or fallopian tubes (the long slender tubes through which eggs pass from the ovaries to the uterus).

- **Stage IIB:** Cancer has spread to other tissue within the pelvis.

- **Stage IIC:** Cancer is found inside one or both ovaries and has spread to the uterus and/or fallopian tubes, or to other tissue within the pelvis. Also, one of the following is true:

  - Cancer is found on the outside surface of one or both ovaries.

  - The capsule (outer covering) of the ovary has ruptured (broken open).

  - Cancer cells are found in the fluid of the peritoneal cavity (the body cavity that contains most of the organs in the abdomen) or in washings of the peritoneum (tissue lining the peritoneal cavity).

Stage III

In stage III, cancer is found in one or both ovaries and has spread outside the pelvis to other parts of the abdomen and/or nearby lymph nodes. Stage III is divided into stage IIIA, stage IIIB, and stage IIIC.

- **Stage IIIA:** The tumor is found in the pelvis only, but cancer cells that can be seen only with a microscope have spread to the surface of the peritoneum (tissue that lines the abdominal wall and covers most of the organs in the abdomen), the small intestines, or the tissue that connects the small intestines to the wall of the abdomen.

- **Stage IIIB:** Cancer has spread to the peritoneum and the cancer in the peritoneum is 2 centimeters or smaller.

- **Stage IIIC:** Cancer has spread to the peritoneum and the cancer in the peritoneum is larger than 2 centimeters and/or cancer has spread to lymph nodes in the abdomen.

Cancer that has spread to the surface of the liver is also considered stage III ovarian cancer.

Stage IV

In stage IV, cancer has spread beyond the abdomen to other parts of the body, such as the lungs or tissue inside the liver. Cancer cells in the fluid around the lungs is also considered stage IV ovarian cancer.

Treatment Option Overview

There are different types of treatment for patients with OGCTs. Some treatments are standard (the currently used treatment), and some are being tested in clinical trials. A treatment clinical trial is a research study meant to help improve current treatments or obtain information on new treatments for patients with cancer. When clinical trials show that a new treatment is better than the standard treatment, the new treatment may become the standard treatment. Patients may want to think about taking part in a clinical trial. Some clinical trials are open only to patients who have not started treatment.

Four types of standard treatment are used:

Surgery

Surgery is the most common treatment of OGCT. A doctor may take out the cancer using one of the following types of surgery.

- **Unilateral salpingo-oophorectomy:** A surgical procedure to remove one ovary and one fallopian tube. Total hysterectomy: A surgical procedure to remove the uterus, including the cervix. If the uterus and cervix are taken out through the vagina, the operation is called a vaginal hysterectomy. If the uterus and cervix are taken out through a large incision (cut) in the abdomen, the operation is called a total abdominal hysterectomy. If the uterus and cervix are taken out through a small incision (cut) in the abdomen using a laparoscope, the operation is called a total laparoscopic hysterectomy.

- **Bilateral salpingo-oophorectomy (BSO):** A surgical procedure to remove both ovaries and both fallopian tubes.

- **Tumor debulking:** A surgical procedure in which as much of the tumor as possible is removed. Some tumors cannot be completely removed.

Even if the doctor removes all the cancer that can be seen at the time of the operation, some patients may be offered chemotherapy or radiation therapy after surgery to kill any cancer cells that are left.

Treatment given after the surgery, to lower the risk that the cancer will come back, is called adjuvant therapy.

After chemotherapy for an OGCT, a second-look laparotomy may be done. This is similar to the laparotomy that is done to find out the stage of the cancer. Second-look laparotomy is a surgical procedure to find out if tumor cells are left after primary treatment. During this procedure, the doctor will take samples of lymph nodes and other tissues in the abdomen to see if any cancer is left. This procedure is not done for dysgerminomas.

Observation

Observation is closely watching a patient's condition without giving any treatment unless signs or symptoms appear or change.

Chemotherapy

Chemotherapy is a cancer treatment that uses drugs to stop the growth of cancer cells, either by killing the cells or by stopping them from dividing. When chemotherapy is taken by mouth or injected into a vein or muscle, the drugs enter the bloodstream and can reach cancer cells throughout the body (systemic chemotherapy). When chemotherapy is placed directly into the cerebrospinal fluid, an organ, or a body cavity such as the abdomen, the drugs mainly affect cancer cells in those areas (regional chemotherapy). Combination chemotherapy is treatment using more than one anticancer drug. The way the chemotherapy is given depends on the type and stage of the cancer being treated.

Radiation Therapy

Radiation therapy is a cancer treatment that uses high-energy X-rays or other types of radiation to kill cancer cells or keep them from growing. There are two types of radiation therapy:

- External radiation therapy uses a machine outside the body to send radiation toward the cancer.

- Internal radiation therapy uses a radioactive substance sealed in needles, seeds, wires, or catheters that are placed directly into or near the cancer.

The way the radiation therapy is given depends on the type and stage of the cancer being treated. External radiation therapy is used to treat OGCTs.

New types of treatment are being tested in clinical trials.

High-Dose Chemotherapy with Bone Marrow Transplant

It is a method of giving very high doses of chemotherapy and replacing blood-forming cells destroyed by the cancer treatment. Stem cells (immature blood cells) are removed from the bone marrow of the patient or a donor and are frozen and stored. After the chemotherapy is completed, the stored stem cells are thawed and given back to the patient through an infusion. These reinfused stem cells grow into (and restore) the body's blood cells.

Section 19.3

Ovarian Epithelial Cancer

This section includes text excerpted from "Ovarian Epithelial, Fallopian Tube, and Primary Peritoneal Cancer Treatment (PDQ®)—Patient Version," National Cancer Institute (NCI), February 20, 2018.

Ovarian epithelial cancer, fallopian tube cancer, and primary peritoneal cancer are diseases in which malignant (cancer) cells form in the tissue covering the ovary or lining the fallopian tube or peritoneum.

The ovaries are a pair of organs in the female reproductive system. They are in the pelvis, one on each side of the uterus (the hollow, pear-shaped organ where a fetus grows). Each ovary is about the size and shape of an almond. The ovaries make eggs and female hormones (chemicals that control the way certain cells or organs work).

The fallopian tubes are a pair of long, slender tubes, one on each side of the uterus. Eggs pass from the ovaries, through the fallopian tubes, to the uterus. Cancer sometimes begins at the end of the fallopian tube near the ovary and spreads to the ovary.

The peritoneum is the tissue that lines the abdominal wall and covers organs in the abdomen. Primary peritoneal cancer is cancer that forms in the peritoneum and has not spread there from another part of the body. Cancer sometimes begins in the peritoneum and spreads to the ovary.

Ovarian epithelial cancer is one type of cancer that affects the ovary. Ovarian epithelial cancer, fallopian tube cancer, and primary peritoneal cancer form in the same type of tissue and are treated the same way.

Women who have a family history of ovarian cancer are at an increased risk of ovarian cancer. Anything that increases your risk of getting a disease is called a risk factor. Having a risk factor does not mean that you will get cancer; not having risk factors doesn't mean that you will not get cancer. Talk with your doctor if you think you may be at risk.

Women who have one first-degree relative (mother, daughter, or sister) with a history of ovarian cancer have an increased risk of ovarian cancer. This risk is higher in women who have one first-degree relative and one second-degree relative (grandmother or aunt) with a history of ovarian cancer. This risk is even higher in women who have two or more first-degree relatives with a history of ovarian cancer.

Some ovarian, fallopian tube, and primary peritoneal cancers are caused by inherited gene mutations (changes). The genes in cells carry the hereditary information that is received from a person's parents. Hereditary ovarian cancer makes up about 20 percent of all cases of ovarian cancer. There are three hereditary patterns: ovarian cancer alone, ovarian and breast cancers, and ovarian and colon cancers.

Fallopian tube cancer and peritoneal cancer may also be caused by certain inherited gene mutations. There are tests that can detect gene mutations. These genetic tests are sometimes done for members of families with a high risk of cancer.

Women with an increased risk of ovarian cancer may consider surgery to lessen the risk. Some women who have an increased risk of ovarian cancer may choose to have a risk-reducing oophorectomy (the removal of healthy ovaries so that cancer cannot grow in them). In high-risk women, this procedure has been shown to greatly decrease the risk of ovarian cancer.

Signs and Symptoms of Ovarian, Fallopian Tube, or Peritoneal Cancer

Signs and symptoms of ovarian, fallopian tube, or peritoneal cancer include pain or swelling in the abdomen. Ovarian, fallopian tube, or peritoneal cancer may not cause early signs or symptoms. When signs or symptoms do appear, the cancer is often advanced. Signs and symptoms may include the following:

- Pain, swelling, or a feeling of pressure in the abdomen or pelvis
- Vaginal bleeding that is heavy or irregular, especially after menopause
- Vaginal discharge that is clear, white, or colored with blood
- A lump in the pelvic area
- Gastrointestinal problems, such as gas, bloating, or constipation

These signs and symptoms also may be caused by other conditions and not by ovarian, fallopian tube, or peritoneal cancer. If the signs or symptoms get worse or do not go away on their own, check with your doctor so that any problem can be diagnosed and treated as early as possible.

Diagnosing Ovarian, Fallopian Tube, or Peritoneal Cancer

Tests that examine the ovaries and pelvic area are used to detect (find), diagnose, and stage ovarian, fallopian tube, and peritoneal cancer. The following tests and procedures may be used to detect, diagnose, and stage ovarian, fallopian tube, and peritoneal cancer:

- **Physical exam and history:** An exam of the body to check general signs of health, including checking for signs of disease, such as lumps or anything else that seems unusual. A history of the patient's health habits and past illnesses and treatments will also be taken.

- **Pelvic exam:** An exam of the vagina, cervix, uterus, fallopian tubes, ovaries, and rectum. A speculum is inserted into the vagina and the doctor or nurse looks at the vagina and cervix for signs of disease. A Pap test of the cervix is usually done. The doctor or nurse also inserts one or two lubricated, gloved fingers of one hand into the vagina and places the other hand over the lower abdomen to feel the size, shape, and position of the uterus and ovaries. The doctor or nurse also inserts a lubricated, gloved finger into the rectum to feel for lumps or abnormal areas.

- **CA 125 (cancer antigen 125) assay:** A test that measures the level of CA 125 in the blood. CA 125 is a substance released by cells into the bloodstream. An increased CA 125 level can be a sign of cancer or another condition such as endometriosis.

- **Ultrasound exam:** A procedure in which high-energy sound waves (ultrasound) are bounced off internal tissues or organs in the abdomen, and make echoes. The echoes form a picture of body tissues called a sonogram. The picture can be printed to be looked at later.

Some patients may have a transvaginal ultrasound.

- **Computerized axial tomography (CAT) or computed tomography (CT) scan:** A procedure that makes a series of detailed pictures of areas inside the body, taken from different angles. The pictures are made by a computer linked to an X-ray machine. A dye may be injected into a vein or swallowed to help the organs or tissues show up more clearly. This procedure is also called computed tomography, computerized tomography, or computerized axial tomography.

- **Positron emission tomography (PET) scan:** A procedure to find malignant tumor cells in the body. A very small amount of radioactive glucose (sugar) is injected into a vein. The PET scanner rotates around the body and makes a picture of where glucose is being used in the body. Malignant tumor cells show up brighter in the picture because they are more active and take up more glucose than normal cells do.

- **Magnetic resonance imaging (MRI):** A procedure that uses a magnet, radio waves, and a computer to make a series of detailed pictures of areas inside the body. This procedure is also called nuclear magnetic resonance imaging (NMRI).

- **Chest X-ray:** An X-ray of the organs and bones inside the chest. An X-ray is a type of energy beam that can go through the body and onto film, making a picture of areas inside the body.

- **Biopsy:** The removal of cells or tissues so they can be viewed under a microscope by a pathologist to check for signs of cancer. The tissue is usually removed during surgery to remove the tumor.

Stages of Ovarian Epithelial, Fallopian Tube, and Primary Peritoneal Cancer

The following stages are used for ovarian epithelial, fallopian tube, and primary peritoneal cancer:

Stage I

In stage I, cancer is found in one or both ovaries or fallopian tubes. Stage I is divided into stage IA, stage IB, and stage IC.

- **Stage IA:** Cancer is found inside a single ovary or fallopian tube.

- **Stage IB:** Cancer is found inside both ovaries or fallopian tubes.

- **Stage IC:** Cancer is found inside one or both ovaries or fallopian tubes and one of the following is true:

  - Cancer is also found on the outside surface of one or both ovaries or fallopian tubes.

  - The capsule (outer covering) of the ovary ruptured (broke open) before or during surgery.

  - Cancer cells are found in the fluid of the peritoneal cavity (the body cavity that contains most of the organs in the abdomen) or in washings of the peritoneum (tissue lining the peritoneal cavity).

Stage II

In stage II, cancer is found in one or both ovaries or fallopian tubes and has spread into other areas of the pelvis, or primary peritoneal cancer is found within the pelvis. Stage II ovarian epithelial and fallopian tube cancers are divided into stage IIA and stage IIB.

- **Stage IIA:** Cancer has spread from where it first formed to the uterus and/or the fallopian tubes and/or the ovaries.

- **Stage IIB:** Cancer has spread from the ovary or fallopian tube to organs in the peritoneal cavity (the space that contains the abdominal organs).

Stage III

In stage III, cancer is found in one or both ovaries or fallopian tubes, or is primary peritoneal cancer, and has spread outside the pelvis to other parts of the abdomen and/or to nearby lymph nodes. Stage III is divided into stage IIIA, stage IIIB, and stage IIIC.

- **Stage IIIA:** In stage IIIA, one of the following is true:
  - Cancer has spread to lymph nodes in the area outside or behind the peritoneum only.
  - Cancer cells that can be seen only with a microscope have spread to the surface of the peritoneum outside the pelvis. Cancer may have spread to nearby lymph nodes.
- **Stage IIIB:** Cancer has spread to the peritoneum outside the pelvis and the cancer in the peritoneum is 2 centimeters or smaller. Cancer may have spread to lymph nodes behind the peritoneum.
- **Stage IIIC:** Cancer has spread to the peritoneum outside the pelvis and the cancer in the peritoneum is larger than 2 centimeters. Cancer may have spread to lymph nodes behind the peritoneum or to the surface of the liver or spleen.

Stage IV

In stage IV, cancer has spread beyond the abdomen to other parts of the body. Stage IV is divided into stage IVA and stage IVB.

- **Stage IVA:** Cancer cells are found in the extra fluid that builds up around the lungs.
- **Stage IVB:** Cancer has spread to organs and tissues outside the abdomen, including lymph nodes in the groin.

Treatment Option Overview

There are different types of treatment for patients with ovarian epithelial cancer. Some treatments are standard, and some are being tested in clinical trials. A treatment clinical trial is a research study meant to help improve current treatments or obtain information on new treatments for patients with cancer. When clinical trials show that a new treatment is better than the treatment currently used as standard treatment, the new treatment may become the standard treatment. Patients with any stage of ovarian cancer may want to think about taking part in a clinical trial. Some clinical trials are open only to patients who have not started treatment.

Three kinds of standard treatment are used:

Surgery

Most patients have surgery to remove as much of the tumor as possible. Different types of surgery may include:

- **Hysterectomy:** Surgery to remove the uterus and, sometimes, the cervix. When only the uterus is removed, it is called a partial hysterectomy. When both the uterus and the cervix are removed, it is called a total hysterectomy. If the uterus and cervix are taken out through the vagina, the operation is called a vaginal hysterectomy. If the uterus and cervix are taken out through a large incision (cut) in the abdomen, the operation is called a total abdominal hysterectomy. If the uterus and cervix are taken out through a small incision (cut) in the abdomen using a laparoscope, the operation is called a total laparoscopic hysterectomy

- **Unilateral salpingo-oophorectomy:** A surgical procedure to remove one ovary and one fallopian tube.

- **Bilateral salpingo-oophorectomy (BSO):** A surgical procedure to remove both ovaries and both fallopian tubes.

- **Omentectomy:** A surgical procedure to remove the omentum (tissue in the peritoneum that contains blood vessels, nerves, lymph vessels, and lymph nodes).

- **Lymph node biopsy:** The removal of all or part of a lymph node. A pathologist views the tissue under a microscope to look for cancer cells.

Chemotherapy

Chemotherapy is a cancer treatment that uses drugs to stop the growth of cancer cells, either by killing the cells or by stopping them from dividing. When chemotherapy is taken by mouth or injected into a vein or muscle, the drugs enter the bloodstream and can reach cancer cells throughout the body (systemic chemotherapy). When chemotherapy is placed directly into the cerebrospinal fluid, an organ, or a body cavity such as the abdomen, the drugs mainly affect cancer cells in those areas (regional chemotherapy).

A type of regional chemotherapy used to treat ovarian cancer is intraperitoneal (IP) chemotherapy. In IP chemotherapy, the anticancer drugs are carried directly into the peritoneal cavity (the space that contains the abdominal organs) through a thin tube. Treatment with more than one anticancer drug is called combination chemotherapy. The way the chemotherapy is given depends on the type and stage of the cancer being treated.

Targeted Therapy

Targeted therapy is a type of treatment that uses drugs or other substances to identify and attack specific cancer cells without harming normal cells. Monoclonal antibody therapy is a type of targeted therapy that uses antibodies made in the laboratory, from a single type of immune system cell. These antibodies can identify substances on cancer cells or normal substances that may help cancer cells grow. The antibodies attach to the substances and kill the cancer cells, block their growth, or keep them from spreading. Monoclonal antibodies are given by infusion. They may be used alone or to carry drugs, toxins, or radioactive material directly to cancer cells.

Bevacizumab is a monoclonal antibody that may be used with chemotherapy to treat ovarian epithelial cancer, fallopian tube cancer, or primary peritoneal cancer that has recurred (come back). Poly (ADP-ribose) polymerase inhibitors (PARP inhibitors) are targeted therapy drugs that block deoxyribonucleic acid (DNA) repair and may cause cancer cells to die. Olaparib, rucaparib, and niraparib are PARP inhibitors that may be used to treat advanced ovarian cancer. Veliparib is a PARP inhibitor that is being studied to treat advanced ovarian cancer.

Angiogenesis inhibitors are targeted therapy drugs that may prevent the growth of new blood vessels that tumors need to grow and may kill cancer cells. Cediranib is an angiogenesis inhibitor being studied in the treatment of recurrent ovarian cancer. New types of treatment are being tested in clinical trials.

Radiation Therapy

Radiation therapy is a cancer treatment that uses high-energy X-rays or other types of radiation to kill cancer cells or keep them from growing. Some women receive a treatment called intraperitoneal radiation therapy, in which radioactive liquid is put directly in the abdomen through a catheter. Intraperitoneal radiation therapy is being studied to treat advanced ovarian cancer.

Immunotherapy

Immunotherapy is a treatment that uses the patient's immune system to fight cancer. Substances made by the body or made in a laboratory are used to boost, direct, or restore the body's natural defenses against cancer. This type of cancer treatment is also called biotherapy or immunotherapy. Vaccine therapy uses a substance to stimulate the immune system to destroy a tumor. Vaccine therapy is being studied to treat advanced ovarian cancer. Patients may want to think about taking part in a clinical trial. For some patients, taking part in a clinical trial may be the best treatment choice. Clinical trials are part of the cancer research process. Clinical trials are done to find out if new cancer treatments are safe and effective or better than the standard treatment.

Section 19.4

Ovarian Low Malignant Potential Tumors

This section includes text excerpted from "Ovarian Low Malignant Potential Tumors Treatment (PDQ®)—Patient Version," National Cancer Institute (NCI), February 2, 2018.

Ovarian low malignant potential tumor is a disease in which abnormal cells form in the tissue covering the ovary. Ovarian low malignant potential tumors have abnormal cells that may become cancer, but usually do not. This disease usually remains in the ovary. When disease is found in one ovary, the other ovary should also be checked carefully for signs of disease.

The ovaries are a pair of organs in the female reproductive system. They are in the pelvis, one on each side of the uterus (the hollow, pear-shaped organ where a fetus grows). Each ovary is about the size and shape of an almond. The ovaries make eggs and female hormones.

Signs and Symptoms of Ovarian Low Malignant Potential Tumor

Signs and symptoms of ovarian low malignant potential tumor include pain or swelling in the abdomen. Ovarian low malignant potential tumor may not cause early signs or symptoms. If you do have signs or symptoms, they may include the following:

- Pain or swelling in the abdomen

- Pain in the pelvis

- Gastrointestinal problems, such as gas, bloating, or constipation

These signs and symptoms may be caused by other conditions. If they get worse or do not go away on their own, check with your doctor. Tests that examine the ovaries are used to detect (find), diagnose, and stage ovarian low malignant potential tumor.

The following tests and procedures may be used:

- **Physical exam and history:** An exam of the body to check general signs of health, including checking for signs of disease, such as lumps or anything else that seems unusual. A history of the patient's health habits and past illnesses and treatments will also be taken.

- **Pelvic exam:** An exam of the vagina, cervix, uterus, fallopian tubes, ovaries, and rectum. A speculum is inserted into the vagina and the doctor or nurse looks at the vagina and cervix for signs of disease. A Pap test of the cervix is usually done. The doctor or nurse also inserts one or two lubricated, gloved fingers of one hand into the vagina and places the other hand over the lower abdomen to feel the size, shape, and position of the uterus and ovaries. The doctor or nurse also inserts a lubricated, gloved finger into the rectum to feel for lumps or abnormal areas.

- **Ultrasound exam:** A procedure in which high-energy sound waves (ultrasound) are bounced off internal tissues or organs and make echoes. The echoes form a picture of body tissues called a sonogram. The picture can be printed to be looked at later.

Other patients may have a transvaginal ultrasound.

- **Computerized axial tomography (CAT) or computed tomography (CT) scan:** A procedure that makes a series of detailed pictures of areas inside the body, taken from different angles. The pictures are made by a computer linked to an X-ray machine. A dye may be injected into a vein or swallowed to help the organs or tissues show up more clearly. This procedure is also called computed tomography, computerized tomography, or computerized axial tomography.

- **CA 125 (cancer antigen 125) assay:** A test that measures the level of CA 125 in the blood. CA 125 is a substance released by cells into the bloodstream. An increased CA 125 level is sometimes a sign of cancer or other condition.

- **Chest X-ray:** An X-ray of the organs and bones inside the chest. An X-ray is a type of energy beam that can go through the body and onto film, making a picture of areas inside the body.

- **Biopsy:** The removal of cells or tissues so they can be viewed under a microscope by a pathologist to check for signs of cancer. The tissue is usually removed during surgery to remove the tumor.

Stages of Ovarian Low Malignant Potential Tumors

After ovarian low malignant potential tumor has been diagnosed, tests are done to find out if abnormal cells have spread within the ovary or to other parts of the body.

The process used to find out whether abnormal cells have spread within the ovary or to other parts of the body is called staging. The information gathered from the staging process determines the stage of the disease. It is important to know the stage in order to plan treatment. Certain tests or procedures are used for staging. Staging laparotomy (a surgical incision made in the wall of the abdomen to remove ovarian tissue) may be used. Most patients are diagnosed with stage I disease.

The following stages are used for ovarian low malignant potential tumor:

Stage I

In stage I, the tumor is found in one or both ovaries. Stage I is divided into stage IA, stage IB, and stage IC.

- **Stage IA:** The tumor is found inside a single ovary.

- **Stage IB:** The tumor is found inside both ovaries.

- **Stage IC:** The tumor is found inside one or both ovaries and one of the following is true:

  - Tumor cells are found on the outside surface of one or both ovaries.

  - The capsule (outer covering) of the ovary has ruptured (broken open).

- Tumor cells are found in the fluid of the peritoneal cavity (the body cavity that contains most of the organs in the abdomen) or in washings of the peritoneum.

Stage II

In stage II, the tumor is found in one or both ovaries and has spread into other areas of the pelvis. Stage II is divided into stage IIA, stage IIB, and stage IIC.

- **Stage IIA:** The tumor has spread to the uterus and/or fallopian tubes (the long slender tubes through which eggs pass from the ovaries to the uterus).

- **Stage IIB:** The tumor has spread to other tissue within the pelvis.

- **Stage IIC:** The tumor is found inside one or both ovaries and has spread to the uterus and/or fallopian tubes, or to other tissue within the pelvis. Also, one of the following is true:

  - Tumor cells are found on the outside surface of one or both ovaries.

  - The capsule (outer covering) of the ovary has ruptured (broken open).

  - Tumor cells are found in the fluid of the peritoneal cavity (the body cavity that contains most of the organs in the abdomen) or in washings of the peritoneum (tissue lining the peritoneal cavity).

Stage III

In stage III, the tumor is found in one or both ovaries and has spread outside the pelvis to other parts of the abdomen and/or nearby lymph nodes. Stage III is divided into stage IIIA, stage IIIB, and stage IIIC.

- **Stage IIIA:** The tumor is found in the pelvis only, but tumor cells that can be seen only with a microscope have spread to the surface of the peritoneum (tissue that lines the abdominal wall and covers most of the organs in the abdomen), the small intestines, or the tissue that connects the small intestines to the wall of the abdomen.

- **Stage IIIB:** The tumor has spread to the peritoneum and the tumor in the peritoneum is 2 centimeters or smaller.

- **Stage IIIC:** The tumor has spread to the peritoneum and the tumor in the peritoneum is larger than 2 centimeters and/or has spread to lymph nodes in the abdomen.

The spread of tumor cells to the surface of the liver is also considered stage III disease.

Stage IV

In stage IV, tumor cells have spread beyond the abdomen to other parts of the body, such as the lungs or tissue inside the liver. Tumor cells in the fluid around the lungs is also considered stage IV disease. Ovarian low malignant potential tumors almost never reach stage IV.

Treatment Option Overview

There are different types of treatment for patients with ovarian low malignant potential tumor. Different types of treatment are available for patients with ovarian low malignant potential tumor. Some treatments are standard (the currently used treatment), and some are being tested in clinical trials. A treatment clinical trial is a research study meant to help improve current treatments or obtain information on new treatments for patients with cancer, tumors, and related conditions. When clinical trials show that a new treatment is better than the standard treatment, the new treatment may become the standard treatment. Patients may want to think about taking part in a clinical trial. Some clinical trials are open only to patients who have not started treatment

Two types of standard treatment are used:

Surgery

The type of surgery (removing the tumor in an operation) depends on the size and spread of the tumor and the woman's plans for having children. Surgery may include the following:

- **Unilateral salpingo-oophorectomy:** Surgery to remove one ovary and one fallopian tube.

- **Bilateral salpingo-oophorectomy (BSO):** Surgery to remove both ovaries and both fallopian tubes.

- **Total hysterectomy and BSO:** Surgery to remove the uterus, cervix, and both ovaries and fallopian tubes. If the uterus and cervix are taken out through the vagina, the operation is called a vaginal hysterectomy. If the uterus and cervix are taken out through a large incision (cut) in the abdomen, the operation is called a total abdominal hysterectomy. If the uterus and cervix are taken out through a small incision (cut) in the abdomen using a laparoscope, the operation is called a total laparoscopic hysterectomy.

- **Partial oophorectomy:** Surgery to remove part of one ovary or part of both ovaries.

- **Omentectomy:** Surgery to remove the omentum (a piece of the tissue lining the abdominal wall).

Even if the doctor removes all disease that can be seen at the time of the operation, the patient may be given chemotherapy after surgery to kill any tumor cells that are left. Treatment given after the surgery, to lower the risk that the tumor will come back, is called adjuvant therapy.

Chemotherapy

Chemotherapy is a cancer treatment that uses drugs to stop the growth of cancer cells, either by killing the cells or by stopping them from dividing. When chemotherapy is taken by mouth or injected into a vein or muscle, the drugs enter the bloodstream and can reach cancer cells throughout the body (systemic chemotherapy). When chemotherapy is placed directly into the cerebrospinal fluid, an organ, or a body cavity such as the abdomen, the drugs mainly affect cancer cells in those areas (regional chemotherapy). The way the chemotherapy is given depends on the type and stage of the cancer being treated.

New types of treatment are being tested in clinical trials. Treatment for ovarian low malignant potential tumors may cause side effects.

Patients may want to think about taking part in a clinical trial. For some patients, taking part in a clinical trial may be the best treatment choice. Clinical trials are part of the medical research process. Clinical trials are done to find out if new treatments are safe and effective or better than the standard treatment.

Section 19.5

Long-Term Oral Contraceptive Use Lowers Risk for Ovarian Cancers

This section includes text excerpted from "Across Many Health Behaviors, Long-Term Oral Contraceptive Use Lowers Risk for Ovarian and Endometrial Cancers," National Cancer Institute (NCI), January 18, 2018.

Oral Contraceptive Usage

Oral contraceptives have been widely used by U.S. women for over 50 years. In addition to preventing pregnancy, these medications have been shown to either increase or decrease a woman's risk of developing certain cancers, though the reasons why are not fully understood. Notably, many questions remain around how oral contraceptive use affects cancer risk in subpopulations of women, such as smokers and overweight women. These groups are already at higher risk for many cancers, so it is especially important to understand how oral contraceptive use changes cancer risks in these women. To address this gap, Division of Cancer Epidemiology and Genetics (DCEG) researchers investigated whether the relationship between oral contraceptive use and risks for ovarian, endometrial, breast, and colorectal cancers change when looking at groups of women who have different health behaviors in the years leading up to and during menopause (for example, smoking, alcohol use, body mass index (BMI), and physical activity).

Long-Term Oral Contraceptive Use and Cancer Risk

Analyzing data from nearly 200,000 women from the National Institutes of Health (NIH)-AARP (American Association of Retired Persons) Diet and Health Study, Kara Michels, Ph.D., Britton Trabert, Ph.D., M.S., and colleagues found that long-term oral contraceptive use (10 years or longer) was associated with reduced risk for ovarian cancer regardless of other health behaviors in later life. Long-term oral contraceptive use also reduced risks for endometrial cancer, but this reduction was strongest for women who were current smokers, obese, or rarely exercised.

Oral contraceptive use was generally not associated with either colorectal cancer or breast cancer. Previous studies have reported that current or recent use of oral contraceptives may slightly increase breast cancer risk. However, the NIH-AARP Diet and Health Study enrolled women who were between 50 and 71 years of age, most of whom were neither current nor recent users of oral contraceptives.

In the future, these findings should be replicated in other populations, particularly among a more diverse group of women. Research to evaluate risks among users of contemporary oral contraceptive medications is also needed. The medications prescribed today are different from those available between the 1960s and 1980s, when most of the study participants would have taken them. The authors note that the results of this analysis indicate that oral contraceptive use may be beneficial for cancer prevention for a range of women with different underlying cancer risk.

Section 19.6

Ovarian Epithelial Tumors Traced to Fallopian Tubes

This section includes text excerpted from "Many Ovarian Cancers May Start in Fallopian Tubes, Study Finds," National Cancer Institute (NCI), November 15, 2017.

Findings from a study provide additional evidence that the most common type of ovarian cancer may originate in the fallopian tubes. Researchers also found that there is a window of several years between the development of abnormal cells, or lesions, in the fallopian tubes and the start of ovarian cancer. The findings "have significant implications for the prevention, early detection, and therapeutic intervention of this disease," the study investigators wrote.

In the study, published October 23 in *Nature Communications*, researchers at the Johns Hopkins Kimmel Cancer Center and Dana–Farber Cancer Institute analyzed multiple tumor samples from nine patients with high-grade serous ovarian carcinomas (HGSOC), the subtype that accounts for approximately 75 percent of ovarian cancers.

The researchers found that most of the genetic alterations seen in ovarian tumors in these patients were present in lesions that had formed years earlier in their fallopian tubes. This finding is important, they wrote, because it could potentially help to enable earlier detection of the disease. Currently, about 70 percent of women with HGSOC are diagnosed with advanced stage disease.

Tracing the Origins of HGSOC

Studies conducted more than a decade ago provided evidence that HGSOCs may not arise from cells of the ovary. Instead, the studies suggested that lesions found in the fallopian tubes, called serous tubal intraepithelial carcinomas (STICs), might be precursors for most HGSOCs, said Christina Annunziata, M.D., Ph.D., clinical director of the Women's Malignancies Branch of National Cancer Institute's (NCI) Center for Cancer Research. Those earlier studies identified STIC lesions in women with *BRCA1* or *BRCA2* mutations who had had prophylactic surgery to remove their fallopian tubes and ovaries to reduce their cancer risk, suggesting that the lesions could be precursors to ovarian cancer.

The study, along with findings from another molecular analysis of STICs published in the same issue of the journal, provide additional evidence that HGSOCs originate from these fallopian tube lesions, Dr. Annunziata said, regardless of whether women have *BRCA* mutations. "We now have a molecular basis to support the original finding," she explained. "It's very exciting."

In the first study, researchers used genomic sequencing to profile all the expressed genes in the genomes of tissue samples from five women with HGSOC who also had STIC lesions and fallopian tube cancer. They also analyzed STIC lesions from four additional patients, three of whom had undergone prophylactic surgery to remove their fallopian tubes and ovaries because of *BRCA* mutations. The fourth patient had fallopian tubes and ovaries removed as well as a hysterectomy because of a pelvic mass.

Using a mathematical model, the researchers then estimated that the average time between the development of the STIC lesions and ovarian cancer was 6.5 years. They found that while the lesions were slower to develop, "in patients with metastatic lesions, the time between the initiation of the ovarian carcinoma and development of metastases appears to have been rapid (average 2 years)," they wrote. This may explain why most cases of HGSOC are in advanced stages at diagnosis and has implications for early detection of the disease, the researchers wrote.

Impact on Ovarian Cancer Prevention

Although the study findings are relevant for the most common type of ovarian cancer, high-grade serous cancers, Dr. Annunziata commented, "(it's important to note that) around 30 percent of ovarian cancers might not originate in the fallopian tubes." Ovarian cancer subtypes other than HGSOC, such as low-grade serous cancers and endometrial cancers, are believed to arise from cells of the ovary itself, "but we don't have these types of extensive molecular analyses to prove that," she said.

This study was also based on a small sample size, the research team acknowledged.

But "if studies in larger groups of women confirm our finding that the fallopian tubes are the site of origin of most ovarian cancer, then this could result in a major change in the way we manage this disease for patients at risk," said lead author Victor Velculescu, M.D., Ph.D., Co-director of Cancer Biology at Johns Hopkins University School of Medicine (JHUSOM), in a press release.

Dr. Annunziata agreed that further studies need to be done to better understand the studies' implications. For example, clinical trials could be done to determine whether removing the fallopian tubes, and not the ovaries, in women who are at high risk for HGSOC is sufficient to reduce their risk of the disease, she said. Removing ovaries causes surgical menopause, which can greatly affect quality of life. Research has also shown that preservation of ovaries provides long-term health benefits by lowering the risk of heart disease and other illnesses.

Trials in the United States and the Netherlands are currently underway to see if removing fallopian tubes and delaying the removal of ovaries should be considered in women with *BRCA* mutations who are at high risk of developing ovarian cancer. The study authors wrote that their findings have implications for women who are not carriers of *BRCA* mutations as well. In fact, other trials are looking at the safety and feasibility of removing fallopian tubes during other gynecologic surgeries, such as hysterectomy, to prevent ovarian cancer in women who are or are not at high risk of developing it.

Section 19.7

Rucaparib Approved as Maintenance Treatment for Some Recurrent Ovarian Cancers

This section includes text excerpted from "Rucaparib Approved as
Maintenance Treatment for Some Recurrent Ovarian Cancers,"
National Cancer Institute (NCI), May 4, 2018.

The U.S. Food and Drug Administration (FDA) has expanded the
approval of the targeted therapy rucaparib (Rubraca) for the treatment
of women with ovarian cancer.

The approval covers the use of rucaparib as a follow-on, or maintenance, treatment for women whose ovarian cancer has returned
after their initial treatment and whose tumors then shrank, at least
partially, during subsequent treatment with a platinum-based chemotherapy. The approval, announced on April 6, also includes women
with fallopian tube or primary peritoneal cancer.

Rucaparib is a type of drug called a poly (ADP-ribose) polymerase
(PARP) inhibitor, which prevents cells from repairing damage to their
deoxyribonucleic acid (DNA). Rucaparib joins olaparib (Lynparza)
and niraparib (Zejula) as the third PARP inhibitor to be approved
as a maintenance therapy for women with recurrent ovarian, fallopian tube, or primary peritoneal cancers that still respond to platinum-based chemotherapies.

What makes the rucaparib approval novel, explained Elise Kohn,
M.D., head of Gynecologic Cancer Therapeutics in National Cancer
Institute's (NCI) Division of Cancer Treatment and Diagnosis (DCTD),
is that it includes the approval of the first companion diagnostic test
measuring possible indicators of PARP sensitivity. The test, called
FoundationFocus CDxBRCA LOH, can help predict which tumors
might be most likely to respond to the treatment.

Under the approval, rucaparib may be prescribed without this test.
However, Dr. Kohn explained, results from it—or from other tests
like it under development—may help patients and their doctors make
decisions about if and what type of maintenance therapy might make

the most sense, also taking into account individual health issues and treatment goals, added Dr. Kohn.

Disrupting DNA Repair in Cancer Cells

Most cells have many molecular mechanisms for repairing DNA, and PARP proteins are part of just one of these mechanisms. That means that drugs like rucaparib, which work by blocking the activity of PARP proteins, are most effective in cancer cells that already have damage to other DNA repair mechanisms, explained Robert Coleman, M.D., of the University of Texas MD Anderson Cancer Center.

Earlier clinical trials of PARP inhibitors found that they worked best in patients with mutations in the *BRCA1* and *BRCA2* genes, both of which play important roles in DNA repair.

However, ongoing research has suggested that PARP inhibitors may also work in tumors with other types of DNA repair defects, including a broad category of defects called homologous recombination deficiency (HRD). The companion diagnostic test approved with rucaparib tests tumors for *BRCA* gene mutations and for HRD.

Less Repair, More Benefit

In the phase 3 randomized trial, called ARIEL3, that led to the new approval for rucaparib, researchers led by Dr. Coleman enrolled 564 women with recurrent ovarian, fallopian tube, or primary peritoneal cancer. ARIEL 3 was funded by Clovis Oncology, Inc., the manufacturer of rucaparib.

All the women in the trial were responding, either completely or partially, to platinum-based chemotherapy. After testing participants' tumors with the companion diagnostic test, the researchers randomly assigned 375 to receive rucaparib, which is given daily as a pill, and 189 to receive a placebo. Women continued treatment until their cancer progressed, they died, or they chose to discontinue treatment because of side effects or other reasons.

Overall, the women who received rucaparib had a longer time before their disease progressed (progression-free survival) than women in the placebo group: 10.8 months, compared with 5.4 months. The benefit of rucaparib was stronger in patients with DNA repair defects, as measured by the companion diagnostic test. Women with HRD tumors but no germline (inherited) *BRCA* mutation who received rucaparib lived for a median of 13.6 months without disease progression. Women with germline *BRCA* mutations treated with rucaparib had a median progression-free survival of 16.6 months.

Serious side effects were more common in the women receiving rucaparib, including anemia, nausea, and headache. These side effects are common in women treated with any of the PARP inhibitors, explained Dr. Kohn. Two patients in the rucaparib group died because of secondary cancers related to treatment, compared with none in the placebo group.

The ARIEL3 researchers are continuing to follow trial participants over time to see whether treatment with rucaparib improves how long women live overall (overall survival).

Future Paths for PARP Inhibition

As clinicians become more comfortable using companion diagnostics to measure HRD and other biomarkers to gauge the potential vulnerability of a tumor to PARP inhibition, "they could end up being important decision-making tools," said Dr. Coleman.

Future trials will likely look at administering PARP maintenance therapy sooner in ovarian cancer treatment, after initial therapy (called primary maintenance), Dr. Coleman explained.

Researchers are also interested in testing PARP inhibitors as an initial, or first-line, treatment in both *BRCA*-positive and *BRCA*-negative ovarian cancers, continued Dr. Coleman.

Research in PARP inhibitors has also been expanded to include combinations with immunotherapies, such as immune checkpoint inhibitors, and with targeted therapies, like cediranib, explained Dr. Kohn. "There's a huge [effort] looking at how to leverage the activity of PARP inhibitors in combination therapies. That's the next step," she said.

Many of these trials are based on new knowledge of DNA repair mechanisms that has been gleaned from studying why some tumors are resistant to PARP inhibition, which in turn has led to the development of new drugs targeting DNA repair, she continued.

"It's a really nice circle that's been a welcome development," concluded Dr. Kohn.

Section 19.8

Aspirin Use May Reduce Ovarian Cancer Risk

This section includes text excerpted from "NIH Study Finds Regular Aspirin Use May Reduce Ovarian Cancer Risk," National Institutes of Health (NIH), February 6, 2014. Reviewed May 2018.

Women who take aspirin daily may reduce their risk of ovarian cancer by 20 percent, according to a study by scientists at the National Cancer Institute (NCI), part of the National Institutes of Health (NIH). However, further research is needed before clinical recommendations can be made.

It has been estimated that over 20,000 women in the United States had ovarian cancer in 2014, and more than 14,000 will die from the disease. Early-stage ovarian cancer may be successfully treated. However, symptoms associated with this disease can mimic more common conditions, such as digestive and bladder disorders, so for this reason and others, it is often not diagnosed until it has reached advanced stages. Late-stage ovarian cancer leaves women with limited treatment options and poor prognoses, making preventive strategies potentially important for controlling this disease.

Chronic or persistent inflammation has been shown to increase the risk of cancer and other diseases. Previous studies have suggested that the anti-inflammatory properties of aspirin and nonaspirin NSAIDs (nonsteroidal anti-inflammatory drugs), may reduce cancer risk overall. However, studies examining whether use of these agents may influence ovarian cancer risk have been largely inconclusive. This is the largest study to date to assess the relationship between these drugs and ovarian cancer risk.

Britton Trabert, Ph.D., and Nicolas Wentzensen, M.D., Ph.D., of NCI's Division of Cancer Epidemiology and Genetics (DCEG), and their colleagues, analyzed data pooled from 12 large epidemiological studies to investigate whether women who used aspirin, nonaspirin NSAIDs, or acetaminophen have a lower risk of ovarian cancer. These 12 studies (nine from the United States) were part of the Ovarian

Cancer Association Consortium (OCAC). The scientists evaluated the benefit of these drugs in nearly 8,000 women with ovarian cancer and close to 12,000 women who did not have the disease.

Among study participants who reported whether or not they used aspirin regularly: 18 percent used aspirin, 24 percent used nonaspirin NSAIDs, and 16 percent used acetaminophen. The researchers determined that participants who reported daily aspirin use had a 20 percent lower risk of ovarian cancer than those who used aspirin less than once per week. For nonaspirin NSAIDs, which include a wide variety of drugs, the picture was less clear: the scientists observed a 10 percent lower ovarian cancer risk among women who used NSAIDs at least once per week compared with those who used NSAIDs less frequently. However, this finding did not fall in a range that was significant statistically. In contrast to the findings for aspirin and NSAIDs, use of acetaminophen, which is not an anti-inflammatory agent, was not associated with reduced ovarian cancer risk.

This study adds to a growing list of malignancies, such as colorectal and other cancers, that appear to be potentially preventable by aspirin usage. "Our study suggests that aspirin regimens, proven to protect against heart attack, may reduce the risk of ovarian cancer as well. However intriguing our results are, they should not influence current clinical practice. Additional studies are needed to explore the delicate balance of risk-benefit for this potential chemopreventive agent, as well as studies to identify the mechanism by which aspirin may reduce ovarian cancer risk," said Trabert.

Adverse side effects of daily aspirin use include upper gastrointestinal bleeding and hemorrhagic stroke. Therefore, a daily aspirin regimen should only be undertaken with a doctor's approval, caution the scientists.

The NCI leads the National Cancer Program and the NIH effort to dramatically reduce cancer and improve the lives of cancer patients and their families, through research into prevention and cancer biology, the development of new interventions, and the training and mentoring of new researchers.

Chapter 20

Uterine Sarcoma Cancer

Uterine sarcoma is a disease in which malignant (cancer) cells form in the muscles of the uterus or other tissues that support the uterus. The uterus is part of the female reproductive system. The uterus is the hollow, pear-shaped organ in the pelvis, where a fetus grows. The cervix is at the lower, narrow end of the uterus, and leads to the vagina. Uterine sarcoma is a very rare kind of cancer that forms in the uterine muscles or in tissues that support the uterus. Uterine sarcoma is different from cancer of the endometrium, a disease in which cancer cells start growing inside the lining of the uterus.

Risk Factors for Uterine Sarcoma

Being exposed to X-rays can increase the risk of uterine sarcoma. Anything that increases your risk of getting a disease is called a risk factor. Having a risk factor does not mean that you will get cancer; not having risk factors doesn't mean that you will not get cancer. Talk with your doctor if you think you may be at risk. Risk factors for uterine sarcoma include the following:

- Past treatment with radiation therapy to the pelvis

- Treatment with tamoxifen for breast cancer. If you are taking this drug, have a pelvic exam every year and report any vaginal bleeding (other than menstrual bleeding) as soon as possible.

This chapter includes text excerpted from "Uterine Sarcoma Treatment (PDQ®)—Patient Version," National Cancer Institute (NCI), October 13, 2017.

Signs and Symptoms of Uterine Sarcoma

Abnormal bleeding from the vagina and other signs and symptoms may be caused by uterine sarcoma or by other conditions. Check with your doctor if you have any of the following:

- Bleeding that is not part of menstrual periods

- Bleeding after menopause

- A mass in the vagina

- Pain or a feeling of fullness in the abdomen

- Frequent urination

Diagnosing Uterine Sarcoma

The following tests and procedures may be used:

- **Physical exam and history:** An exam of the body to check general signs of health, including checking for signs of disease, such as lumps or anything else that seems unusual. A history of the patient's health habits and past illnesses and treatments will also be taken.

- **Pelvic exam:** An exam of the vagina, cervix, uterus, fallopian tubes, ovaries, and rectum. A speculum is inserted into the vagina and the doctor or nurse looks at the vagina and cervix for signs of disease. A Pap (Papanicolaou) test of the cervix is usually done. The doctor or nurse also inserts one or two lubricated, gloved fingers of one hand into the vagina and places the other hand over the lower abdomen to feel the size, shape, and position of the uterus and ovaries. The doctor or nurse also inserts a lubricated, gloved finger into the rectum to feel for lumps or abnormal areas.

- **Pap test:** A procedure to collect cells from the surface of the cervix and vagina. A piece of cotton, a brush, or a small wooden stick is used to gently scrape cells from the cervix and vagina. The cells are viewed under a microscope to find out if they are abnormal. This procedure is also called a Pap smear. Because uterine sarcoma begins inside the uterus, this cancer may not show up on the Pap test.

- **Transvaginal ultrasound exam:** A procedure used to examine the vagina, uterus, fallopian tubes, and bladder. An ultrasound transducer (probe) is inserted into the vagina and used to bounce high-energy sound waves (ultrasound) off internal tissues or organs and make echoes. The echoes form a picture of body tissues called a sonogram. The doctor can identify tumors by looking at the sonogram.

- **Dilatation and curettage (D&C):** A procedure to remove samples of tissue from the inner lining of the uterus. The cervix is dilated and a curette (spoon-shaped instrument) is inserted into the uterus to remove tissue. The tissue samples are checked under a microscope for signs of disease. This procedure is also called a D&C.

- **Endometrial biopsy:** The removal of tissue from the endometrium (inner lining of the uterus) by inserting a thin, flexible tube through the cervix and into the uterus. The tube is used to gently scrape a small amount of tissue from the endometrium and then remove the tissue samples. A pathologist views the tissue under a microscope to look for cancer cells.

Stages of Uterine Sarcoma

After uterine sarcoma has been diagnosed, tests are done to find out if cancer cells have spread within the uterus or to other parts of the body. The process used to find out if cancer has spread within the uterus or to other parts of the body is called staging. The information gathered from the staging process determines the stage of the disease. It is important to know the stage in order to plan treatment. The following procedures may be used in the staging process:

- **Blood chemistry studies:** A procedure in which a blood sample is checked to measure the amounts of certain substances released into the blood by organs and tissues in the body. An unusual (higher or lower than normal) amount of a substance can be a sign of disease.

- **CA 125 (cancer antigen 125) assay:** A test that measures the level of CA 125 in the blood. CA 125 is a substance released by cells into the bloodstream. An increased CA 125 level is sometimes a sign of cancer or other condition.

- **Chest X-ray:** An X-ray of the organs and bones inside the chest. An X-ray is a type of energy beam that can go through the body and onto film, making a picture of areas inside the body.

- **Transvaginal ultrasound exam:** A procedure used to examine the vagina, uterus, fallopian tubes, and bladder. An ultrasound transducer (probe) is inserted into the vagina and used to bounce high-energy sound waves (ultrasound) off internal tissues or organs and make echoes. The echoes form a picture of body tissues called a sonogram. The doctor can identify tumors by looking at the sonogram.

- **Computerized axial tomography (CAT) or computed tomography (CT) scan:** A procedure that makes a series of detailed pictures of areas inside the body, such as the abdomen and pelvis, taken from different angles. The pictures are made by a computer linked to an X-ray machine. A dye may be injected into a vein or swallowed to help the organs or tissues to show up more clearly. This procedure is also called computed tomography, computerized tomography, or computerized axial tomography.

- **Cystoscopy:** A procedure to look inside the bladder and urethra to check for abnormal areas. A cystoscope is inserted through the urethra into the bladder. A cystoscope is a thin, tube-like instrument with a light and a lens for viewing. It may also have a tool to remove tissue samples, which are checked under a microscope for signs of cancer.

Uterine sarcoma may be diagnosed, staged, and treated in the same surgery. Surgery is used to diagnose, stage, and treat uterine sarcoma. During this surgery, the doctor removes as much of the cancer as possible. The following procedures may be used to diagnose, stage, and treat uterine sarcoma:

- **Laparotomy:** A surgical procedure in which an incision (cut) is made in the wall of the abdomen to check the inside of the abdomen for signs of disease. The size of the incision depends on the reason the laparotomy is being done. Sometimes organs are removed or tissue samples are taken and checked under a microscope for signs of disease.

- **Abdominal and pelvic washings:** A procedure in which a saline solution is placed into the abdominal and pelvic body cavities. After a short time, the fluid is removed and viewed under a microscope to check for cancer cells.

- **Total abdominal hysterectomy:** A surgical procedure to remove the uterus and cervix through a large incision (cut) in the abdomen.

- **Bilateral salpingo-oophorectomy (BSO):** Surgery to remove both ovaries and both fallopian tubes.

- **Lymphadenectomy:** A surgical procedure in which lymph nodes are removed and checked under a microscope for signs of cancer. For a regional lymphadenectomy, some of the lymph nodes in the tumor area are removed. For a radical lymphadenectomy, most or all of the lymph nodes in the tumor area are removed. This procedure is also called lymph node dissection.

Stage I

In stage I, cancer is found in the uterus only. Stage I is divided into stages IA and IB, based on how far the cancer has spread.

- **Stage IA:** Cancer is in the endometrium only or less than halfway through the myometrium (muscle layer of the uterus).

- **Stage IB:** Cancer has spread halfway or more into the myometrium.

Stage II

In stage II, cancer has spread into connective tissue of the cervix, but has not spread outside the uterus.

Stage III

In stage III, cancer has spread beyond the uterus and cervix, but has not spread beyond the pelvis. Stage III is divided into stages IIIA, IIIB, and IIIC, based on how far the cancer has spread within the pelvis.

- **Stage IIIA:** Cancer has spread to the outer layer of the uterus and/or to the fallopian tubes, ovaries, and ligaments of the uterus.

- **Stage IIIB:** Cancer has spread to the vagina or to the parametrium (connective tissue and fat around the uterus).

- **Stage IIIC:** Cancer has spread to lymph nodes in the pelvis and/or around the aorta (largest artery in the body, which carries blood away from the heart).

Stage IV

In stage IV, cancer has spread beyond the pelvis. Stage IV is divided into stages IVA and IVB, based on how far the cancer has spread.

- **Stage IVA:** Cancer has spread to the bladder and/or bowel wall.

- **Stage IVB:** Cancer has spread to other parts of the body beyond the pelvis, including the abdomen and/or lymph nodes in the groin.

Treatment Option Overview

Different types of treatments are available for patients with uterine sarcoma. Some treatments are standard (the currently used treatment), and some are being tested in clinical trials. A treatment clinical trial is a research study meant to help improve current treatments or obtain information on new treatments for patients with cancer. When clinical trials show that a new treatment is better than the standard treatment, the new treatment may become the standard treatment. Patients may want to think about taking part in a clinical trial. Some clinical trials are open only to patients who have not started treatment.

Surgery

Surgery is the most common treatment for uterine sarcoma. Even if the doctor removes all the cancer that can be seen at the time of the surgery, some patients may be given chemotherapy or radiation therapy after surgery to kill any cancer cells that are left. Treatment given after the surgery, to lower the risk that the cancer will come back, is called adjuvant therapy.

Radiation Therapy

Radiation therapy is a cancer treatment that uses high energy X-rays or other types of radiation to kill cancer cells or keep them from growing. There are two types of radiation therapy:

- External radiation therapy uses a machine outside the body to send radiation toward the cancer.

- Internal radiation therapy uses a radioactive substance sealed in needles, seeds, wires, or catheters that are placed directly into or near the cancer.

The way the radiation therapy is given depends on the type and stage of the cancer being treated. External and internal radiation therapy are used to treat uterine sarcoma, and may also be used as palliative therapy to relieve symptoms and improve quality of life.

Chemotherapy

Chemotherapy is a cancer treatment that uses drugs to stop the growth of cancer cells, either by killing the cells or by stopping them from dividing. When chemotherapy is taken by mouth or injected into a vein or muscle, the drugs enter the bloodstream and can reach cancer cells throughout the body (systemic chemotherapy). When chemotherapy is placed directly into the cerebrospinal fluid (CSF), an organ, or a body cavity such as the abdomen, the drugs mainly affect cancer cells in those areas (regional chemotherapy). The way the chemotherapy is given depends on the type and stage of the cancer being treated.

Hormone Therapy

Hormone therapy is a cancer treatment that removes hormones or blocks their action and stops cancer cells from growing. Hormones are substances produced by glands in the body and circulated in the bloodstream. Some hormones can cause certain cancers to grow. If tests show the cancer cells have places where hormones can attach (receptors), drugs, surgery, or radiation therapy is used to reduce the production of hormones or block them from working.

Clinical Trial

For some patients, taking part in a clinical trial may be the best treatment choice. Clinical trials are part of the cancer research process. Clinical trials are done to find out if new cancer treatments are safe and effective or better than the standard treatment. Many of today's standard treatments for cancer are based on earlier clinical trials. Patients who take part in a clinical trial may receive the standard treatment or be among the first to receive a new treatment.

Patients who take part in clinical trials also help improve the way cancer will be treated in the future. Even when clinical trials do not lead to effective new treatments, they often answer important questions and help move research forward. Patients can enter clinical trials before, during, or after starting their cancer treatment. Some clinical trials only include patients who have not yet received treatment. Other trials test treatments for patients whose cancer has not gotten better. There are also clinical trials that test new ways to stop cancer from recurring (coming back) or reduce the side effects of cancer treatment.

Follow-Up Tests May Be Needed

Some of the tests that were done to diagnose the cancer or to find out the stage of the cancer may be repeated. Some tests will be repeated in order to see how well the treatment is working. Decisions about whether to continue, change, or stop treatment may be based on the results of these tests. Some of the tests will continue to be done from time to time after treatment has ended. The results of these tests can show if your condition has changed or if the cancer has recurred (come back). These tests are sometimes called follow-up tests or check-ups.

Chapter 21

Vaginal Cancer

Vaginal cancer is a disease in which malignant (cancer) cells form in the vagina. The vagina is the canal leading from the cervix (the opening of uterus) to the outside of the body. At birth, a baby passes out of the body through the vagina (also called the birth canal).

Vaginal cancer is not common. There are two main types of vaginal cancer:

- **Squamous cell carcinoma:** Cancer that forms in squamous cells, the thin, flat cells lining the vagina. Squamous cell vaginal cancer spreads slowly and usually stays near the vagina, but may spread to the lungs, liver, or bone. This is the most common type of vaginal cancer.

- **Adenocarcinoma:** Cancer that begins in glandular cells. Glandular cells in the lining of the vagina make and release fluids such as mucus. Adenocarcinoma is more likely than squamous cell cancer to spread to the lungs and lymph nodes. A rare type of adenocarcinoma is linked to being exposed to diethylstilbestrol (DES) before birth. Adenocarcinomas that are not linked with being exposed to DES are most common in women after menopause.

Age and being exposed to the drug DES before birth affect a woman's risk of vaginal cancer. Anything that increases your risk of getting

---

This chapter includes text excerpted from "Vaginal Cancer Treatment (PDQ®)—Patient Version," National Cancer Institute (NCI), March 9, 2018.

a disease is called a risk factor. Having a risk factor does not mean that you will get cancer; not having risk factors doesn't mean that you will not get cancer. Talk with your doctor if you think you may be at risk.

Risk Factors for Vaginal Cancer

Risk factors for vaginal cancer include the following:

- Being aged 60 or older

- Being exposed to DES while in the mother's womb. In the 1950s, the drug DES was given to some pregnant women to prevent miscarriage (premature birth of a fetus that cannot survive). Women who were exposed to DES before birth have an increased risk of vaginal cancer. Some of these women develop a rare form of vaginal cancer called clear cell adenocarcinoma.

- Having human papillomavirus (HPV) infection

- Having a history of abnormal cells in the cervix or cervical cancer

- Having a history of abnormal cells in the uterus or cancer of the uterus

- Having had a hysterectomy for health problems that affect the uterus

Signs and Symptoms of Vaginal Cancer

Vaginal cancer often does not cause early signs or symptoms. It may be found during a routine pelvic exam and Pap (Papanicolaou) test. Signs and symptoms may be caused by vaginal cancer or by other conditions. Check with your doctor if you have any of the following:

- Bleeding or discharge not related to menstrual periods

- Pain during sexual intercourse

- Pain in the pelvic area

- A lump in the vagina

- Pain when urinating

- Constipation

Diagnosing Vaginal Cancer

The following tests and procedures may be used:

- **Physical exam and history:** An exam of the body to check general signs of health, including checking for signs of disease, such as lumps or anything else that seems unusual. A history of the patient's health habits and past illnesses and treatments will also be taken.

- **Pelvic exam:** An exam of the vagina, cervix, uterus, fallopian tubes, ovaries, and rectum. A speculum is inserted into the vagina and the doctor or nurse looks at the vagina and cervix for signs of disease. A Pap test of the cervix is usually done. The doctor or nurse also inserts one or two lubricated, gloved fingers of one hand into the vagina and places the other hand over the lower abdomen to feel the size, shape, and position of the uterus and ovaries. The doctor or nurse also inserts a lubricated, gloved finger into the rectum to feel for lumps or abnormal areas.

- **Pap test:** A procedure to collect cells from the surface of the cervix and vagina. A piece of cotton, a brush, or a small wooden stick is used to gently scrape cells from the cervix and vagina. The cells are viewed under a microscope to find out if they are abnormal. This procedure is also called a Pap smear.

- **Colposcopy:** A procedure in which a colposcope (a lighted, magnifying instrument) is used to check the vagina and cervix for abnormal areas. Tissue samples may be taken using a curette (spoon-shaped instrument) or a brush and checked under a microscope for signs of disease.

- **Biopsy:** The removal of cells or tissues from the vagina and cervix so they can be viewed under a microscope by a pathologist to check for signs of cancer. If a Pap test shows abnormal cells in the vagina, a biopsy may be done during a colposcopy.

Stages of Vaginal Cancer

After vaginal cancer has been diagnosed, tests are done to find out if cancer cells have spread within the vagina or to other parts of the body. The process used to find out if cancer has spread within the vagina or to other parts of the body is called staging. The information gathered from the staging process determines the stage of the disease.

241

It is important to know the stage in order to plan treatment. The following procedures may be used in the staging process:

- **Chest X-ray:** An X-ray of the organs and bones inside the chest. An X-ray is a type of energy beam that can go through the body and onto film, making a picture of areas inside the body.

- **Computerized axial tomography (CAT) or computed tomography (CT) scan:** A procedure that makes a series of detailed pictures of areas inside the body, taken from different angles. The pictures are made by a computer linked to an X-ray machine. A dye may be injected into a vein or swallowed to help the organs or tissues show up more clearly. This procedure is also called computed tomography, computerized tomography, or computerized axial tomography.

- **Magnetic resonance imaging (MRI):** A procedure that uses a magnet, radio waves, and a computer to make a series of detailed pictures of areas inside the body. This procedure is also called nuclear magnetic resonance imaging (NMRI).

- **Positron emission tomography (PET) scan:** A procedure to find malignant tumor cells in the body. A small amount of radioactive glucose (sugar) is injected into a vein. The PET scanner rotates around the body and makes a picture of where glucose is being used in the body. Malignant tumor cells show up brighter in the picture because they are more active and take up more glucose than normal cells do.

- **Cystoscopy:** A procedure to look inside the bladder and urethra to check for abnormal areas. A cystoscope is inserted through the urethra into the bladder. A cystoscope is a thin, tube-like instrument with a light and a lens for viewing. It may also have a tool to remove tissue samples, which are checked under a microscope for signs of cancer.

- **Ureteroscopy:** A procedure to look inside the ureters to check for abnormal areas. A ureteroscope is inserted through the bladder and into the ureters. A ureteroscope is a thin, tube-like instrument with a light and a lens for viewing. It may also have a tool to remove tissue to be checked under a microscope for signs of disease. A ureteroscopy and cystoscopy may be done during the same procedure.

- **Proctoscopy:** A procedure to look inside the rectum to check for abnormal areas. A proctoscope is inserted through the rectum. A proctoscope is a thin, tube-like instrument with a light and a lens for viewing. It may also have a tool to remove tissue to be checked under a microscope for signs of disease.

- **Biopsy:** A biopsy may be done to find out if cancer has spread to the cervix. A sample of tissue is removed from the cervix and viewed under a microscope. A biopsy that removes only a small amount of tissue is usually done in the doctor's office. A cone biopsy (removal of a larger, cone-shaped piece of tissue from the cervix and cervical canal) is usually done in the hospital. A biopsy of the vulva may also be done to see if cancer has spread there.

Stage I

In stage I, cancer is found in the vaginal wall only.

Stage II

In stage II, cancer has spread through the wall of the vagina to the tissue around the vagina. Cancer has not spread to the wall of the pelvis.

Stage III

In stage III, cancer has spread to the wall of the pelvis.

Stage IV

Stage IV is divided into stage IVA and stage IVB:

- **Stage IVA:** Cancer may have spread to one or more of the following areas:
  - The lining of the bladder
  - The lining of the rectum
  - Beyond the area of the pelvis that has the bladder, uterus, ovaries, and cervix

- **Stage IVB:** Cancer has spread to parts of the body that are not near the vagina, such as the lung or bone.

Treatment Option Overview

Different types of treatments are available for patients with vaginal cancer. Some treatments are standard (the currently used treatment), and some are being tested in clinical trials. A treatment clinical trial is a research study meant to help improve current treatments or obtain information on new treatments for patients with cancer. When clinical trials show that a new treatment is better than the standard treatment, the new treatment may become the standard treatment. Patients may want to think about taking part in a clinical trial. Some clinical trials are open only to patients who have not started treatment.

Surgery

Surgery is the most common treatment of vaginal cancer. The following surgical procedures may be used:

- **Laser surgery:** A surgical procedure that uses a laser beam (a narrow beam of intense light) as a knife to make bloodless cuts in tissue or to remove a surface lesion such as a tumor.

- **Wide local excision:** A surgical procedure that takes out the cancer and some of the healthy tissue around it.

- **Vaginectomy:** A surgery to remove all or part of the vagina.

- **Total hysterectomy:** Surgery to remove the uterus, including the cervix. If the uterus and cervix are taken out through the vagina, the operation is called a vaginal hysterectomy. If the uterus and cervix are taken out through a large incision (cut) in the abdomen, the operation is called a total abdominal hysterectomy. If the uterus and cervix are taken out through a small incision in the abdomen using a laparoscope, the operation is called a total laparoscopic hysterectomy (TLH).

- **Lymph node dissection:** A surgical procedure in which lymph nodes are removed and a sample of tissue is checked under a microscope for signs of cancer. This procedure is also called lymphadenectomy. If the cancer is in the upper vagina, the pelvic lymph nodes may be removed. If the cancer is in the lower vagina, lymph nodes in the groin may be removed.

- **Pelvic exenteration:** Surgery to remove the lower colon, rectum, bladder, cervix, vagina, and ovaries. Nearby lymph nodes are also removed. Artificial openings (stoma) are made for urine and stool to flow from the body into a collection bag.

Skin grafting may follow surgery, to repair or reconstruct the vagina. Skin grafting is a surgical procedure in which skin is moved from one part of the body to another. A piece of healthy skin is taken from a part of the body that is usually hidden, such as the buttock or thigh, and used to repair or rebuild the area treated with surgery.

Even if the doctor removes all the cancer that can be seen at the time of the surgery, some patients may be given radiation therapy after surgery to kill any cancer cells that are left. Treatment given after the surgery, to lower the risk that the cancer will come back, is called adjuvant therapy.

Radiation Therapy

Radiation therapy is a cancer treatment that uses high-energy X-rays or other types of radiation to kill cancer cells or keep them from growing. There are two types of radiation therapy:

- External radiation therapy uses a machine outside the body to send radiation toward the cancer.

- Internal radiation therapy uses a radioactive substance sealed in needles, seeds, wires, or catheters that are placed directly into or near the cancer.

The way the radiation therapy is given depends on the type and stage of the cancer being treated. External and internal radiation therapy are used to treat vaginal cancer, and may also be used as palliative therapy to relieve symptoms and improve quality of life.

Chemotherapy

Chemotherapy is a cancer treatment that uses drugs to stop the growth of cancer cells, either by killing the cells or by stopping them from dividing. When chemotherapy is taken by mouth or injected into a vein or muscle, the drugs enter the bloodstream and can affect cancer cells throughout the body (systemic chemotherapy). When chemotherapy is placed directly into the cerebrospinal fluid (CSF), an organ, or a body cavity such as the abdomen, the drugs mainly affect cancer cells in those areas (regional chemotherapy). The way the chemotherapy is given depends on the type and stage of the cancer being treated. Topical chemotherapy for squamous cell vaginal cancer may be applied to the vagina in a cream or lotion.

Clinical Trial

For some patients, taking part in a clinical trial may be the best treatment choice. Clinical trials are part of the cancer research process. Clinical trials are done to find out if new cancer treatments are safe and effective or better than the standard treatment. Many of today's standard treatments for cancer are based on earlier clinical trials. Patients who take part in a clinical trial may receive the standard treatment or be among the first to receive a new treatment.

Patients who take part in clinical trials also help improve the way cancer will be treated in the future. Even when clinical trials do not lead to effective new treatments, they often answer important questions and help move research forward. Patients can enter clinical trials before, during, or after starting their cancer treatment. Some clinical trials only include patients who have not yet received treatment. Other trials test treatments for patients whose cancer has not gotten better. There are also clinical trials that test new ways to stop cancer from recurring (coming back) or reduce the side effects of cancer treatment.

Follow-Up Tests May Be Needed

Some of the tests that were done to diagnose the cancer or to find out the stage of the cancer may be repeated. Some tests will be repeated in order to see how well the treatment is working. Decisions about whether to continue, change, or stop treatment may be based on the results of these tests.

Chapter 22

Vulvar Cancer

Vulvar cancer is a rare disease in which malignant (cancer) cells form in the tissues of the vulva. Vulvar cancer forms in a woman's external genitalia. The vulva includes:

- Inner and outer lips of the vagina

- Clitoris (sensitive tissue between the lips)

- Opening of the vagina and its glands

- Mons pubis (the rounded area in front of the pubic bones that becomes covered with hair at puberty)

- Perineum (the area between the vulva and the anus)

Vulvar cancer most often affects the outer vaginal lips. Less often, cancer affects the inner vaginal lips, clitoris, or vaginal glands. Vulvar cancer usually forms slowly over a number of years. Abnormal cells can grow on the surface of the vulvar skin for a long time. This condition is called vulvar intraepithelial neoplasia (VIN). Because it is possible for VIN to become vulvar cancer, it is very important to get treatment.

Risk Factors of Vulvar Cancer

Vulvar intraepithelial neoplasia or HPV infection can affect the risk of vulvar cancer. Anything that increases your risk of getting a

This chapter includes text excerpted from "Vulvar Cancer Treatment (PDQ®)—Patient Version," National Cancer Institute (NCI), October 13, 2017.

disease is called a risk factor. Having a risk factor does not mean that you will get cancer; not having risk factors doesn't mean that you will not get cancer. Talk with your doctor if you think you may be at risk. Risk factors for vulvar cancer include the following:

- Having vulvar intraepithelial neoplasia (VIN)

- Having human papillomavirus (HPV) infection

- Having a history of genital warts

Other possible risk factors include the following:

- Having many sexual partners

- Having first sexual intercourse at a young age

- Having a history of abnormal Pap (Papanicolaou) tests (Pap smears)

Signs of Vulvar Cancer

Vulvar cancer often does not cause early signs or symptoms. Signs and symptoms may be caused by vulvar cancer or by other conditions. Check with your doctor if you have any of the following:

- A lump or growth on the vulva

- Changes in the vulvar skin, such as color changes or growths that look like a wart or ulcer

- Itching in the vulvar area, that does not go away

- Bleeding not related to menstruation (periods)

- Tenderness in the vulvar area

Diagnosing Vulvar Cancer

The following tests and procedures may be used:

- **Physical exam and history.** An exam of the body to check general signs of health, including checking the vulva for signs of disease, such as lumps or anything else that seems unusual. A history of the patient's health habits and past illnesses and treatments will also be taken.

- **Biopsy.** The removal of samples of cells or tissues from the vulva so they can be viewed under a microscope by a pathologist to check for signs of cancer.

Stages of Vulvar Cancer

After vulvar cancer has been diagnosed, tests are done to find out if cancer cells have spread within the vulva or to other parts of the body. The process used to find out if cancer has spread within the vulva or to other parts of the body is called staging. The information gathered from the staging process determines the stage of the disease. It is important to know the stage in order to plan treatment. The following tests and procedures may be used in the staging process:

- **Pelvic exam.** An exam of the vagina, cervix, uterus, fallopian tubes, ovaries, and rectum. A speculum is inserted into the vagina and the doctor or nurse looks at the vagina and cervix for signs of disease. A Pap test of the cervix is usually done. The doctor or nurse also inserts one or two lubricated, gloved fingers of one hand into the vagina and places the other hand over the lower abdomen to feel the size, shape, and position of the uterus and ovaries. The doctor or nurse also inserts a lubricated, gloved finger into the rectum to feel for lumps or abnormal areas.

- **Colposcopy.** A procedure in which a colposcope (a lighted, magnifying instrument) is used to check the vagina and cervix for abnormal areas. Tissue samples may be taken using a curette (spoon-shaped instrument) or a brush and checked under a microscope for signs of disease.

- **Cystoscopy.** A procedure to look inside the bladder and urethra to check for abnormal areas. A cystoscope is inserted through the urethra into the bladder. A cystoscope is a thin, tube-like instrument with a light and a lens for viewing. It may also have a tool to remove tissue samples, which are checked under a microscope for signs of cancer.

- **Proctoscopy.** A procedure to look inside the rectum and anus to check for abnormal areas. A proctoscope is inserted into the anus and rectum. A proctoscope is a thin, tube-like instrument with a light and a lens for viewing. It may also have a tool to remove tissue samples, which are checked under a microscope for signs of cancer.

- **X-rays.** An X-ray is a type of energy beam that can go through the body and onto film, making a picture of areas inside the body. To stage vulvar cancer, X-rays may be taken of the organs and bones inside the chest, and the pelvic bones.

- **Intravenous pyelogram (IVP).** A series of X-rays of the kidneys, ureters, and bladder to find out if cancer has spread to these organs. A contrast dye is injected into a vein. As the contrast dye moves through the kidneys, ureters and bladder, X-rays are taken to see if there are any blockages. This procedure is also called intravenous urography.

- **Computerized axial tomography (CAT) or computed tomography (CT) scan.** A procedure that makes a series of detailed pictures of areas inside the body, taken from different angles. The pictures are made by a computer linked to an X-ray machine. A dye may be injected into a vein or swallowed to help the organs or tissues show up more clearly. This procedure is also called computed tomography, computerized tomography, or computerized axial tomography.

- **Magnetic resonance imaging (MRI).** A procedure that uses a magnet, radio waves, and a computer to make a series of detailed pictures of areas inside the body. This procedure is also called nuclear magnetic resonance imaging (NMRI).

- **Positron emission tomography (PET) scan.** A procedure to find malignant tumor cells in the body. A small amount of radioactive glucose (sugar) is injected into a vein. The PET scanner rotates around the body and makes a picture of where glucose is being used in the body. Malignant tumor cells show up brighter in the picture because they are more active and take up more glucose than normal cells do.

- **Sentinel lymph node biopsy.** The removal of the sentinel lymph node during surgery. The sentinel lymph node is the first lymph node to receive lymphatic drainage from a tumor. It is the first lymph node the cancer is likely to spread to from the tumor. A radioactive substance and/or blue dye is injected near the tumor. The substance or dye flows through the lymph ducts to the lymph nodes. The first lymph node to receive the substance or dye is removed. A pathologist views the tissue under a microscope to look for cancer cells. If cancer cells are not found, it may not be necessary to remove more lymph nodes. Sentinel lymph node biopsy may be done during surgery to remove the tumor for early-stage vulvar cancer.

The following stages are used for vulvar cancer:

Stage I

In stage I, cancer has formed. The tumor is found only in the vulva or perineum (area between the rectum and the vagina). Stage I is divided into stages IA and IB.

- In stage IA, the tumor is 2 centimeters or smaller and has spread 1 millimeter or less into the tissue of the vulva. Cancer has not spread to the lymph nodes.

- In stage IB, the tumor is larger than 2 centimeters or has spread more than 1 millimeter into the tissue of the vulva. Cancer has not spread to the lymph nodes.

Stage II

In stage II, the tumor is any size and has spread into the lower part of the urethra, the lower part of the vagina, or the anus. Cancer has not spread to the lymph nodes

Stage III

In stage III, the tumor is any size and may have spread into the lower part of the urethra, the lower part of the vagina, or the anus. Cancer has spread to one or more nearby lymph nodes. Stage III is divided into stages IIIA, IIIB, and IIIC.

- In stage IIIA, cancer is found in 1 or 2 lymph nodes that are smaller than 5 millimeters or in one lymph node that is 5 millimeters or larger.

- In stage IIIB, cancer is found in 2 or more lymph nodes that are 5 millimeters or larger, or in 3 or more lymph nodes that are smaller than 5 millimeters.

- In stage IIIC, cancer is found in lymph nodes and has spread to the outside surface of the lymph nodes.

Stage IV

In stage IV, the tumor has spread into the upper part of the urethra, the upper part of the vagina, or to other parts of the body. Stage IV is divided into stages IVA and IVB.

In stage IVA:

- cancer has spread into the lining of the upper urethra, the upper vagina, the bladder, or the rectum, or has attached to the pelvic bone; or

- cancer has spread to nearby lymph nodes and the lymph nodes are not moveable or have formed an ulcer.

In stage IVB, cancer has spread to lymph nodes in the pelvis or to other parts of the body.

Treatment Option Overview

Different types of treatments are available for patients with vulvar cancer. Some treatments are standard (the currently used treatment), and some are being tested in clinical trials. A treatment clinical trial is a research study meant to help improve current treatments or obtain information on new treatments for patients with cancer. When clinical trials show that a new treatment is better than the standard treatment, the new treatment may become the standard treatment. Patients may want to think about taking part in a clinical trial. Some clinical trials are open only to patients who have not started treatment.

Surgery

Surgery is the most common treatment for vulvar cancer. The goal of surgery is to remove all the cancer without any loss of the woman's sexual function. One of the following types of surgery may be done:

- **Laser surgery:** A surgical procedure that uses a laser beam (a narrow beam of intense light) as a knife to make bloodless cuts in tissue or to remove a surface lesion such as a tumor.

- **Wide local excision:** A surgical procedure to remove the cancer and some of the normal tissue around the cancer.

- **Radical local excision:** A surgical procedure to remove the cancer and a large amount of normal tissue around it. Nearby lymph nodes in the groin may also be removed.

- **Ultrasound surgical aspiration:** A surgical procedure to break the tumor up into small pieces using very fine vibrations. The small pieces of tumor are washed away and removed by suction. This procedure causes less damage to nearby tissue.

- **Vulvectomy:** A surgical procedure to remove part or all of the vulva:

  - **Skinning vulvectomy:** The top layer of vulvar skin where the cancer is found is removed. Skin grafts from other parts of the body may be needed to cover the area where the skin was removed.

  - **Modified radical vulvectomy:** Surgery to remove part of the vulva. Nearby lymph nodes may also be removed.

  - **Radical vulvectomy:** Surgery to remove the entire vulva. Nearby lymph nodes are also removed.

- **Pelvic exenteration:** A surgical procedure to remove the lower colon, rectum, and bladder. The cervix, vagina, ovaries, and nearby lymph nodes are also removed. Artificial openings (stoma) are made for urine and stool to flow from the body into a collection bag.

Even if the doctor removes all the cancer that can be seen at the time of the surgery, some patients may have chemotherapy or radiation therapy after surgery to kill any cancer cells that are left. Treatment given after the surgery, to lower the risk that the cancer will come back, is called adjuvant therapy.

Radiation Therapy

Radiation therapy is a cancer treatment that uses high-energy X-rays or other types of radiation to kill cancer cells or keep them from growing. There are two types of radiation therapy:

- External radiation therapy uses a machine outside the body to send radiation toward the cancer.

- Internal radiation therapy uses a radioactive substance sealed in needles, seeds, wires, or catheters that are placed directly into or near the cancer.

The way the radiation therapy is given depends on the type and stage of the cancer being treated. External and internal radiation therapy are used to treat vulvar cancer, and external radiation therapy may also be used as palliative therapy to relieve symptoms and improve quality of life.

Chemotherapy

Chemotherapy is a cancer treatment that uses drugs to stop the growth of cancer cells, either by killing the cells or by stopping the cells from dividing. When chemotherapy is taken by mouth or injected into a vein or muscle, the drugs enter the bloodstream and can reach cancer cells throughout the body (systemic chemotherapy). When chemotherapy is placed directly into the cerebrospinal fluid, an organ, a body cavity such as the abdomen, or onto the skin, the drugs mainly affect cancer cells in those areas (regional chemotherapy). The way the chemotherapy is given depends on the type and stage of the cancer being treated. Topical chemotherapy for vulvar cancer may be applied to the skin in a cream or lotion.

Biologic Therapy

Biologic therapy is a treatment that uses the patient's immune system to fight cancer. Substances made by the body or made in a laboratory are used to boost, direct, or restore the body's natural defenses against cancer. This type of cancer treatment is also called biotherapy or immunotherapy. Imiquimod is a biologic therapy that may be used to treat vulvar lesions and is applied to the skin in a cream.

Follow-Up Tests May Be Needed

Some of the tests that were done to diagnose the cancer or to find out the stage of the cancer may be repeated. Some tests will be repeated in order to see how well the treatment is working. Decisions about whether to continue, change, or stop treatment may be based on the results of these tests. Some of the tests will continue to be done from time to time after treatment has ended. The results of these tests can show if your condition has changed or if the cancer has recurred (come back). These tests are sometimes called follow-up tests or check-ups. It is important to have regular follow-up exams to check for recurrent vulvar cancer.

Part Four

Other Cancers of Special Concern to Women

Chapter 23

Anal Cancer

Anal cancer is a disease in which malignant (cancer) cells form in the tissues of the anus. The anus is the end of the large intestine, below the rectum, through which stool (solid waste) leaves the body. The anus is formed partly from the outer skin layers of the body and partly from the intestine. Two ring-like muscles, called sphincter muscles, open and close the anal opening and let stool pass out of the body. The anal canal, the part of the anus between the rectum and the anal opening, is about 1–1½ inches long. The skin around the outside of the anus is called the perianal area. Tumors in this area are skin tumors, not anal cancer.

Risk Factors for Anal Cancer

Human papillomavirus (HPV) increases the risk of developing anal cancer. Risk factors include the following:

- Being infected with HPV
- Having many sexual partners
- Having receptive anal intercourse (anal sex)
- Being older than 50 years
- Frequent anal redness, swelling, and soreness

This chapter includes text excerpted from "Anal Cancer Treatment (PDQ®)— Patient Version," National Cancer Institute (NCI), January 25, 2018.

- Having anal fistulas (abnormal openings)
- Tobacco use

Signs of Anal Cancer

These and other signs and symptoms may be caused by anal cancer or by other conditions. Check with your doctor if you have any of the following:

- Bleeding from the anus or rectum
- Pain or pressure in the area around the anus
- Itching or discharge from the anus
- A lump near the anus
- A change in bowel habits

Diagnosing Anal Cancer

The following tests and procedures may be used:

- **Physical exam and history:** An exam of the body to check general signs of health, including checking for signs of disease, such as lumps or anything else that seems unusual. A history of the patient's health habits and past illnesses and treatments will also be taken.

- **Digital rectal examination (DRE):** An exam of the anus and rectum. The doctor or nurse inserts a lubricated, gloved finger into the lower part of the rectum to feel for lumps or anything else that seems unusual.

- **Anoscopy:** An exam of the anus and lower rectum using a short, lighted tube called an anoscope.

- **Proctoscopy:** An exam of the rectum using a short, lighted tube called a proctoscope.

- **Endo-anal or endorectal ultrasound:** A procedure in which an ultrasound transducer (probe) is inserted into the anus or rectum and used to bounce high-energy sound waves (ultrasound) off internal tissues or organs and make echoes. The echoes form a picture of body tissues called a sonogram.

- **Biopsy:** The removal of cells or tissues so they can be viewed under a microscope by a pathologist to check for signs of cancer.

If an abnormal area is seen during the anoscopy, a biopsy may be done at that time.

Stages of Anal Cancer

After anal cancer has been diagnosed, tests are done to find out if cancer cells have spread within the anus or to other parts of the body. The process used to find out if cancer has spread within the anus or to other parts of the body is called staging. The information gathered from the staging process determines the stage of the disease. It is important to know the stage in order to plan treatment. The following tests may be used in the staging process:

- **Computerized axial tomography (CAT) scan:** A procedure that makes a series of detailed pictures of areas inside the body, such as the abdomen or chest, taken from different angles. The pictures are made by a computer linked to an X-ray machine. A dye may be injected into a vein or swallowed to help the organs or tissues show up more clearly. This procedure is also called computed tomography, computerized tomography, or computerized axial tomography. For anal cancer, a CT scan of the pelvis and abdomen may be done.

- **Chest X-ray:** An X-ray of the organs and bones inside the chest. An X-ray is a type of energy beam that can go through the body and onto film, making a picture of areas inside the body.

- **Magnetic resonance imaging (MRI):** A procedure that uses a magnet, radio waves, and a computer to make a series of detailed pictures of areas inside the body. This procedure is also called nuclear magnetic resonance imaging (NMRI).

- **Positron emission tomography (PET) scan:** A procedure to find malignant tumor cells in the body. A small amount of radioactive glucose (sugar) is injected into a vein. The PET scanner rotates around the body and makes a picture of where glucose is being used in the body. Malignant tumor cells show up brighter in the picture because they are more active and take up more glucose than normal cells do.

- **Pelvic exam:** An exam of the vagina, cervix, uterus, fallopian tubes, ovaries, and rectum. A speculum is inserted into the vagina and the doctor or nurse looks at the vagina and cervix for signs of disease. A Pap (Papanicolaou) test of the cervix is usually done. The doctor or nurse also inserts one or two lubricated, gloved fingers of one hand into the vagina and places the other hand over the lower abdomen to feel the size, shape, and position of the uterus and ovaries. The doctor or nurse also inserts a lubricated, gloved finger into the rectum to feel for lumps or abnormal areas.

Stage 0

In stage 0, abnormal cells are found in the mucosa (innermost layer) of the anus. These abnormal cells may become cancer and spread into nearby normal tissue. Stage 0 is also called high-grade squamous intraepithelial lesion (HSIL).

Stage I

In stage I, cancer has formed and the tumor is 2 centimeters or smaller.

Stage II

Stage II anal cancer is divided into stages IIA and IIB.

- In stage IIA, the tumor is larger than 2 centimeters but not larger than 5 centimeters.

- In stage IIB, the tumor is larger than 5 centimeters.

Stage III

Stage III anal cancer is divided into stages IIIA, IIIB, and IIIC.

- In stage IIIA, the tumor is 5 centimeters or smaller and has spread to lymph nodes near the anus or groin.

- In stage IIIB, the tumor is any size and has spread to nearby organs, such as the vagina, urethra, or bladder. Cancer has not spread to lymph nodes.

- In stage IIIC, the tumor is any size and may have spread to nearby organs. Cancer has spread to lymph nodes near the anus or groin.

Stage IV

In stage IV, the tumor is any size. Cancer may have spread to lymph nodes or nearby organs and has spread to other parts of the body, such as the liver or lungs.

Treatment Option Overview

Different types of treatments are available for patients with anal cancer. Some treatments are standard (the currently used treatment), and some are being tested in clinical trials. A treatment clinical trial is a research study meant to help improve current treatments or obtain information on new treatments for patients with cancer. When clinical trials show that a new treatment is better than the standard treatment, the new treatment may become the standard treatment. Patients may want to think about taking part in a clinical trial. Some clinical trials are open only to patients who have not started treatment.

Three types of standard treatment are used:

Radiation Therapy

Radiation therapy is a cancer treatment that uses high-energy X-rays or other types of radiation to kill cancer cells or keep them from growing. There are two types of radiation therapy:

- External radiation therapy uses a machine outside the body to send radiation toward the cancer.

- Internal radiation therapy uses a radioactive substance sealed in needles, seeds, wires, or catheters that are placed directly into or near the cancer.

The way the radiation therapy is given depends on the type and stage of the cancer being treated. External and internal radiation therapy are used to treat anal cancer.

Chemotherapy

Chemotherapy is a cancer treatment that uses drugs to stop the growth of cancer cells, either by killing the cells or by stopping the cells from dividing. When chemotherapy is taken by mouth or injected into a vein or muscle, the drugs enter the bloodstream and can reach cancer cells throughout the body (systemic chemotherapy). When chemotherapy is placed directly into the cerebrospinal fluid, an organ, or a body cavity such as the abdomen, the drugs mainly affect cancer cells in those areas (regional chemotherapy). The way the chemotherapy is given depends on the type and stage of the cancer being treated.

Surgery

- **Local resection:** A surgical procedure in which the tumor is cut from the anus along with some of the healthy tissue around it. Local resection may be used if the cancer is small and has not spread. This procedure may save the sphincter muscles so the patient can still control bowel movements. Tumors that form in the lower part of the anus can often be removed with local resection.

- **Abdominoperineal resection:** A surgical procedure in which the anus, the rectum, and part of the sigmoid colon are removed through an incision made in the abdomen. The doctor sews the end of the intestine to an opening, called a stoma, made in the surface of the abdomen so body waste can be collected in a disposable bag outside of the body. This is called a colostomy. Lymph nodes that contain cancer may also be removed during this operation.

Human Immunodeficiency Virus (HIV) Can Affect Treatment of Anal Cancer

Cancer therapy can further damage the already weakened immune systems of patients who have the human immunodeficiency virus (HIV). For this reason, patients who have anal cancer and HIV are usually treated with lower doses of anticancer drugs and radiation than patients who do not have HIV.

Follow-Up Tests May Be Needed

Some of the tests that were done to diagnose the cancer or to find out the stage of the cancer may be repeated. Some tests will be repeated in order to see how well the treatment is working. Decisions about whether to continue, change, or stop treatment may be based on the results of these tests. Some of the tests will continue to be done from time to time after treatment has ended. The results of these tests can show if your condition has changed or if the cancer has recurred (come back). These tests are sometimes called follow-up tests or check-ups.

Chapter 24

Colorectal Cancer

Chapter Contents

Section 24.1

Cancers of the Colon and Rectum

This section includes text excerpted from "What Is
Colorectal Cancer?" Centers for Disease Control and
Prevention (CDC), April 25, 2016.

What Is Colorectal Cancer?

Colorectal cancer is cancer that occurs in the colon or rectum. Sometimes it is called colon cancer, for short. As the drawing shows, the
colon is the large intestine or large bowel. The rectum is the passage-
way that connects the colon to the anus. Sometimes abnormal growths,
called polyps, form in the colon or rectum. Over time, some polyps
may turn into cancer. Screening tests can find polyps so they can be
removed before turning into cancer. Screening also helps find colorectal
cancer at an early stage, when treatment often leads to a cure.

What Are the Risk Factors for Colorectal Cancer?

Your risk of getting colorectal cancer increases as you get older.
More than 90 percent of cases occur in people who are 50 years old or
older. Other risk factors include having:

- Inflammatory bowel disease (IBD) such as Crohn's disease or
  ulcerative colitis

- A personal or family history of colorectal cancer or colorectal
  polyps

- A genetic syndrome such as familial adenomatous polyposis
  (FAP) or hereditary nonpolyposis colorectal cancer (HNPCC)
  (Lynch syndrome)

Lifestyle factors that may contribute to an increased risk of colorectal cancer include:

- Lack of regular physical activity

- A diet low in fruit and vegetables

- A low-fiber and high-fat diet
- Overweight and obesity
- Alcohol consumption
- Tobacco use

What Can I Do to Reduce My Risk of Colorectal Cancer?

Almost all colorectal cancers begin as precancerous polyps (abnormal growths) in the colon or rectum. Such polyps can be present in the colon for years before invasive cancer develops. They may not cause any symptoms. Colorectal cancer screening can find precancerous polyps so they can be removed before they turn into cancer. In this way, colorectal cancer is prevented. Screening can also find colorectal cancer early, when there is a greater chance that treatment will be most effective and lead to a cure.

Research is underway to find out if changes to your diet can reduce your colorectal cancer risk. Medical experts don't agree on the role of diet in preventing colorectal cancer, but often recommend a diet low in animal fats and high in fruits, vegetables, and whole grains to reduce the risk of other chronic diseases, such as coronary artery disease and diabetes. This diet also may reduce the risk of colorectal cancer. Also, researchers are examining the role of certain medicines and supplements in preventing colorectal cancer.

The U.S. Preventive Services Task Force (USPSTF) found that taking low-dose aspirin can help prevent cardiovascular disease and colorectal cancer in some adults, depending on age and risk factors. Some studies suggest that people may reduce their risk of developing colorectal cancer by increasing physical activity, limiting alcohol consumption, and avoiding tobacco. Overall, the most effective way to reduce your risk of colorectal cancer is by having regular colorectal cancer screening tests beginning at age 50.

What Are the Symptoms of Colorectal Cancer?

Colorectal polyps and colorectal cancer don't always cause symptoms, especially at first. Someone could have polyps or colorectal cancer and not know it. That is why getting screened regularly for colorectal cancer is so important.

If you have symptoms, they may include:

- Blood in or on your stool (bowel movement)

- Stomach pain, aches, or cramps that don't go away

- Losing weight and you don't know why

If you have any of these symptoms, talk to your doctor. They may be caused by something other than cancer. The only way to know what is causing them is to see your doctor.

What Is Colorectal Cancer Screening?

A screening test is used to look for a disease when a person doesn't have symptoms. When a person has symptoms, diagnostic tests are used to find out the cause of the symptoms. Colorectal cancer almost always develops from precancerous polyps (abnormal growths) in the colon or rectum. Screening tests can find precancerous polyps, so that they can be removed before they turn into cancer. Screening tests can also find colorectal cancer early, when treatment works best.

Screening Guidelines

Regular screening, beginning at age 50, is the key to preventing colorectal cancer. The USPSTF recommends that adults age 50–75 be screened for colorectal cancer. The USPSTF recommends that adults age 76–85 ask their doctor if they should be screened.

When Should I Begin to Get Screened?

You should begin screening for colorectal cancer soon after turning 50, then continue getting screened at regular intervals. However, you may need to be tested earlier than 50, or more often than other people, if:

- You or a close relative have had colorectal polyps or colorectal cancer

- You have an inflammatory bowel disease such as Crohn's disease or ulcerative colitis

- You have a genetic syndrome such as familial adenomatous polyposis (FAP) or hereditary nonpolyposis colorectal cancer (Lynch syndrome)

If you think you are at increased risk for colorectal cancer, speak with your doctor about:

- When to begin screening
- Which test is right for you
- How often to get tested

Free or Low-Cost Screening

Six states in Centers for Disease Control and Prevention's (CDC) Colorectal Cancer Control Program (CRCCP) provide colorectal cancer screening to some people. Those eligible are low-income men and women aged 50–64 years who are underinsured or uninsured for screening, when resources are available and there is no other payment option. Colorectal cancer screening tests may be covered by your health insurance policy without a deductible or co-pay.

Section 24.2

Staging and Treating Cancer of the Colon

This section includes text excerpted from "Colon Cancer Treatment (PDQ®)—Patient Version," National Cancer Institute (NCI), December 7, 2017.

Stages of Colon Cancer

After colon cancer has been diagnosed, tests are done to find out if cancer cells have spread within the colon or to other parts of the body. The process used to find out if cancer has spread within the colon or to other parts of the body is called staging. The information gathered from the staging process determines the stage of the disease. It is important to know the stage in order to plan treatment.

The following tests and procedures may be used in the staging process:

- **Computerized axial tomography (CAT) scan.** A procedure that makes a series of detailed pictures of areas inside the body, such as the abdomen or chest, taken from different angles. The pictures are made by a computer linked to an X-ray machine. A dye may be injected into a vein or swallowed to help the organs or tissues show up more clearly. This procedure is also called computed tomography, computerized tomography, or computerized axial tomography.

- **Magnetic resonance imaging (MRI).** A procedure that uses a magnet, radio waves, and a computer to make a series of detailed pictures of areas inside the colon. A substance called gadolinium is injected into the patient through a vein. The gadolinium collects around the cancer cells so they show up brighter in the picture. This procedure is also called nuclear magnetic resonance imaging (NMRI).

- **Positron emission tomography (PET) scan.** A procedure to find malignant tumor cells in the body. A small amount of radioactive glucose (sugar) is injected into a vein. The PET scanner rotates around the body and makes a picture of where glucose is being used in the body. Malignant tumor cells show up brighter in the picture because they are more active and take up more glucose than normal cells do.

- **Chest X-ray.** An X-ray of the organs and bones inside the chest. An X-ray is a type of energy beam that can go through the body and onto film, making a picture of areas inside the body.

- **Surgery.** A procedure to remove the tumor and see how far it has spread through the colon.

- **Lymph node biopsy.** The removal of all or part of a lymph node. A pathologist views the tissue under a microscope to look for cancer cells.

- **Complete blood count (CBC).** A procedure in which a sample of blood is drawn and checked for the following:

  - The number of red blood cells (RBCs), white blood cells (WBCs), and platelets.

  - The amount of hemoglobin (the protein that carries oxygen) in the red blood cells.

  - The portion of the blood sample made up of red blood cells.

- **Carcinoembryonic antigen (CEA) assay.** A test that measures the level of CEA in the blood. CEA is released into the bloodstream from both cancer cells and normal cells. When found in higher than normal amounts, it can be a sign of colon cancer or other conditions.

Stage 0 (Carcinoma in Situ)

In stage 0, abnormal cells are found in the mucosa (innermost layer) of the colon wall. These abnormal cells may become cancer and spread. Stage 0 is also called carcinoma in situ.

Stage I

In stage I, cancer has formed in the mucosa (innermost layer) of the colon wall and has spread to the submucosa (layer of tissue under the mucosa). Cancer may have spread to the muscle layer of the colon wall.

Stage II

Stage II colon cancer is divided into stage IIA, stage IIB, and stage IIC.

- **Stage IIA:** Cancer has spread through the muscle layer of the colon wall to the serosa (outermost layer) of the colon wall.

- **Stage IIB:** Cancer has spread through the serosa (outermost layer) of the colon wall but has not spread to nearby organs.

- **Stage IIC:** Cancer has spread through the serosa (outermost layer) of the colon wall to nearby organs.

Stage III

Stage III colon cancer is divided into stage IIIA, stage IIIB, and stage IIIC.

In stage IIIA:

- Cancer has spread through the mucosa (innermost layer) of the colon wall to the submucosa (layer of tissue under the mucosa) and may have spread to the muscle layer of the colon wall. Cancer has spread to at least one but not more than 3 nearby lymph nodes or cancer cells have formed in tissues near the lymph nodes.

- Cancer has spread through the mucosa (innermost layer) of the colon wall to the submucosa (layer of tissue under the mucosa).

269

Cancer has spread to at least 4 but not more than 6 nearby lymph nodes.

In stage IIIB:

- Cancer has spread through the muscle layer of the colon wall to the serosa (outermost layer) of the colon wall or has spread through the serosa but not to nearby organs. Cancer has spread to at least one but not more than 3 nearby lymph nodes or cancer cells have formed in tissues near the lymph nodes.

- Cancer has spread to the muscle layer of the colon wall or to the serosa (outermost layer) of the colon wall. Cancer has spread to at least 4 but not more than 6 nearby lymph nodes.

- Cancer has spread through the mucosa (innermost layer) of the colon wall to the submucosa (layer of tissue under the mucosa) and may have spread to the muscle layer of the colon wall. Cancer has spread to 7 or more nearby lymph nodes.

In stage IIIC:

- Cancer has spread through the serosa (outermost layer) of the colon wall but has not spread to nearby organs. Cancer has spread to at least 4 but not more than 6 nearby lymph nodes.

- Cancer has spread through the muscle layer of the colon wall to the serosa (outermost layer) of the colon wall or has spread through the serosa but has not spread to nearby organs. Cancer has spread to 7 or more nearby lymph nodes.

- Cancer has spread through the serosa (outermost layer) of the colon wall and has spread to nearby organs. Cancer has spread to one or more nearby lymph nodes or cancer cells have formed in tissues near the lymph nodes.

Stage IV

Stage IV colon cancer is divided into stage IVA and stage IVB.

- **Stage IVA:** Cancer may have spread through the colon wall and may have spread to nearby organs or lymph nodes. Cancer has spread to one organ that is not near the colon, such as the liver, lung, or ovary, or to a distant lymph node.

- **Stage IVB:** Cancer may have spread through the colon wall and may have spread to nearby organs or lymph nodes. Cancer has spread to more than one organ that is not near the colon or into the lining of the abdominal wall.

Treatment Option Overview

Different types of treatment are available for patients with colon cancer. Some treatments are standard (the currently used treatment), and some are being tested in clinical trials. A treatment clinical trial is a research study meant to help improve current treatments or obtain information on new treatments for patients with cancer. When clinical trials show that a new treatment is better than the standard treatment, the new treatment may become the standard treatment. Patients may want to think about taking part in a clinical trial. Some clinical trials are open only to patients who have not started treatment.

Six types of standard treatment are used:

Surgery

Surgery (removing the cancer in an operation) is the most common treatment for all stages of colon cancer. A doctor may remove the cancer using one of the following types of surgery:

- **Local excision:** If the cancer is found at a very early stage, the doctor may remove it without cutting through the abdominal wall. Instead, the doctor may put a tube with a cutting tool through the rectum into the colon and cut the cancer out. This is called a local excision. If the cancer is found in a polyp (a small bulging area of tissue), the operation is called a polypectomy.

- **Resection of the colon with anastomosis:** If the cancer is larger, the doctor will perform a partial colectomy (removing the cancer and a small amount of healthy tissue around it). The doctor may then perform an anastomosis (sewing the healthy parts of the colon together). The doctor will also usually remove lymph nodes near the colon and examine them under a microscope to see whether they contain cancer.

- **Resection of the colon with colostomy:** If the doctor is not able to sew the 2 ends of the colon back together, a stoma (an opening) is made on the outside of the body for waste to pass through. This procedure is called a colostomy. A bag is placed around the stoma to collect the waste. Sometimes the colostomy is needed only until the lower colon has healed, and then it can

271

be reversed. If the doctor needs to remove the entire lower colon, however, the colostomy may be permanent.

Even if the doctor removes all the cancer that can be seen at the time of the operation, some patients may be given chemotherapy or radiation therapy after surgery to kill any cancer cells that are left. Treatment given after the surgery, to lower the risk that the cancer will come back, is called adjuvant therapy.

Radiofrequency Ablation

Radiofrequency ablation is the use of a special probe with tiny electrodes that kill cancer cells. Sometimes the probe is inserted directly through the skin and only local anesthesia is needed. In other cases, the probe is inserted through an incision in the abdomen. This is done in the hospital with general anesthesia.

Cryosurgery

Cryosurgery is a treatment that uses an instrument to freeze and destroy abnormal tissue. This type of treatment is also called cryotherapy.

Chemotherapy

Chemotherapy is a cancer treatment that uses drugs to stop the growth of cancer cells, either by killing the cells or by stopping them from dividing. When chemotherapy is taken by mouth or injected into a vein or muscle, the drugs enter the bloodstream and can reach cancer cells throughout the body (systemic chemotherapy). When chemotherapy is placed directly into the cerebrospinal fluid, an organ, or a body cavity such as the abdomen, the drugs mainly affect cancer cells in those areas (regional chemotherapy).

Chemoembolization of the hepatic artery may be used to treat cancer that has spread to the liver. This involves blocking the hepatic artery (the main artery that supplies blood to the liver) and injecting anticancer drugs between the blockage and the liver. The liver's arteries then deliver the drugs throughout the liver. Only a small amount of the drug reaches other parts of the body. The blockage may be temporary or permanent, depending on what is used to block the artery. The liver continues to receive some blood from the hepatic portal vein, which carries blood from the stomach and intestine.

The way the chemotherapy is given depends on the type and stage of the cancer being treated.

Radiation Therapy

Radiation therapy is a cancer treatment that uses high-energy X-rays or other types of radiation to kill cancer cells or keep them from growing. There are two types of radiation therapy:

- External radiation therapy uses a machine outside the body to send radiation toward the cancer.

- Internal radiation therapy uses a radioactive substance sealed in needles, seeds, wires, or catheters that are placed directly into or near the cancer.

The way the radiation therapy is given depends on the type and stage of the cancer being treated. External radiation therapy is used as palliative therapy to relieve symptoms and improve quality of life.

Targeted Therapy

Targeted therapy is a type of treatment that uses drugs or other substances to identify and attack specific cancer cells without harming normal cells.

Types of targeted therapies used in the treatment of colon cancer include the following:

- **Monoclonal antibodies (mAbs):** Monoclonal antibodies are made in the laboratory from a single type of immune system cell. These antibodies can identify substances on cancer cells or normal substances that may help cancer cells grow. The antibodies attach to the substances and kill the cancer cells, block their growth, or keep them from spreading. Monoclonal antibodies are given by infusion. They may be used alone or to carry drugs, toxins, or radioactive material directly to cancer cells.

    - Bevacizumab and ramucirumab are types of monoclonal antibodies that bind to a protein called vascular endothelial growth factor (VEGF). This may prevent the growth of new blood vessels that tumors need to grow.

    - Cetuximab and panitumumab are types of monoclonal antibodies that bind to a protein called epidermal growth factor receptor (EGFR) on the surface of some types of cancer cells. This may stop cancer cells from growing and dividing.

- **Angiogenesis inhibitors:** Angiogenesis inhibitors stop the growth of new blood vessels that tumors need to grow.

  - Ziv-aflibercept is a vascular endothelial growth factor trap that blocks an enzyme needed for the growth of new blood vessels in tumors.

  - Regorafenib is used to treat colorectal cancer that has spread to other parts of the body and has not gotten better with other treatment. It blocks the action of certain proteins, including vascular endothelial growth factor. This may help keep cancer cells from growing and may kill them. It may also prevent the growth of new blood vessels that tumors need to grow.

Follow-Up Tests May Be Needed

Some of the tests that were done to diagnose the cancer or to find out the stage of the cancer may be repeated. Some tests will be repeated in order to see how well the treatment is working. Decisions about whether to continue, change, or stop treatment may be based on the results of these tests. Some of the tests will continue to be done from time to time after treatment has ended. The results of these tests can show if your condition has changed or if the cancer has recurred (come back). These tests are sometimes called follow-up tests or check-ups.

Section 24.3

Staging and Treating Cancer of the Rectum

This section includes text excerpted from "Rectal Cancer Treatment (PDQ®)—Patient Version," National Cancer Institute (NCI), February 16, 2018.

Stages of Rectal Cancer

After rectal cancer has been diagnosed, tests are done to find out if cancer cells have spread within the rectum or to other parts of the body. The process used to find out whether cancer has spread within the rectum or to other parts of the body is called staging. The information gathered from the staging process determines the stage of the disease. It is important to know the stage in order to plan treatment.

The following tests and procedures may be used in the staging process:

- **Chest X-ray:** An X-ray of the organs and bones inside the chest. An X-ray is a type of energy beam that can go through the body and onto film, making a picture of areas inside the body.

- **Colonoscopy:** A procedure to look inside the rectum and colon for polyps (small pieces of bulging tissue). abnormal areas, or cancer. A colonoscope is a thin, tube-like instrument with a light and a lens for viewing. It may also have a tool to remove polyps or tissue samples, which are checked under a microscope for signs of cancer.

- **Computerized axial tomography (CAT) scan:** A procedure that makes a series of detailed pictures of areas inside the body, such as the abdomen, pelvis, or chest, taken from different angles. The pictures are made by a computer linked to an X-ray machine. A dye may be injected into a vein or swallowed to help the organs or tissues show up more clearly. This procedure is also called computed tomography, computerized tomography, or computerized axial tomography.

- **Magnetic resonance imaging (MRI):** A procedure that uses a magnet, radio waves, and a computer to make a series of detailed pictures of areas inside the body. This procedure is also called nuclear magnetic resonance imaging (NMRI).

- **Positron emission tomography (PET) scan:** A procedure to find malignant tumor cells in the body. A small amount of radioactive glucose (sugar) is injected into a vein. The PET scanner rotates around the body and makes a picture of where glucose is being used in the body. Malignant tumor cells show up brighter in the picture because they are more active and take up more glucose than normal cells do.

- **Endorectal ultrasound:** A procedure used to examine the rectum and nearby organs. An ultrasound transducer (probe) is inserted into the rectum and used to bounce high-energy sound waves (ultrasound) off internal tissues or organs and make echoes. The echoes form a picture of body tissues called a sonogram. The doctor can identify tumors by looking at the sonogram. This procedure is also called transrectal ultrasound.

Stage 0 (Carcinoma in Situ)

In stage 0, abnormal cells are found in the mucosa (innermost layer) of the rectum wall. These abnormal cells may become cancer and spread. Stage 0 is also called carcinoma in situ.

Stage I

In stage I, cancer has formed in the mucosa (innermost layer) of the rectum wall and has spread to the submucosa (layer of tissue under the mucosa). Cancer may have spread to the muscle layer of the rectum wall.

Stage II

Stage II rectal cancer is divided into stage IIA, stage IIB, and stage IIC.

- **Stage IIA:** Cancer has spread through the muscle layer of the rectum wall to the serosa (outermost layer) of the rectum wall.

- **Stage IIB:** Cancer has spread through the serosa (outermost layer) of the rectum wall but has not spread to nearby organs.

- **Stage IIC:** Cancer has spread through the serosa (outermost layer) of the rectum wall to nearby organs.

Stage III

Stage III rectal cancer is divided into stage IIIA, stage IIIB, and stage IIIC.

Stage IIIA

- Cancer has spread through the mucosa (innermost layer) of the rectum wall to the submucosa (layer of tissue under the mucosa) and may have spread to the muscle layer of the rectum wall. Cancer has spread to at least one but not more than 3 nearby lymph nodes or cancer cells have formed in tissues near the lymph nodes.

- Cancer has spread through the mucosa (innermost layer) of the rectum wall to the submucosa (layer of tissue under the mucosa). Cancer has spread to at least 4 but not more than 6 nearby lymph nodes.

Stage IIIB

- Cancer has spread through the muscle layer of the rectum wall to the serosa (outermost layer) of the rectum wall or has spread through the serosa but not to nearby organs. Cancer has spread to at least one but not more than 3 nearby lymph nodes or cancer cells have formed in tissues near the lymph nodes.

- Cancer has spread to the muscle layer of the rectum wall or to the serosa (outermost layer) of the rectum wall. Cancer has spread to at least 4 but not more than 6 nearby lymph nodes.

- Cancer has spread through the mucosa (innermost layer) of the rectum wall to the submucosa (layer of tissue under the mucosa) and may have spread to the muscle layer of the rectum wall. Cancer has spread to 7 or more nearby lymph nodes.

Stage IIIC

- Cancer has spread through the serosa (outermost layer) of the rectum wall but has not spread to nearby organs. Cancer has spread to at least 4 but not more than 6 nearby lymph nodes.

- Cancer has spread through the muscle layer of the rectum wall to the serosa (outermost layer) of the rectum wall or has spread through the serosa but has not spread to nearby organs. Cancer has spread to 7 or more nearby lymph nodes.

- Cancer has spread through the serosa (outermost layer) of the rectum wall and has spread to nearby organs. Cancer has spread to one or more nearby lymph nodes or cancer cells have formed in tissues near the lymph nodes.

Stage IV

Stage IV rectal cancer is divided into stage IVA and stage IVB.

- **Stage IVA:** Cancer may have spread through the rectum wall and may have spread to nearby organs or lymph nodes. Cancer has spread to one organ that is not near the rectum, such as the liver, lung, or ovary, or to a distant lymph node.

- **Stage IVB:** Cancer may have spread through the rectum wall and may have spread to nearby organs or lymph nodes. Cancer has spread to more than one organ that is not near the rectum or into the lining of the abdominal wall.

Treatment Option Overview

Different types of treatment are available for patients with rectal cancer. Some treatments are standard (the currently used treatment), and some are being tested in clinical trials. A treatment clinical trial is a research study meant to help improve current treatments or obtain information on new treatments for patients with cancer. When clinical trials show that a new treatment is better than the standard treatment, the new treatment may become the standard treatment. Patients may want to think about taking part in a clinical trial. Some clinical trials are open only to patients who have not started treatment.

Five types of standard treatment are used:

Surgery

Surgery is the most common treatment for all stages of rectal cancer. The cancer is removed using one of the following types of surgery:

- **Polypectomy:** If the cancer is found in a polyp (a small piece of bulging tissue), the polyp is often removed during a colonoscopy.

- **Local excision:** If the cancer is found on the inside surface of the rectum and has not spread into the wall of the rectum, the cancer and a small amount of surrounding healthy tissue is removed.

- **Resection:** If the cancer has spread into the wall of the rectum, the section of the rectum with cancer and nearby healthy tissue is removed. Sometimes the tissue between the rectum and the abdominal wall is also removed. The lymph nodes near the rectum are removed and checked under a microscope for signs of cancer.

- **Radiofrequency ablation:** The use of a special probe with tiny electrodes that kill cancer cells. Sometimes the probe is inserted directly through the skin and only local anesthesia is needed. In other cases, the probe is inserted through an incision in the abdomen. This is done in the hospital with general anesthesia.

- **Cryosurgery:** A treatment that uses an instrument to freeze and destroy abnormal tissue. This type of treatment is also called cryotherapy.

- **Pelvic exenteration:** If the cancer has spread to other organs near the rectum, the lower colon, rectum, and bladder are removed. The cervix, vagina, ovaries, and nearby lymph nodes may be removed.

After the cancer is removed, the surgeon will either:

- do an anastomosis (sew the healthy parts of the rectum together, sew the remaining rectum to the colon, or sew the colon to the anus);

or

- make a stoma (an opening) from the rectum to the outside of the body for waste to pass through. This procedure is done if the cancer is too close to the anus and is called a colostomy. A bag is placed around the stoma to collect the waste. Sometimes the colostomy is needed only until the rectum has healed, and then it can be reversed. If the entire rectum is removed, however, the colostomy may be permanent.

Radiation therapy and/or chemotherapy may be given before surgery to shrink the tumor, make it easier to remove the cancer, and help with bowel control after surgery. Treatment given before surgery is called neoadjuvant therapy. Even if all the cancer that can be seen at the time of the operation is removed, some patients may be given radiation therapy and/or chemotherapy after surgery to kill any cancer cells that are left. Treatment given after the surgery, to lower the risk that the cancer will come back, is called adjuvant therapy.

Radiation Therapy

Radiation therapy is a cancer treatment that uses high-energy X-rays or other types of radiation to kill cancer cells or keep them from growing. There are two types of radiation therapy:

- External radiation therapy uses a machine outside the body to send radiation toward the cancer.

- Internal radiation therapy uses a radioactive substance sealed in needles, seeds, wires, or catheters that are placed directly into or near the cancer.

The way the radiation therapy is given depends on the type and stage of the cancer being treated. External radiation therapy is used to treat rectal cancer.

Short-course preoperative radiation therapy (SCRT) is used in some types of rectal cancer. This treatment uses fewer and lower doses of radiation than standard treatment, followed by surgery several days after the last dose.

Chemotherapy

Chemotherapy is a cancer treatment that uses drugs to stop the growth of cancer cells, either by killing the cells or by stopping the cells from dividing. When chemotherapy is taken by mouth or injected into a vein or muscle, the drugs enter the bloodstream and can reach cancer cells throughout the body (systemic chemotherapy). When chemotherapy is placed directly in the cerebrospinal fluid, an organ, or a body cavity such as the abdomen, the drugs mainly affect cancer cells in those areas (regional chemotherapy).

Chemoembolization of the hepatic artery is a type of regional chemotherapy that may be used to treat cancer that has spread to the liver. This is done by blocking the hepatic artery (the main artery that supplies blood to the liver) and injecting anticancer drugs between the blockage and the liver. The liver's arteries then carry the drugs into the liver. Only a small amount of the drug reaches other parts of the body. The blockage may be temporary or permanent, depending on what is used to block the artery. The liver continues to receive some blood from the hepatic portal vein, which carries blood from the stomach and intestine.

The way the chemotherapy is given depends on the type and stage of the cancer being treated.

Active Surveillance

Active surveillance is closely following a patient's condition without giving any treatment unless there are changes in test results. It is used to find early signs that the condition is getting worse. In active surveillance, patients are given certain exams and tests to check if the cancer is growing. When the cancer begins to grow, treatment is given to cure the cancer. Tests include the following:

- Digital rectal exam (DRE)
- MRI
- Endoscopy
- Sigmoidoscopy
- CT scan
- Carcinoembryonic antigen (CEA) assay

Targeted Therapy

Targeted therapy is a type of treatment that uses drugs or other substances to identify and attack specific cancer cells without harming normal cells.

Types of targeted therapies used in the treatment of rectal cancer include the following:

- **Monoclonal antibodies (mAbs):** Monoclonal antibody therapy is a type of targeted therapy being used for the treatment of rectal cancer. Monoclonal antibody therapy uses antibodies made in the laboratory from a single type of immune system cell. These antibodies can identify substances on cancer cells or normal substances that may help cancer cells grow. The antibodies attach to the substances and kill the cancer cells, block their growth, or keep them from spreading. Monoclonal antibodies are given by infusion. They may be used alone or to carry drugs, toxins, or radioactive material directly to cancer cells.

  - Bevacizumab and ramucirumab are types of monoclonal antibodies that bind to a protein called vascular endothelial growth factor (VEGF). This may prevent the growth of new blood vessels that tumors need to grow.

  - Cetuximab and panitumumab are types of monoclonal antibodies that bind to a protein called epidermal growth factor receptor (EGFR) on the surface of some types of cancer cells. This may stop cancer cells from growing and dividing.

- **Angiogenesis inhibitors:** Angiogenesis inhibitors stop the growth of new blood vessels that tumors need to grow.

  - Ziv-aflibercept is a vascular endothelial growth factor trap that blocks an enzyme needed for the growth of new blood vessels in tumors.

  - Regorafenib is used to treat colorectal cancer that has spread to other parts of the body and has not gotten better with other treatment. It blocks the action of certain proteins, including vascular endothelial growth factor. This may help keep cancer cells from growing and may kill them. It may also prevent the growth of new blood vessels that tumors need to grow.

Follow-Up Tests May Be Needed

Some of the tests that were done to diagnose the cancer or to find out the stage of the cancer may be repeated. Some tests will be repeated in order to see how well the treatment is working. Decisions about whether to continue, change, or stop treatment may be based on the results of these tests.

Chapter 25

Gallbladder and Bile Duct Cancers

Chapter Contents

Section 25.1

Gallbladder Cancer

This section includes text excerpted from "Gallbladder
Cancer Treatment (PDQ®)—Patient Version," National
Cancer Institute (NCI), March 22, 2018.

Gallbladder cancer is a disease in which malignant (cancer) cells form in the tissues of the gallbladder. It is a rare disease in which malignant (cancer) cells are found in the tissues of the gallbladder. The gallbladder is a pear-shaped organ that lies just under the liver in the upper abdomen. The gallbladder stores bile, a fluid made by the liver to digest fat. When food is being broken down in the stomach and intestines, bile is released from the gallbladder through a tube called the common bile duct, which connects the gallbladder and liver to the first part of the small intestine.

The wall of the gallbladder has four main layers of tissue.

- Mucosal (inner) layer

- Muscle layer

- Connective tissue layer

- Serosal (outer) layer

Primary gallbladder cancer starts in the inner layer and spreads through the outer layers as it grows. Being female can increase the risk of developing gallbladder cancer. Anything that increases your chance of getting a disease is called a risk factor. Having a risk factor does not mean that you will get cancer; not having risk factors doesn't mean that you will not get cancer. Talk with your doctor if you think you may be at risk. Risk factors for gallbladder cancer include the following:

- Being female

- Being Native American

Signs and Symptoms of Gallbladder Cancer

These and other signs and symptoms may be caused by gallbladder cancer or by other conditions. Check with your doctor if you have any of the following:

- Jaundice (yellowing of the skin and whites of the eyes)
- Pain above the stomach
- Fever
- Nausea and vomiting
- Bloating
- Lumps in the abdomen

Gallbladder cancer is difficult to detect (find) and diagnose for the following reasons:

- There are no signs or symptoms in the early stages of gallbladder cancer.
- The symptoms of gallbladder cancer, when present, are like the symptoms of many other illnesses.
- The gallbladder is hidden behind the liver.

Gallbladder cancer is sometimes found when the gallbladder is removed for other reasons. Patients with gallstones rarely develop gallbladder cancer.

Diagnosing Gallbladder Cancer

Tests that examine the gallbladder and nearby organs are used to detect (find), diagnose, and stage gallbladder cancer. Procedures that make pictures of the gallbladder and the area around it help diagnose gallbladder cancer and show how far the cancer has spread. The process used to find out if cancer cells have spread within and around the gallbladder is called staging. In order to plan treatment, it is important to know if the gallbladder cancer can be removed by surgery. Tests and procedures to detect, diagnose, and stage gallbladder cancer are usually done at the same time. The following tests and procedures may be used:

- **Physical exam and history:** An exam of the body to check general signs of health, including checking for signs of disease, such as lumps or anything else that seems unusual. A history of the patient's health habits and past illnesses and treatments will also be taken.

- **Liver function tests:** A procedure in which a blood sample is checked to measure the amounts of certain substances released into the blood by the liver. A higher than normal amount of a substance can be a sign of liver disease that may be caused by gallbladder cancer.

- **Blood chemistry studies:** A procedure in which a blood sample is checked to measure the amounts of certain substances released into the blood by organs and tissues in the body. An unusual (higher or lower than normal) amount of a substance can be a sign of disease.

- **Computed tomography (CT) scan:** A procedure that makes a series of detailed pictures of areas inside the body, such as the chest, abdomen, and pelvis, taken from different angles. The pictures are made by a computer linked to an X-ray machine. A dye may be injected into a vein or swallowed to help the organs or tissues show up more clearly. This procedure is also called computed tomography, computerized tomography, or computerized axial tomography.

- **Ultrasound exam:** A procedure in which high-energy sound waves (ultrasound) are bounced off internal tissues or organs and make echoes. The echoes form a picture of body tissues called a sonogram. An abdominal ultrasound is done to diagnose gallbladder cancer.

- **Percutaneous transhepatic cholangiography (PTC):** A procedure used to X-ray the liver and bile ducts. A thin needle is inserted through the skin below the ribs and into the liver. Dye is injected into the liver or bile ducts and an X-ray is taken. If a blockage is found, a thin, flexible tube called a stent is sometimes left in the liver to drain bile into the small intestine or a collection bag outside the body.

- **Endoscopic retrograde cholangiopancreatography (ERCP):** A procedure used to X-ray the ducts (tubes) that carry bile from the liver to the gallbladder and from the gallbladder to the small intestine. Sometimes gallbladder cancer causes these ducts to narrow and block or slow the flow of bile, causing jaundice. An endoscope (a thin, lighted tube) is passed through the mouth, esophagus, and stomach into the first part of the small intestine. A catheter (a smaller tube) is then inserted through the endoscope into the bile ducts. A dye is injected through the catheter into the ducts and an X-ray is taken. If the ducts are blocked by a tumor, a fine tube may be inserted into the duct to unblock it. This tube (or stent) may be left in place to keep the duct open. Tissue samples may also be taken.

- **Magnetic resonance imaging (MRI) with gadolinium:** A procedure that uses a magnet, radio waves, and a computer to make a series of detailed pictures of areas inside the body. A substance called gadolinium is injected into a vein. The gadolinium collects around the cancer cells so they show up brighter in the picture. This procedure is also called nuclear magnetic resonance imaging (NMRI).

- **Endoscopic ultrasound (EUS):** A procedure in which an endoscope is inserted into the body, usually through the mouth or rectum. An endoscope is a thin, tube-like instrument with a light and a lens for viewing. A probe at the end of the endoscope is used to bounce high-energy sound waves (ultrasound) off internal tissues or organs and make echoes. The echoes form a picture of body tissues called a sonogram. This procedure is also called endosonography.

- **Laparoscopy:** A surgical procedure to look at the organs inside the abdomen to check for signs of disease. Small incisions (cuts) are made in the wall of the abdomen and a laparoscope (a thin, lighted tube) is inserted into one of the incisions. Other instruments may be inserted through the same or other incisions to perform procedures such as removing organs or taking tissue samples for biopsy. The laparoscopy helps to find out if the cancer is within the gallbladder only or has spread to nearby tissues and if it can be removed by surgery.

- **Biopsy:** The removal of cells or tissues so they can be viewed under a microscope by a pathologist to check for signs of cancer. The biopsy may be done after surgery to remove the tumor. If the tumor clearly cannot be removed by surgery, the biopsy may be done using a fine needle to remove cells from the tumor.

Stages of Gallbladder Cancer

Tests and procedures to stage gallbladder cancer are usually done at the same time as diagnosis.

Stage 0 (Carcinoma in Situ)

In stage 0, abnormal cells are found in the mucosa (innermost layer) of the gallbladder wall. These abnormal cells may become cancer and spread into nearby normal tissue. Stage 0 is also called carcinoma in situ.

Stage I

In stage I, cancer has formed in the mucosa (innermost layer) of the gallbladder wall and may have spread to the muscle layer of the gallbladder wall.

Stage II

Stage II is divided into stages IIA and IIB, depending on where the cancer has spread in the gallbladder.

In stage IIA, cancer has spread through the muscle layer to the connective tissue layer of the gallbladder wall on the side of the gallbladder that is not near the liver.

In stage IIB, cancer has spread through the muscle layer to the connective tissue layer of the gallbladder wall on the same side as the liver. Cancer has not spread to the liver.

Stage III

Stage III is divided into stages IIIA and IIIB, depending on where the cancer has spread.

In stage IIIA, cancer has spread through the connective tissue layer of the gallbladder wall and one or more of the following is true:

- Cancer has spread to the serosa (layer of tissue that covers the gallbladder).

- Cancer has spread to the liver.

- Cancer has spread to one nearby organ or structure (such as the stomach, small intestine, colon, pancreas, or the bile ducts outside the liver).

In stage IIIB, cancer has formed in the mucosa (innermost layer) of the gallbladder wall and may have spread to the muscle, connective tissue, or serosa (layer of tissue that covers the gallbladder) and may have also spread to the liver or to one nearby organ or structure (such as the stomach, small intestine, colon, pancreas, or the bile ducts outside the liver). Cancer has spread to one to three nearby lymph nodes.

Stage IV

Stage IV is divided into stages IVA and IVB.

In stage IVA, cancer has spread to the portal vein or hepatic artery or to two or more organs or structures other than the liver. Cancer may have spread to one to three nearby lymph nodes.

In stage IVB, cancer may have spread to nearby organs or structures:

- to four or more nearby lymph nodes; or

- to other parts of the body, such as the peritoneum and liver.

Treatment Option Overview

There are different types of treatment for patients with gallbladder cancer. Some treatments are standard (the currently used treatment), and some are being tested in clinical trials. A treatment clinical trial is a research study meant to help improve current treatments or obtain information on new treatments for patients with cancer. When clinical trials show that a new treatment is better than the standard treatment, the new treatment may become the standard treatment. Patients may want to think about taking part in a clinical trial. Some clinical trials are open only to patients who have not started treatment.

Three types of standard treatment are used:

Surgery

Gallbladder cancer may be treated with a cholecystectomy, surgery to remove the gallbladder and some of the tissues around it. Nearby lymph nodes may be removed. A laparoscope is sometimes used to guide gallbladder surgery. The laparoscope is attached to a video camera and inserted through an incision (port) in the abdomen. Surgical instruments are inserted through other ports to perform the surgery. Because there is a risk that gallbladder cancer cells may spread to these ports, tissue surrounding the port sites may also be removed.

If the cancer has spread and cannot be removed, the following types of palliative surgery may relieve symptoms:

- **Biliary bypass:** If the tumor is blocking the bile duct and bile is building up in the gallbladder, a biliary bypass may be done. During this operation, the doctor will cut the gallbladder or bile duct in the area before the blockage and sew it to the small intestine to create a new pathway around the blocked area.

- **Endoscopic stent placement:** If the tumor is blocking the bile duct, surgery may be done to put in a stent (a thin tube) to drain bile that has built up in the area. The doctor may place the stent through a catheter that drains the bile into a bag on the outside of the body or the stent may go around the blocked area and drain the bile into the small intestine.

- **Percutaneous transhepatic biliary drainage (PTBD):** A procedure done to drain bile when there is a blockage and endoscopic stent placement is not possible. An X-ray of the liver and bile ducts is done to locate the blockage. Images made by ultrasound are used to guide placement of a stent, which is left in the liver to drain bile into the small intestine or a collection bag outside the body. This procedure may be done to relieve jaundice before surgery.

Radiation Therapy

Radiation therapy is a cancer treatment that uses high-energy X-rays or other types of radiation to kill cancer cells or keep them from growing. There are two types of radiation therapy:

- External radiation therapy uses a machine outside the body to send radiation toward the cancer.

- Internal radiation therapy uses a radioactive substance sealed in needles, seeds, wires, or catheters that are placed directly into or near the cancer.

The way the radiation therapy is given depends on the type and stage of the cancer being treated. External radiation therapy is used to treat gallbladder cancer.

Chemotherapy

Chemotherapy is a cancer treatment that uses drugs to stop the growth of cancer cells, either by killing the cells or by stopping the cells from dividing. When chemotherapy is taken by mouth or injected into a vein or muscle, the drugs enter the bloodstream and can reach cancer cells throughout the body (systemic chemotherapy). When chemotherapy is placed directly into the cerebrospinal fluid, an organ, or a body cavity such as the abdomen, the drugs mainly affect cancer cells in those areas (regional chemotherapy). The way the chemotherapy is given depends on the type and stage of the cancer being treated.

New types of treatment are being tested in clinical trials.

Radiation Sensitizers

Clinical trials are studying ways to improve the effect of radiation therapy on tumor cells, including the following:

- **Hyperthermia therapy:** A treatment in which body tissue is exposed to high temperatures to damage and kill cancer cells or to make cancer cells more sensitive to the effects of radiation therapy and certain anticancer drugs.

- **Radiosensitizers:** Drugs that make tumor cells more sensitive to radiation therapy. Giving radiation therapy together with radiosensitizers may kill more tumor cells.

Treatment for gallbladder cancer may cause side effects. Patients may want to think about taking part in a clinical trial. For some patients, taking part in a clinical trial may be the best treatment choice. Clinical trials are part of the cancer research process. Clinical trials are done to find out if new cancer treatments are safe and effective or better than the standard treatment. Many treatments for cancer are based on earlier clinical trials. Patients who take part in a clinical trial may receive the standard treatment or be among the first to receive a new treatment.

Section 25.2

Bile Duct Cancer

This section includes text excerpted from "Bile Duct Cancer (Cholangiocarcinoma) Treatment (PDQ®)—Patient Version," National Cancer Institute (NCI), March 22, 2018.

A network of tubes, called ducts, connects the liver, gallbladder, and small intestine. This network begins in the liver where many small ducts collect bile (a fluid made by the liver to break down fats during digestion). The small ducts come together to form the right and left hepatic ducts, which lead out of the liver. The two ducts join outside the liver and form the common hepatic duct. The cystic duct connects the gallbladder to the common hepatic duct. Bile from the liver passes through the hepatic ducts, common hepatic duct, and cystic duct and is stored in the gallbladder.

When food is being digested, bile stored in the gallbladder is released and passes through the cystic duct to the common bile duct and into the small intestine. Bile duct cancer is also called cholangiocarcinoma.

There are two types of bile duct cancer:

- **Intrahepatic bile duct cancer.** This type of cancer forms in the bile ducts inside the liver. Only a small number of bile duct cancers are intrahepatic. Intrahepatic bile duct cancers are also called intrahepatic cholangiocarcinomas.

- **Extrahepatic bile duct cancer.** The extrahepatic bile duct is made up of the hilum region and the distal region. Cancer can form in either region:

  - **Perihilar bile duct cancer:** This type of cancer is found in the hilum region, the area where the right and left bile ducts exit the liver and join to form the common hepatic duct. Perihilar bile duct cancer is also called a Klatskin tumor or perihilar cholangiocarcinoma.

  - **Distal extrahepatic bile duct cancer:** This type of cancer is found in the distal region. The distal region is made up of the common bile duct which passes through the pancreas and ends in the small intestine. Distal extrahepatic bile duct cancer is also called extrahepatic cholangiocarcinoma.

Risk Factors for Bile Duct Cancer

Colitis or certain liver diseases can increase the risk of bile duct cancer. Anything that increases your risk of getting a disease is called a risk factor. Having a risk factor does not mean that you will get cancer; not having risk factors doesn't mean that you will not get cancer. People who think they may be at risk should discuss this with their doctor.

Risk factors for bile duct cancer include the following conditions:

- Primary sclerosing cholangitis (PSC) (a progressive disease in which the bile ducts become blocked by inflammation and scarring)

- Chronic ulcerative colitis
- Cysts in the bile ducts (cysts block the flow of bile and can cause swollen bile ducts, inflammation, and infection)
- Infection with a Chinese liver fluke parasite

Signs of Bile Duct Cancer

These and other signs and symptoms may be caused by bile duct cancer or by other conditions. Check with your doctor if you have any of the following:

- Jaundice (yellowing of the skin or whites of the eyes)
- Dark urine
- Clay-colored stool
- Pain in the abdomen
- Fever
- Itchy skin
- Nausea and vomiting
- Weight loss for an unknown reason

Diagnosing Bile Duct Cancer

Procedures that make pictures of the bile ducts and the nearby area help diagnose bile duct cancer and show how far the cancer has spread. The process used to find out if cancer cells have spread within and around the bile ducts or to distant parts of the body is called staging.

In order to plan treatment, it is important to know if the bile duct cancer can be removed by surgery. Tests and procedures to detect, diagnose, and stage bile duct cancer are usually done at the same time.

The following tests and procedures may be used:

Physical exam and history. An exam of the body to check general signs of health, including checking for signs of disease, such as lumps or anything else that seems unusual. A history of the patient's health habits and past illnesses and treatments will also be taken.

Liver function tests. A procedure in which a blood sample is checked to measure the amounts of bilirubin and alkaline phosphatase released into the blood by the liver. A higher than normal amount of

293

these substances can be a sign of liver disease that may be caused by bile duct cancer.

Laboratory tests. Medical procedures that test samples of tissue, blood, urine, or other substances in the body. These tests help to diagnose disease, plan and check treatment, or monitor the disease over time.

Carcinoembryonic antigen (CEA) and cancer antigen (CA) 19-9 tumor marker test. A procedure in which a sample of blood, urine, or tissue is checked to measure the amounts of certain substances made by organs, tissues, or tumor cells in the body. Certain substances are linked to specific types of cancer when found in increased levels in the body. These are called tumor markers. Higher than normal levels of carcinoembryonic antigen (CEA) and CA 19-9 may mean there is bile duct cancer.

Ultrasound exam. A procedure in which high-energy sound waves (ultrasound) are bounced off internal tissues or organs, such as the abdomen, and make echoes. The echoes form a picture of body tissues called a sonogram. The picture can be printed to be looked at later.

Computed tomography (CT) scan. A procedure that makes a series of detailed pictures of areas inside the body, such as the abdomen, taken from different angles. The pictures are made by a computer linked to an X-ray machine. A dye may be injected into a vein or swallowed to help the organs or tissues show up more clearly. This procedure is also called computed tomography, computerized tomography, or computerized axial tomography.

Magnetic resonance imaging (MRI). A procedure that uses a magnet, radio waves, and a computer to make a series of detailed pictures of areas inside the body. This procedure is also called nuclear magnetic resonance imaging (NMRI).

Magnetic resonance cholangiopancreatography (MRCP). A procedure that uses a magnet, radio waves, and a computer to make a series of detailed pictures of areas inside the body such as the liver, bile ducts, gallbladder, pancreas, and pancreatic duct.

Different procedures may be used to obtain a sample of tissue and diagnose bile duct cancer. Cells and tissues are removed during a biopsy so they can be viewed under a microscope by a pathologist to check for signs of cancer. Different procedures may be used to obtain the sample of cells and tissue. The type of procedure used depends on whether the patient is well enough to have surgery.

Types of biopsy procedures include the following:

- **Laparoscopy.** A surgical procedure to look at the organs inside the abdomen, such as the bile ducts and liver, to check for signs of cancer. Small incisions (cuts) are made in the wall of the abdomen and a laparoscope (a thin, lighted tube) is inserted into one of the incisions. Other instruments may be inserted through the same or other incisions to perform procedures such as taking tissue samples to be checked for signs of cancer.

- **Percutaneous transhepatic cholangiography (PTC).** A procedure used to X-ray the liver and bile ducts. A thin needle is inserted through the skin below the ribs and into the liver. Dye is injected into the liver or bile ducts and an X-ray is taken. A sample of tissue is removed and checked for signs of cancer. If the bile duct is blocked, a thin, flexible tube called a stent may be left in the liver to drain bile into the small intestine or a collection bag outside the body. This procedure may be used when a patient cannot have surgery.

- **Endoscopic retrograde cholangiopancreatography (ERCP).** A procedure used to X-ray the ducts (tubes) that carry bile from the liver to the gallbladder and from the gallbladder to the small intestine. Sometimes bile duct cancer causes these ducts to narrow and block or slow the flow of bile, causing jaundice. An endoscope is passed through the mouth and stomach and into the small intestine. Dye is injected through the endoscope (thin, tube-like instrument with a light and a lens for viewing) into the bile ducts and an X-ray is taken. A sample of tissue is removed and checked for signs of cancer. If the bile duct is blocked, a thin tube may be inserted into the duct to unblock it. This tube (or stent) may be left in place to keep the duct open. This procedure may be used when a patient cannot have surgery.

- **Endoscopic ultrasound (EUS).** A procedure in which an endoscope is inserted into the body, usually through the mouth or rectum. An endoscope is a thin, tube-like instrument with a light and a lens for viewing. A probe at the end of the endoscope is used to bounce high-energy sound waves (ultrasound) off internal tissues or organs and make echoes. The echoes form a picture of body tissues called a sonogram. A sample of tissue is removed and checked for signs of cancer. This procedure is also called endosonography.

Stages of Bile Duct Cancer

Intrahepatic Bile Duct Cancer

Stage 0: In stage 0 intrahepatic bile duct cancer, abnormal cells are found in the innermost layer of tissue lining the intrahepatic bile duct. These abnormal cells may become cancer and spread into nearby normal tissue. Stage 0 is also called carcinoma in situ.

Stage I: Stage I intrahepatic bile duct cancer is divided into stages IA and IB.

- In stage IA, cancer has formed in an intrahepatic bile duct and the tumor is 5 centimeters or smaller.

- In stage IB, cancer has formed in an intrahepatic bile duct and the tumor is larger than 5 centimeters.

Stage II: In stage II intrahepatic bile duct cancer, either of the following is found:

- the tumor has spread through the wall of an intrahepatic bile duct and into a blood vessel.

- more than one tumor has formed in the intrahepatic bile duct and may have spread into a blood vessel.

Stage III: Stage III intrahepatic bile duct cancer is divided into stages IIIA and IIIB.

- In stage IIIA, the tumor has spread through the capsule (outer lining) of the liver.

- In stage IIIB, cancer has spread to organs or tissues near the liver, such as the duodenum, colon, stomach, common bile duct, abdominal wall, diaphragm, or the part of the vena cava behind the liver, or the cancer has spread to nearby lymph nodes.

Stage IV: In stage IV intrahepatic bile duct cancer, cancer has spread to other parts of the body, such as the bone, lungs, distant lymph nodes, or tissue lining the wall of the abdomen and most organs in the abdomen.

Perihilar Bile Duct Cancer

Stage 0: In stage 0 perihilar bile duct cancer, abnormal cells are found in the innermost layer of tissue lining the perihilar bile duct. These abnormal cells may become cancer and spread into nearby normal tissue. Stage 0 is also called carcinoma in situ or high-grade dysplasia.

Stage I: In stage I perihilar bile duct cancer, cancer has formed in the innermost layer of tissue lining the perihilar bile duct and has spread into the muscle layer or fibrous tissue layer of the perihilar bile duct wall.

Stage II: In stage II perihilar bile duct cancer, cancer has spread through the wall of the perihilar bile duct to nearby fatty tissue or to liver tissue.

Stage III: Stage III perihilar bile duct cancer is divided into stages IIIA, IIIB, and IIIC.

- **Stage IIIA:** Cancer has spread to branches on one side of the hepatic artery or of the portal vein.

- **Stage IIIB:** Cancer has spread to one or more of the following:

  - The main part of the portal vein or its branches on both sides

  - The common hepatic artery

  - The right hepatic duct and the left branch of the hepatic artery or of the portal vein

  - The left hepatic duct and the right branch of the hepatic artery or of the portal vein

- **Stage IIIC:** Cancer has spread to 1–3 nearby lymph nodes.

Stage IV: Stage IV perihilar bile duct cancer is divided into stages IVA and IVB.

- **Stage IVA:** Cancer has spread to 4 or more nearby lymph nodes.

- **Stage IVB:** Cancer has spread to other parts of the body, such as the liver, lung, bone, brain, skin, distant lymph nodes, or tissue lining the wall of the abdomen and most organs in the abdomen.

Distal Extrahepatic Bile Duct Cancer

Stage 0: In stage 0 distal extrahepatic bile duct cancer, abnormal cells are found in the innermost layer of tissue lining the distal extrahepatic bile duct. These abnormal cells may become cancer and spread into nearby normal tissue. Stage 0 is also called carcinoma in situ or high-grade dysplasia.

- **Stage I:** In stage I distal extrahepatic bile duct cancer, cancer has formed and spread fewer than 5 millimeters into the wall of the distal extrahepatic bile duct.

- **Stage II:** In stage II distal extrahepatic bile duct cancer is divided into stages IIA and IIB.

  - **Stage IIA:** Cancer has spread:

    - Fewer than 5 millimeters into the wall of the distal extrahepatic bile duct and has spread to 1–3 nearby lymph nodes.

    - 5–12 millimeters into the wall of the distal extrahepatic bile duct.

  - **Stage IIB:** Cancer has spread 5 millimeters or more into the wall of the distal extrahepatic bile duct. Cancer may have spread to 1–3 nearby lymph nodes.

- **Stage III:** Stage III distal extrahepatic bile duct cancer is divided into stages IIIA and IIIB.

  - **Stage IIIA:** Cancer has spread into the wall of the distal extrahepatic bile duct and to 4 or more nearby lymph nodes.

  - **Stage IIIB:** Cancer has spread to the large vessels that carry blood to the organs in the abdomen. Cancer may have spread to 1 or more nearby lymph nodes.

- **Stage IV:** In stage IV distal extrahepatic bile duct cancer, cancer has spread to other parts of the body, such as the liver, lungs, or tissue lining the wall of the abdomen and most organs in the abdomen.

Treatment Option Overview

Different types of treatments are available for patients with bile duct cancer. Some treatments are standard (the currently used treatment), and some are being tested in clinical trials. A treatment clinical trial is a research study meant to help improve current treatments or obtain information on new treatments for patients with cancer. When clinical trials show that a new treatment is better than the standard treatment, the new treatment may become the standard treatment. Patients may want to think about taking part in a clinical trial. Some clinical trials are open only to patients who have not started treatment.

Three types of standard treatment are used:

Surgery

The following types of surgery are used to treat bile duct cancer:

- **Removal of the bile duct:** A surgical procedure to remove part of the bile duct if the tumor is small and in the bile duct only. Lymph nodes are removed and tissue from the lymph nodes is viewed under a microscope to see if there is cancer.

- **Partial hepatectomy:** A surgical procedure in which the part of the liver where cancer is found is removed. The part removed may be a wedge of tissue, an entire lobe, or a larger part of the liver, along with some normal tissue around it.

- **Whipple procedure:** A surgical procedure in which the head of the pancreas, the gallbladder, part of the stomach, part of the small intestine, and the bile duct are removed. Enough of the pancreas is left to make digestive juices and insulin.

After the doctor removes all the cancer that can be seen at the time of the surgery, some patients may be given chemotherapy or radiation therapy after surgery to kill any cancer cells that are left. Treatment given after the surgery, to lower the risk that the cancer will come back, is called adjuvant therapy. It is not yet known whether chemotherapy or radiation therapy given after surgery helps keep the cancer from coming back.

The following types of palliative surgery may be done to relieve symptoms caused by a blocked bile duct and improve quality of life:

- **Biliary bypass:** If cancer is blocking the bile duct and bile is building up in the gallbladder, a biliary bypass may be done. During this operation, the doctor will cut the gallbladder or bile duct in the area before the blockage and sew it to the part of the bile duct that is past the blockage or to the small intestine to create a new pathway around the blocked area.

- **Endoscopic stent placement:** If the tumor is blocking the bile duct, surgery may be done to put in a stent (a thin tube) to drain bile that has built up in the area. The doctor may place the stent through a catheter that drains the bile into a bag on the outside of the body or the stent may go around the blocked area and drain the bile into the small intestine.

- **Percutaneous transhepatic biliary drainage (PTBD):** A procedure used to X-ray the liver and bile ducts. A thin needle is inserted through the skin below the ribs and into the liver. Dye is injected into the liver or bile ducts and an X-ray is taken. If the bile duct is blocked, a thin, flexible tube called a stent may be left in the liver to drain bile into the small intestine or a collection bag outside the body.

Radiation Therapy

Radiation therapy is a cancer treatment that uses high-energy X-rays or other types of radiation to kill cancer cells or keep them from growing. There are two types of radiation therapy:

- External radiation therapy uses a machine outside the body to send radiation toward the cancer.

- Internal radiation therapy uses a radioactive substance sealed in needles, seeds, wires, or catheters that are placed directly into or near the cancer.

External and internal radiation therapy are used to treat bile duct cancer.

It is not yet known whether external radiation therapy helps in the treatment of resectable bile duct cancer. In unresectable, metastatic, or recurrent bile duct cancer, new ways to improve the effect of external radiation therapy on cancer cells are being studied:

- **Hyperthermia therapy:** A treatment in which body tissue is exposed to high temperatures to make cancer cells more sensitive to the effects of radiation therapy and certain anticancer drugs.

- **Radiosensitizers:** Drugs that make cancer cells more sensitive to radiation therapy. Combining radiation therapy with radiosensitizers may kill more cancer cells.

Chemotherapy

Chemotherapy is a cancer treatment that uses drugs to stop the growth of cancer cells, either by killing the cells or by stopping them from dividing. When chemotherapy is taken by mouth or injected into a vein or muscle, the drugs enter the bloodstream and can reach cancer cells throughout the body (systemic chemotherapy). When chemotherapy is placed directly into the cerebrospinal fluid, an organ, or a body cavity such as the abdomen, the drugs mainly affect cancer cells in those areas (regional chemotherapy).

Systemic chemotherapy is used to treat unresectable, metastatic, or recurrent bile duct cancer. It is not yet known whether systemic chemotherapy helps in the treatment of resectable bile duct cancer.

In unresectable, metastatic, or recurrent bile duct cancer, intra-arterial embolization is being studied. It is a procedure in which the blood supply to a tumor is blocked after anticancer drugs are given in blood vessels near the tumor. Sometimes, the anticancer drugs are attached to small beads that are injected into an artery that feeds the tumor. The beads block blood flow to the tumor as they release the drug. This allows a higher amount of drug to reach the tumor for a longer period of time, which may kill more cancer cells.

Chapter 26

Lung Cancer

Chapter Contents

Section 26.1

What You Need to Know about Lung Cancer

This section includes text excerpted from "What Is Lung Cancer?"
Centers for Disease Control and Prevention (CDC), August 28, 2014.
Reviewed May 2018.

What Is Lung Cancer?

Cancer is a disease in which cells in the body grow out of control. When cancer starts in the lungs, it is called lung cancer. Lung cancer begins in the lungs and may spread to lymph nodes or other organs in the body, such as the brain. Cancer from other organs also may spread to the lungs. When cancer cells spread from one organ to another, they are called metastases. Lung cancers usually are grouped into two main types called small cell and nonsmall cell. These types of lung cancer grow differently and are treated differently. Nonsmall cell lung cancer is more common than small cell lung cancer.

What Are the Risk Factors for Lung Cancer?

Research has found several risk factors that may increase your chances of getting lung cancer.

Smoking

Cigarette smoking is the number one risk factor for lung cancer. In the United States, cigarette smoking is linked to about 80–90 percent of lung cancers. Using other tobacco products such as cigars or pipes also increases the risk for lung cancer. Tobacco smoke is a toxic mix of more than 7,000 chemicals. Many are poisons. At least 70 are known to cause cancer in people or animals.

People who smoke cigarettes are 15–30 times more likely to get lung cancer or die from lung cancer than people who do not smoke. Even smoking a few cigarettes a day or smoking occasionally increases the risk of lung cancer. The more years a person smokes and the more cigarettes smoked each day, the more risk goes up.

People who quit smoking have a lower risk of lung cancer than if they had continued to smoke, but their risk is higher than the risk for people who never smoked. Quitting smoking at any age can lower the risk of lung cancer.

Cigarette smoking can cause cancer almost anywhere in the body. Cigarette smoking causes cancer of the mouth and throat, esophagus, stomach, colon, rectum, liver, pancreas, voice box (larynx), trachea, bronchus, kidney and renal pelvis, urinary bladder, and cervix, and causes acute myeloid leukemia.

Secondhand Smoke

Smoke from other people's cigarettes, pipes, or cigars (secondhand smoke) also causes lung cancer. When a person breathes in secondhand smoke, it is like he or she is smoking. In the United States, two out of five adults who don't smoke and half of the children are exposed to secondhand smoke, and about 7,300 people who never smoked die from lung cancer due to secondhand smoke every year.

Radon

Radon is a naturally occurring gas that comes from rocks and dirt and can get trapped in houses and buildings. It cannot be seen, tasted, or smelled. According to the U.S. Environmental Protection Agency (EPA), radon causes about 20,000 cases of lung cancer each year, making it the second leading cause of lung cancer. Nearly one out of every 15 homes in the United States is thought to have high radon levels. The EPA recommends testing homes for radon and using proven ways to lower high radon levels.

Other Substances

Examples of substances found at some workplaces that increase risk include asbestos, arsenic, diesel exhaust, and some forms of silica and chromium. For many of these substances, the risk of getting lung cancer is even higher for those who smoke.

Personal or Family History of Lung Cancer

If you are a lung cancer survivor, there is a risk that you may develop another lung cancer, especially if you smoke. Your risk of lung cancer may be higher if your parents, brothers or sisters, or children have had lung cancer. This could be true because they also smoke, or they live or work in the same place where they are exposed to radon and other substances that can cause lung cancer.

Radiation Therapy to the Chest

Cancer survivors who had radiation therapy to the chest are at higher risk of lung cancer.

Diet

Scientists are studying many different foods and dietary supplements to see whether they change the risk of getting lung cancer. They do know that smokers who take beta-carotene supplements have increased risk of lung cancer.

Also, arsenic in drinking water (primarily from private wells) can increase the risk of lung cancer.

What Are the Symptoms of Lung Cancer?

Different people have different symptoms for lung cancer. Some people have symptoms related to the lungs. Some people whose lung cancer has spread to other parts of the body (metastasized) have symptoms specific to that part of the body. Some people just have general symptoms of not feeling well. Most people with lung cancer don't have symptoms until the cancer is advanced. Lung cancer symptoms may include:

- Coughing that gets worse or doesn't go away

- Chest pain

- Shortness of breath

- Wheezing

- Coughing up blood

- Feeling very tired all the time

- Weight loss with no known cause

Other changes that can sometimes occur with lung cancer may include repeated bouts of pneumonia and swollen or enlarged lymph nodes (glands) inside the chest in the area between the lungs. These symptoms can happen with other illnesses, too. If you have some of these symptoms, talk to your doctor, who can help find the cause.

What Can I Do to Reduce My Risk of Lung Cancer?

You can help lower your risk of lung cancer in the following ways:

- **Don't smoke.** Cigarette smoking causes about 90 percent of lung cancer deaths in the United States. The most important thing you can do to prevent lung cancer is to not start smoking, or to quit if you smoke.

- **Avoid secondhand smoke.** Smoke from other people's cigarettes, cigars, or pipes is called secondhand smoke. Make your home and car smoke-free.

- **Get your home tested for radon.** The EPA recommends that all homes be tested for radon.

- **Be careful at work.** Health and safety guidelines in the workplace can help workers avoid carcinogens—things that can cause cancer.

What Screening Tests Are There?

Screening means testing for a disease when there are no symptoms or history of that disease. Doctors recommend a screening test to find a disease early, when treatment may work better. The only recommended screening test for lung cancer is low-dose computed tomography (also called a low-dose CT scan, or LDCT). In this test, an X-ray machine scans the body and uses low doses of radiation to make detailed pictures of the lungs.

Who Should Be Screened?

The U.S. Preventive Services Task Force (USPSTF) recommends yearly lung cancer screening with LDCT for people who:

- Have a history of heavy smoking

- Smoke now or have quit within the past 15 years

- Are between 55 and 80 years old

Heavy smoking means a smoking history of 30 pack years or more. A pack year is smoking an average of one pack of cigarettes per day for one year. For example, a person could have a 30 pack-year history by smoking one pack a day for 30 years or two packs a day for 15 years.

Risks of Screening

Lung cancer screening has at least three risks:

- A lung cancer screening test can suggest that a person has lung cancer when no cancer is present. This is called a false-positive result. False-positive results can lead to follow-up tests and surgeries that are not needed and may have more risks.

- A lung cancer screening test can find cases of cancer that may never have caused a problem for the patient. This is called overdiagnosis. Overdiagnosis can lead to treatment that is not needed.

- Radiation from repeated low-dose computed tomography (LDCT) tests can cause cancer in otherwise healthy people.

That is why lung cancer screening is recommended only for adults who have no symptoms but who are at high risk for developing the disease because of their smoking history and age.

If you are thinking about getting screened, talk to your doctor. If lung cancer screening is right for you, your doctor can refer you to a high-quality treatment facility.

The best way to reduce your risk of lung cancer is to not smoke and to avoid secondhand smoke. Lung cancer screening is not a substitute for quitting smoking.

When Should Screening Stop?

The Task Force recommends that yearly lung cancer screening stop when the person being screened:

- Turns 81 years old

- Has not smoked in 15 years

- Develops a health problem that makes him or her unwilling or unable to have surgery if lung cancer is found

What Are the Types of Lung Cancer?

There two main types of lung cancer are small cell lung cancer (SCLC) and nonsmall cell lung cancer (NSCLC). These categories refer to what the cancer cells look like under a microscope. Nonsmall cell lung cancer is more common than small cell lung cancer.

Section 26.2

Staging and Treating Small Cell Lung Cancer

This section includes text excerpted from "Small Cell Lung Cancer Treatment (PDQ®)—Patient Version," National Cancer Institute (NCI), March 30, 2018.

Stages of Small Cell Lung Cancer

After small cell lung cancer has been diagnosed, tests are done to find out if cancer cells have spread within the chest or to other parts of the body. The process used to find out if cancer has spread within the chest or to other parts of the body is called staging. The information gathered from the staging process determines the stage of the disease. It is important to know the stage in order to plan treatment. Some of the tests used to diagnose small cell lung cancer are also used to stage the disease.

Other tests and procedures that may be used in the staging process include the following:

- **Magnetic resonance imaging (MRI) of the brain:** A procedure that uses a magnet, radio waves, and a computer to make a series of detailed pictures of areas inside the body. This procedure is also called nuclear magnetic resonance imaging (NMRI).

- **Computed tomography (CT) scan:** A procedure that makes a series of detailed pictures of areas inside the body, such as the brain, chest or upper abdomen, taken from different angles. The pictures are made by a computer linked to an X-ray machine. A dye may be injected into a vein or swallowed to help the organs or tissues show up more clearly. This procedure is also called computed tomography, computerized tomography, or computerized axial tomography.

- **Positron emission tomography (PET) scan:** A procedure to find malignant tumor cells in the body. A small amount of radioactive glucose (sugar) is injected into a vein. The PET scanner rotates around the body and makes a picture of where glucose is being used in the body. Malignant tumor cells show up brighter in the picture because they are more active and take up more glucose than normal cells do. A PET scan and CT scan may be done at the same time. This is called a PET-CT.

- **Bone scan:** A procedure to check if there are rapidly dividing cells, such as cancer cells, in the bone. A very small amount of radioactive material is injected into a vein and travels through the bloodstream. The radioactive material collects in the bones with cancer and is detected by a scanner.

The following stages are used for small cell lung cancer:

Limited-Stage Small Cell Lung Cancer

In limited-stage, cancer is in the lung where it started and may have spread to the area between the lungs or to the lymph nodes above the collarbone.

Extensive-Stage Small Cell Lung Cancer

In extensive-stage, cancer has spread beyond the lung or the area between the lungs or the lymph nodes above the collarbone to other places in the body.

Treatment Option Overview

Different types of treatment are available for patients with small cell lung cancer. Some treatments are standard (the currently used treatment), and some are being tested in clinical trials. A treatment clinical trial is a research study meant to help improve current treatments or obtain information on new treatments for patients with cancer. When clinical trials show that a new treatment is better than the standard treatment, the new treatment may become the standard treatment. Patients may want to think about taking part in a clinical trial. Some clinical trials are open only to patients who have not started treatment.

Five types of standard treatment are used:

Surgery

Surgery may be used if the cancer is found in one lung and in nearby lymph nodes only. Because this type of lung cancer is usually found in both lungs, surgery alone is not often used. During surgery, the doctor will also remove lymph nodes to find out if they have cancer in them. Sometimes, surgery may be used to remove a sample of lung tissue to find out the exact type of lung cancer.

Even if the doctor removes all the cancer that can be seen at the time of the operation, some patients may be given chemotherapy or radiation therapy after surgery to kill any cancer cells that are left. Treatment given after the surgery, to lower the risk that the cancer will come back, is called adjuvant therapy.

Chemotherapy

Chemotherapy is a cancer treatment that uses drugs to stop the growth of cancer cells, either by killing the cells or by stopping them from dividing. When chemotherapy is taken by mouth or injected into a vein or muscle, the drugs enter the bloodstream and can reach cancer cells throughout the body (systemic chemotherapy). When chemotherapy is placed directly into the cerebrospinal fluid, an organ, or a body cavity such as the abdomen, the drugs mainly affect cancer cells in those areas (regional chemotherapy). The way the chemotherapy is given depends on the type and stage of the cancer being treated.

Radiation Therapy

Radiation therapy is a cancer treatment that uses high-energy X-rays or other types of radiation to kill cancer cells or keep them from growing. There are two types of radiation therapy:

- External radiation therapy uses a machine outside the body to send radiation toward the cancer.

- Internal radiation therapy uses a radioactive substance sealed in needles, seeds, wires, or catheters that are placed directly into or near the cancer.

The way the radiation therapy is given depends on the type and stage of the cancer being treated. External radiation therapy is used to treat small cell lung cancer, and may also be used as palliative therapy to relieve symptoms and improve quality of life. Radiation therapy to the brain to lessen the risk that cancer will spread to the brain may also be given.

Laser Therapy

Laser therapy is a cancer treatment that uses a laser beam (a narrow beam of intense light) to kill cancer cells.

Endoscopic Stent Placement

An endoscope is a thin, tube-like instrument used to look at tissues inside the body. An endoscope has a light and a lens for viewing and may be used to place a stent in a body structure to keep the structure open. An endoscopic stent can be used to open an airway blocked by abnormal tissue.

Section 26.3

Staging and Treating Nonsmall Cell Lung Cancer

This section includes text excerpted from "Non-Small Cell Lung Cancer Treatment (PDQ®)—Patient Version," National Cancer Institute (NCI), March 30, 2018.

Stages of Nonsmall Cell Lung Cancer

After lung cancer has been diagnosed, tests are done to find out if cancer cells have spread within the lungs or to other parts of the body. The process used to find out if cancer has spread within the lungs or to other parts of the body is called staging. The information gathered from the staging process determines the stage of the disease. It is important to know the stage in order to plan treatment. Some of the tests used to diagnose nonsmall cell lung cancer are also used to stage the disease.

Other tests and procedures that may be used in the staging process include the following:

- **Magnetic resonance imaging (MRI):** A procedure that uses a magnet, radio waves, and a computer to make a series of detailed pictures of areas inside the body, such as the brain. This procedure is also called nuclear magnetic resonance imaging (NMRI).

- **Computed tomography (CT) scan:** A procedure that makes a series of detailed pictures of areas inside the body, such as the brain and abdomen, taken from different angles. The pictures are made by a computer linked to an X-ray machine. A dye may be injected into a vein or swallowed to help the organs or tissues show up more clearly. This procedure is also called computed tomography, computerized tomography, or computerized axial tomography.

- **Positron emission tomography (PET) scan:** A procedure to find malignant tumor cells in the body. A small amount of radioactive glucose (sugar) is injected into a vein. The PET scanner rotates around the body and makes a picture of where glucose is being used in the body. Malignant tumor cells show up brighter in the picture because they are more active and take up more glucose than normal cells do.

- **Radionuclide bone scan:** A procedure to check if there are rapidly dividing cells, such as cancer cells, in the bone. A very small amount of radioactive material is injected into a vein and travels through the bloodstream. The radioactive material collects in the bones and is detected by a scanner.

- **Pulmonary function test (PFT):** A test to see how well the lungs are working. It measures how much air the lungs can hold and how quickly air moves into and out of the lungs. It also measures how much oxygen is used and how much carbon dioxide is given off during breathing. This is also called lung function test.

- **Endoscopic ultrasound (EUS):** A procedure in which an endoscope is inserted into the body. An endoscope is a thin, tube-like instrument with a light and a lens for viewing. A probe at the end of the endoscope is used to bounce high-energy sound waves (ultrasound) off internal tissues or organs and make echoes. The echoes form a picture of body tissues called a sonogram. This procedure is also called endosonography. EUS may be used to guide fine needle aspiration (FNA) biopsy of the lung, lymph nodes, or other areas.

- **Mediastinoscopy:** A surgical procedure to look at the organs, tissues, and lymph nodes between the lungs for abnormal areas. An incision (cut) is made at the top of the breastbone and a mediastinoscope is inserted into the chest. A mediastinoscope is a thin, tube-like instrument with a light and a lens for viewing. It may also have a tool to remove tissue or lymph node samples, which are checked under a microscope for signs of cancer.

- **Anterior mediastinotomy:** A surgical procedure to look at the organs and tissues between the lungs and between the breastbone and heart for abnormal areas. An incision (cut) is made next to the breastbone and a mediastinoscope is inserted into the chest. A mediastinoscope is a thin, tube-like instrument with a light and a lens for viewing. It may also have a tool to remove tissue or lymph node samples, which are checked under a microscope for signs of cancer. This is also called the Chamberlain procedure.

- **Lymph node biopsy:** The removal of all or part of a lymph node. A pathologist views the tissue under a microscope to look for cancer cells.

- **Bone marrow aspiration and biopsy:** The removal of bone marrow, blood, and a small piece of bone by inserting a hollow needle into the hipbone or breastbone. A pathologist views the bone marrow, blood, and bone under a microscope to look for signs of cancer.

Occult (Hidden) Stage

In the occult (hidden) stage, cancer cannot be seen by imaging or bronchoscopy. Cancer cells are found in sputum (mucus coughed up from the lungs) or bronchial washing (a sample of cells taken from inside the airways that lead to the lung). Cancer may have spread to other parts of the body.

Stage 0 (Carcinoma in Situ)

In stage 0, abnormal cells are found in the lining of the airways. These abnormal cells may become cancer and spread into nearby normal tissue. Stage 0 is also called carcinoma in situ.

Stage I

In stage I, cancer has formed. Stage I is divided into stages IA and IB:

- **Stage IA:** The tumor is in the lung only and is 3 centimeters or smaller.

- **Stage IB:** Cancer has not spread to the lymph nodes and one or more of the following is true:

  - The tumor is larger than 3 centimeters but not larger than 5 centimeters.

- Cancer has spread to the main bronchus and is at least 2 centimeters below where the trachea joins the bronchus.

- Cancer has spread to the innermost layer of the membrane that covers the lung.

- Part of the lung has collapsed or developed pneumonitis (inflammation of the lung) in the area where the trachea joins the bronchus.

Stage II

Stage II is divided into stages IIA and IIB. Stage IIA and IIB are each divided into two sections depending on the size of the tumor, where the tumor is found, and whether there is cancer in the lymph nodes.

Stage IIA

1. Cancer has spread to lymph nodes on the same side of the chest as the tumor. The lymph nodes with cancer are within the lung or near the bronchus. Also, one or more of the following is true:

   - The tumor is not larger than 5 centimeters.

   - Cancer has spread to the main bronchus and is at least 2 centimeters below where the trachea joins the bronchus.

   - Cancer has spread to the innermost layer of the membrane that covers the lung.

   - Part of the lung has collapsed or developed pneumonitis (inflammation of the lung) in the area where the trachea joins the bronchus.

   or

2. Cancer has not spread to lymph nodes and one or more of the following is true:

   - The tumor is larger than 5 centimeters but not larger than 7 centimeters.

   - Cancer has spread to the main bronchus and is at least 2 centimeters below where the trachea joins the bronchus.

   - Cancer has spread to the innermost layer of the membrane that covers the lung.

- Part of the lung has collapsed or developed pneumonitis (inflammation of the lung) in the area where the trachea joins the bronchus.

Stage IIB

1. Cancer has spread to nearby lymph nodes on the same side of the chest as the tumor. The lymph nodes with cancer are within the lung or near the bronchus. Also, one or more of the following is true:

   - The tumor is larger than 5 centimeters but not larger than 7 centimeters.
   - Cancer has spread to the main bronchus and is at least 2 centimeters below where the trachea joins the bronchus.
   - Cancer has spread to the innermost layer of the membrane that covers the lung.
   - Part of the lung has collapsed or developed pneumonitis (inflammation of the lung) in the area where the trachea joins the bronchus.

   or

2. Cancer has not spread to lymph nodes and one or more of the following is true:

   - The tumor is larger than 7 centimeters.
   - Cancer has spread to the main bronchus (and is less than 2 centimeters below where the trachea joins the bronchus), the chest wall, the diaphragm, or the nerve that controls the diaphragm.
   - Cancer has spread to the membrane around the heart or lining the chest wall.
   - The whole lung has collapsed or developed pneumonitis (inflammation of the lung).
   - There are one or more separate tumors in the same lobe of the lung.

Stage III

Stage IIIA

Stage IIIA is divided into three sections depending on the size of the tumor, where the tumor is found, and which lymph nodes have cancer (if any).

1. Cancer has spread to lymph nodes on the same side of the chest as the tumor. The lymph nodes with cancer are near the sternum (chest bone) or where the bronchus enters the lung. Also:

   - The tumor may be any size.

   - Part of the lung (where the trachea joins the bronchus) or the whole lung may have collapsed or developed pneumonitis (inflammation of the lung).

   - There may be one or more separate tumors in the same lobe of the lung.

   - Cancer may have spread to any of the following:

      - Main bronchus, but not the area where the trachea joins the bronchus

      - Chest wall

      - Diaphragm and the nerve that controls it

      - Membrane around the lung or lining the chest wall

      - Membrane around the heart

   or

2. Cancer has spread to lymph nodes on the same side of the chest as the tumor. The lymph nodes with cancer are within the lung or near the bronchus. Also:

   - The tumor may be any size.

   - The whole lung may have collapsed or developed pneumonitis (inflammation of the lung).

   - There may be one or more separate tumors in any of the lobes of the lung with cancer.

   - Cancer may have spread to any of the following:

      - Main bronchus, but not the area where the trachea joins the bronchus

      - Chest wall

      - Diaphragm and the nerve that controls it

      - Membrane around the lung or lining the chest wall

      - Heart or the membrane around it

- Major blood vessels that lead to or from the heart
- Trachea
- Esophagus
- Nerve that controls the larynx (voice box)
- Sternum (chest bone) or backbone
- Carina (where the trachea joins the bronchi)

or

3. Cancer has not spread to the lymph nodes and the tumor may be any size. Cancer has spread to any of the following:

- Heart
- Major blood vessels that lead to or from the heart
- Trachea
- Esophagus
- Nerve that controls the larynx (voice box)
- Sternum (chest bone) or backbone
- Carina (where the trachea joins the bronchi)

Stage IIIB

Stage IIIB is divided into two sections depending on the size of the tumor, where the tumor is found, and which lymph nodes have cancer.

1. Cancer has spread to lymph nodes above the collarbone or to lymph nodes on the opposite side of the chest as the tumor. Also:

- The tumor may be any size.
- Part of the lung (where the trachea joins the bronchus) or the whole lung may have collapsed or developed pneumonitis (inflammation of the lung).
- There may be one or more separate tumors in any of the lobes of the lung with cancer.
- Cancer may have spread to any of the following:
  - Main bronchus
  - Chest wall

- Diaphragm and the nerve that controls it
- Membrane around the lung or lining the chest wall
- Heart or the membrane around it
- Major blood vessels that lead to or from the heart
- Trachea
- Esophagus
- Nerve that controls the larynx (voice box)
- Sternum (chest bone) or backbone
- Carina (where the trachea joins the bronchi)

or

2. Cancer has spread to lymph nodes on the same side of the chest as the tumor. The lymph nodes with cancer are near the sternum (chest bone) or where the bronchus enters the lung. Also:

- The tumor may be any size.
- There may be separate tumors in different lobes of the same lung.
- Cancer has spread to any of the following:
  - Heart
  - Major blood vessels that lead to or from the heart
  - Trachea
  - Esophagus
  - Nerve that controls the larynx (voice box)
  - Sternum (chest bone) or backbone
  - Carina (where the trachea joins the bronchi)

Stage IV

In stage IV, the tumor may be any size and cancer may have spread to lymph nodes. One or more of the following is true:

- There are one or more tumors in both lungs.
- Cancer is found in fluid around the lungs or the heart.

319

- Cancer has spread to other parts of the body, such as the brain, liver, adrenal glands, kidneys, or bone.

Treatment Option Overview

Different types of treatments are available for patients with non-small cell lung cancer. Some treatments are standard (the currently used treatment), and some are being tested in clinical trials. A treatment clinical trial is a research study meant to help improve current treatments or obtain information on new treatments for patients with cancer. When clinical trials show that a new treatment is better than the standard treatment, the new treatment may become the standard treatment. Patients may want to think about taking part in a clinical trial. Some clinical trials are open only to patients who have not started treatment.

Nine types of standard treatment are used:

Surgery

Four types of surgery are used to treat lung cancer:

- **Wedge resection:** Surgery to remove a tumor and some of the normal tissue around it. When a slightly larger amount of tissue is taken, it is called a segmental resection.

- **Lobectomy:** Surgery to remove a whole lobe (section) of the lung.

- **Pneumonectomy:** Surgery to remove one whole lung.

- **Sleeve resection:** Surgery to remove part of the bronchus.

Even if the doctor removes all the cancer that can be seen at the time of the surgery, some patients may be given chemotherapy or radiation therapy after surgery to kill any cancer cells that are left. Treatment given after the surgery, to lower the risk that the cancer will come back, is called adjuvant therapy.

Radiation Therapy

Radiation therapy is a cancer treatment that uses high-energy X-rays or other types of radiation to kill cancer cells or keep them from growing. There are two types of radiation therapy:

- External radiation therapy uses a machine outside the body to send radiation toward the cancer.

- Internal radiation therapy uses a radioactive substance sealed in needles, seeds, wires, or catheters that are placed directly into or near the cancer.

Stereotactic body radiation therapy (SBRT) is a type of external radiation therapy. Special equipment is used to place the patient in the same position for each radiation treatment. Once a day for several days, a radiation machine aims a larger than usual dose of radiation directly at the tumor. By having the patient in the same position for each treatment, there is less damage to nearby healthy tissue. This procedure is also called stereotactic external-beam radiation therapy (EBRT) and stereotaxic radiation therapy.

Stereotactic radiosurgery (SRS) is a type of external radiation therapy used to treat lung cancer that has spread to the brain. A rigid head frame is attached to the skull to keep the head still during the radiation treatment. A machine aims a single large dose of radiation directly at the tumor in the brain. This procedure does not involve surgery. It is also called stereotaxic radiosurgery, radiosurgery, and radiation surgery.

For tumors in the airways, radiation is given directly to the tumor through an endoscope.

The way the radiation therapy is given depends on the type and stage of the cancer being treated. It also depends on where the cancer is found. External and internal radiation therapy are used to treat nonsmall cell lung cancer.

Chemotherapy

Chemotherapy is a cancer treatment that uses drugs to stop the growth of cancer cells, either by killing the cells or by stopping them from dividing. When chemotherapy is taken by mouth or injected into a vein or muscle, the drugs enter the bloodstream and can reach cancer cells throughout the body (systemic chemotherapy). When chemotherapy is placed directly into the cerebrospinal fluid, an organ, or a body cavity such as the abdomen, the drugs mainly affect cancer cells in those areas (regional chemotherapy). The way the chemotherapy is given depends on the type and stage of the cancer being treated.

Targeted Therapy

Targeted therapy is a type of treatment that uses drugs or other substances to attack specific cancer cells. Targeted therapies usually cause less harm to normal cells than chemotherapy or radiation therapy do. Monoclonal antibodies (mAbs) and tyrosine kinase inhibitors (TKIs) are the two main types of targeted therapy being used to treat advanced, metastatic, or recurrent nonsmall cell lung cancer.

Monoclonal Antibodies

Monoclonal antibody therapy is a cancer treatment that uses antibodies made in the laboratory from a single type of immune system cell. These antibodies can identify substances on cancer cells or normal substances in the blood or tissues that may help cancer cells grow. The antibodies attach to the substances and kill the cancer cells, block their growth, or keep them from spreading. Monoclonal antibodies are given by infusion. They may be used alone or to carry drugs, toxins, or radioactive material directly to cancer cells.

There are different types of monoclonal antibody therapy:

- **Vascular endothelial growth factor (VEGF) inhibitor therapy:** Cancer cells make a substance called VEGF, which causes new blood vessels to form (angiogenesis) and helps the cancer grow. VEGF inhibitors block VEGF and stop new blood vessels from forming. This may kill cancer cells because they need new blood vessels to grow. Bevacizumab and ramucirumab are VEGF inhibitors and angiogenesis inhibitors.

- **Epidermal growth factor receptor (EGFR) inhibitor therapy:** EGFRs are proteins found on the surface of certain cells, including cancer cells. Epidermal growth factor attaches to the EGFR on the surface of the cell and causes the cells to grow and divide. EGFR inhibitors block the receptor and stop the epidermal growth factor from attaching to the cancer cell. This stops the cancer cell from growing and dividing. Cetuximab and necitumumab are EGFR inhibitors.

- **Immune checkpoint inhibitor therapy:** PD-1 is a protein on the surface of T cells that helps keep the body's immune responses in check. When PD-1 attaches to another protein called PDL-1 on a cancer cell, it stops the T cell from killing the cancer cell. PD-1 inhibitors attach to PDL-1 and allow the T cells to kill cancer cells. Nivolumab, pembrolizumab, and atezolizumab are types of immune checkpoint inhibitors.

Tyrosine Kinase Inhibitors (TKIs)

Tyrosine kinase inhibitors are small-molecule drugs that go through the cell membrane and work inside cancer cells to block signals that cancer cells need to grow and divide. Some tyrosine kinase inhibitors also have angiogenesis inhibitor effects.

There are different types of tyrosine kinase inhibitors:

- **Epidermal growth factor receptor (EGFR) tyrosine kinase inhibitors:** EGFRs are proteins found on the surface and inside certain cells, including cancer cells. Epidermal growth factor attaches to the EGFR inside the cell and sends signals to the tyrosine kinase area of the cell, which tells the cell to grow and divide. EGFR tyrosine kinase inhibitors stop these signals and stop the cancer cell from growing and dividing. Erlotinib, gefitinib, and afatinib are types of EGFR tyrosine kinase inhibitors. Some of these drugs work better when there is also a mutation (change) in the *EGFR* gene.

- **Kinase inhibitors that affect cells with certain gene changes:** Certain changes in the *ALK* and *ROS1* genes cause too much protein to be made. Blocking these proteins may stop the cancer from growing and spreading. Crizotinib is used to stop proteins from being made by the *ALK* and *ROS1* gene. Ceritinib is used to stop proteins from being made by the *ALK* gene.

Laser Therapy

Laser therapy is a cancer treatment that uses a laser beam (a narrow beam of intense light) to kill cancer cells.

Photodynamic Therapy (PDT)

Photodynamic therapy (PDT) is a cancer treatment that uses a drug and a certain type of laser light to kill cancer cells. A drug that is not active until it is exposed to light is injected into a vein. The drug collects more in cancer cells than in normal cells. Fiber-optic tubes are then used to carry the laser light to the cancer cells, where the drug becomes active and kills the cells. Photodynamic therapy causes little damage to healthy tissue. It is used mainly to treat tumors on or just under the skin or in the lining of internal organs. When the tumor is in the airways, PDT is given directly to the tumor through an endoscope.

Cryosurgery

Cryosurgery is a treatment that uses an instrument to freeze and destroy abnormal tissue, such as carcinoma in situ. This type of treatment is also called cryotherapy. For tumors in the airways, cryosurgery is done through an endoscope.

Electrocautery

Electrocautery is a treatment that uses a probe or needle heated by an electric current to destroy abnormal tissue. For tumors in the airways, electrocautery is done through an endoscope.

Watchful Waiting

Watchful waiting is closely monitoring a patient's condition without giving any treatment until signs or symptoms appear or change. This may be done in certain rare cases of nonsmall cell lung cancer.

Chapter 27

Pancreatic Cancer

Pancreatic cancer is a disease in which malignant (cancer) cells form in the tissues of the pancreas. The pancreas is a gland about 6 inches long that is shaped like a thin pear lying on its side. The wider end of the pancreas is called the head, the middle section is called the body, and the narrow end is called the tail. The pancreas lies between the stomach and the spine.

The pancreas has two main jobs in the body:

- To make juices that help digest (break down) food

- To make hormones, such as insulin and glucagon, that help control blood sugar levels. Both of these hormones help the body use and store the energy it gets from food

The digestive juices are made by exocrine pancreas cells and the hormones are made by endocrine pancreas cells. About 95 percent of pancreatic cancers begin in exocrine cells.

Risk Factors for Pancreatic Cancer

Smoking and health history can affect the risk of pancreatic cancer. Anything that increases your risk of getting a disease is called a risk factor. Having a risk factor does not mean that you will get cancer; not having risk factors doesn't mean that you will not get cancer. Talk with your doctor if you think you may be at risk.

This chapter includes text excerpted from "Pancreatic Cancer Treatment (PDQ®)—Patient Version," National Cancer Institute (NCI), March 30, 2018.

Risk factors for pancreatic cancer include the following:

- Tobacco use

- Being very overweight

- Having a personal history of diabetes or chronic pancreatitis

- Having a family history of pancreatic cancer or pancreatitis

- Having certain hereditary conditions, such as:

  - Multiple endocrine neoplasia type 1 (MEN1) syndrome

  - Hereditary nonpolyposis colon cancer (HNPCC; Lynch syndrome)

  - von Hippel-Lindau syndrome (VHL)

  - Peutz-Jeghers syndrome (PJS)

  - Hereditary breast and ovarian cancer syndrome

  - Familial atypical multiple mole melanoma (FAMMM) syndrome

Signs and Symptoms of Pancreatic Cancer

Pancreatic cancer may not cause early signs or symptoms. Signs and symptoms may be caused by pancreatic cancer or by other conditions. Check with your doctor if you have any of the following:

- Jaundice (yellowing of the skin and whites of the eyes)

- Light-colored stools

- Dark urine

- Pain in the upper or middle abdomen and back

- Weight loss for no known reason

- Loss of appetite

- Feeling very tired

Diagnosing Pancreatic Cancer

Pancreatic cancer is difficult to detect and diagnose for the following reasons:

- There aren't any noticeable signs or symptoms in the early stages of pancreatic cancer.

- The signs and symptoms of pancreatic cancer, when present, are like the signs and symptoms of many other illnesses.

- The pancreas is hidden behind other organs such as the stomach, small intestine, liver, gallbladder, spleen, and bile ducts.

Tests to Detect Pancreatic Cancer

Pancreatic cancer is usually diagnosed with tests and procedures that make pictures of the pancreas and the area around it. The process used to find out if cancer cells have spread within and around the pancreas is called staging. Tests and procedures to detect, diagnose, and stage pancreatic cancer are usually done at the same time. In order to plan treatment, it is important to know the stage of the disease and whether or not the pancreatic cancer can be removed by surgery.

The following tests and procedures may be used:

- **Physical exam and history.** An exam of the body to check general signs of health, including checking for signs of disease, such as lumps or anything else that seems unusual. A history of the patient's health habits and past illnesses and treatments will also be taken.

- **Blood chemistry studies.** A procedure in which a blood sample is checked to measure the amounts of certain substances, such as bilirubin, released into the blood by organs and tissues in the body. An unusual (higher or lower than normal) amount of a substance can be a sign of disease.

- **Tumor marker test.** A procedure in which a sample of blood, urine, or tissue is checked to measure the amounts of certain substances, such as CA 19-9, and carcinoembryonic antigen (CEA), made by organs, tissues, or tumor cells in the body. Certain substances are linked to specific types of cancer when found in increased levels in the body. These are called tumor markers.

- **Magnetic resonance imaging (MRI).** A procedure that uses a magnet, radio waves, and a computer to make a series of detailed pictures of areas inside the body. This procedure is also called nuclear magnetic resonance imaging (NMRI).

- **Computerized axial tomography (CAT) scan.** A procedure that makes a series of detailed pictures of areas inside the

327

body, taken from different angles. The pictures are made by a computer linked to an X-ray machine. A dye may be injected into a vein or swallowed to help the organs or tissues show up more clearly. This procedure is also called computed tomography, computerized tomography, or computerized axial tomography. A spiral or helical CT scan makes a series of very detailed pictures of areas inside the body using an X-ray machine that scans the body in a spiral path.

- **Positron emission tomography (PET) scan.** A procedure to find malignant tumor cells in the body. A small amount of radioactive glucose (sugar) is injected into a vein. The PET scanner rotates around the body and makes a picture of where glucose is being used in the body. Malignant tumor cells show up brighter in the picture because they are more active and take up more glucose than normal cells do. A PET scan and CT scan may be done at the same time. This is called a PET-CT.

- **Abdominal ultrasound.** An ultrasound exam used to make pictures of the inside of the abdomen. The ultrasound transducer is pressed against the skin of the abdomen and directs high-energy sound waves (ultrasound) into the abdomen. The sound waves bounce off the internal tissues and organs and make echoes. The transducer receives the echoes and sends them to a computer, which uses the echoes to make pictures called sonograms. The picture can be printed to be looked at later.

- **Endoscopic ultrasound (EUS).** A procedure in which an endoscope is inserted into the body, usually through the mouth or rectum. An endoscope is a thin, tube-like instrument with a light and a lens for viewing. A probe at the end of the endoscope is used to bounce high-energy sound waves (ultrasound) off internal tissues or organs and make echoes. The echoes form a picture of body tissues called a sonogram. This procedure is also called endosonography.

- **Endoscopic retrograde cholangiopancreatography (ERCP).** A procedure used to X-ray the ducts (tubes) that carry bile from the liver to the gallbladder and from the gallbladder to the small intestine. Sometimes pancreatic cancer causes these ducts to narrow and block or slow the flow of bile, causing jaundice. An endoscope (a thin, lighted tube) is passed through the mouth, esophagus, and stomach into the first part of the small intestine. A catheter (a smaller tube) is then inserted through the endoscope into the pancreatic ducts. A dye is injected through the catheter into the ducts and an X-ray is taken. If the ducts are blocked by a tumor, a fine tube may be inserted into the duct to unblock it. This tube (or stent) may be left in place to keep the duct open. Tissue samples may also be taken.

- **Percutaneous transhepatic cholangiography (PTC).** A procedure used to X-ray the liver and bile ducts. A thin needle is inserted through the skin below the ribs and into the liver. Dye is injected into the liver or bile ducts and an X-ray is taken. If a blockage is found, a thin, flexible tube called a stent is sometimes left in the liver to drain bile into the small intestine or a collection bag outside the body. This test is done only if ERCP cannot be done.

- **Laparoscopy.** A surgical procedure to look at the organs inside the abdomen to check for signs of disease. Small incisions (cuts) are made in the wall of the abdomen and a laparoscope (a thin, lighted tube) is inserted into one of the incisions. The laparoscope may have an ultrasound probe at the end in order to bounce high-energy sound waves off internal organs, such as the pancreas. This is called laparoscopic ultrasound. Other instruments may be inserted through the same or other incisions to perform procedures such as taking tissue samples from the pancreas or a sample of fluid from the abdomen to check for cancer.

- **Biopsy.** The removal of cells or tissues so they can be viewed under a microscope by a pathologist to check for signs of cancer. There are several ways to do a biopsy for pancreatic cancer. A fine needle or a core needle may be inserted into the pancreas during an X-ray or ultrasound to remove cells. Tissue may also be removed during a laparoscopy or surgery to remove the tumor.

Stages of Pancreatic Cancer

Tests and procedures to stage pancreatic cancer are usually done at the same time as diagnosis. The process used to find out if cancer has spread within the pancreas or to other parts of the body is called staging. The information gathered from the staging process determines the stage of the disease. It is important to know the stage of the disease in order to plan treatment. The results of some of the tests used to diagnose pancreatic cancer are often also used to stage the disease.

Stage 0 (Carcinoma in Situ)

In stage 0, abnormal cells are found in the lining of the pancreas. These abnormal cells may become cancer and spread into nearby normal tissue. Stage 0 is also called carcinoma in situ.

Stage I

In stage I, cancer has formed and is found in the pancreas only. Stage I is divided into stage IA and stage IB, based on the size of the tumor.

- **Stage IA:** The tumor is 2 centimeters or smaller.
- **Stage IB:** The tumor is larger than 2 centimeters.

Stage II

In stage II, cancer may have spread to nearby tissue and organs, and may have spread to lymph nodes near the pancreas. Stage II is divided into stage IIA and stage IIB, based on where the cancer has spread.

- **Stage IIA:** Cancer has spread to nearby tissue and organs but has not spread to nearby lymph nodes.
- **Stage IIB:** Cancer has spread to nearby lymph nodes and may have spread to nearby tissue and organs.

Stage III

In stage III, cancer has spread to the major blood vessels near the pancreas and may have spread to nearby lymph nodes.

Stage IV

In stage IV, cancer may be of any size and has spread to distant organs, such as the liver, lung, and peritoneal cavity. It may have also spread to organs and tissues near the pancreas or to lymph nodes.

Treatment Option Overview

Different types of treatment are available for patients with pancreatic cancer. Some treatments are standard (the currently used treatment), and some are being tested in clinical trials. A treatment clinical trial is a research study meant to help improve current treatments or obtain information on new treatments for patients with cancer. When clinical trials show that a new treatment is better than the standard treatment, the new treatment may become the standard treatment. Patients may want to think about taking part in a clinical trial. Some clinical trials are open only to patients who have not started treatment.

Surgery

One of the following types of surgery may be used to take out the tumor:

- **Whipple procedure:** A surgical procedure in which the head of the pancreas, the gallbladder, part of the stomach, part of the small intestine, and the bile duct are removed. Enough of the pancreas is left to produce digestive juices and insulin.

- **Total pancreatectomy:** This operation removes the whole pancreas, part of the stomach, part of the small intestine, the common bile duct, the gallbladder, the spleen, and nearby lymph nodes.

- **Distal pancreatectomy:** Surgery to remove the body and the tail of the pancreas. The spleen may also be removed if cancer has spread to the spleen.

If the cancer has spread and cannot be removed, the following types of palliative surgery may be done to relieve symptoms and improve quality of life:

- **Biliary bypass:** If cancer is blocking the bile duct and bile is building up in the gallbladder, a biliary bypass may be done. During this operation, the doctor will cut the gallbladder or bile duct in the area before the blockage and sew it to the small intestine to create a new pathway around the blocked area.

- **Endoscopic stent placement:** If the tumor is blocking the bile duct, surgery may be done to put in a stent (a thin tube) to drain bile that has built up in the area. The doctor may place the stent through a catheter that drains the bile into a bag on the outside of the body or the stent may go around the blocked area and drain the bile into the small intestine.

- **Gastric bypass:** If the tumor is blocking the flow of food from the stomach, the stomach may be sewn directly to the small intestine so the patient can continue to eat normally.

Radiation Therapy

Radiation therapy is a cancer treatment that uses high-energy X-rays or other types of radiation to kill cancer cells or keep them from growing. There are two types of radiation therapy:

- External radiation therapy uses a machine outside the body to send radiation toward the cancer.
- Internal radiation therapy uses a radioactive substance sealed in needles, seeds, wires, or catheters that are placed directly into or near the cancer.

The way the radiation therapy is given depends on the type and stage of the cancer being treated. External radiation therapy is used to treat pancreatic cancer.

Chemotherapy

Chemotherapy is a cancer treatment that uses drugs to stop the growth of cancer cells, either by killing the cells or by stopping them from dividing. When chemotherapy is taken by mouth or injected into a vein or muscle, the drugs enter the bloodstream and can reach cancer cells throughout the body (systemic chemotherapy). When chemotherapy is placed directly into the cerebrospinal fluid, an organ, or a body cavity such as the abdomen, the drugs mainly affect cancer cells in those areas (regional chemotherapy). Combination chemotherapy is treatment using more than one anticancer drug. The way the chemotherapy is given depends on the type and stage of the cancer being treated.

Chemoradiation Therapy

Chemoradiation therapy combines chemotherapy and radiation therapy to increase the effects of both.

Targeted Therapy

Targeted therapy is a type of treatment that uses drugs or other substances to identify and attack specific cancer cells without harming normal cells. Tyrosine kinase inhibitors (TKIs) are targeted therapy drugs that block signals needed for tumors to grow. Erlotinib is a type of TKI used to treat pancreatic cancer.

Follow-Up Tests May Be Needed

Some of the tests that were done to diagnose the cancer or to find out the stage of the cancer may be repeated. Some tests will be repeated in order to see how well the treatment is working. Decisions about whether to continue, change, or stop treatment may be based on the results of these tests. Some of the tests will continue to be done from time to time after treatment has ended. The results of these tests can show if your condition has changed or if the cancer has recurred (come back). These tests are sometimes called follow-up tests or check-ups.

Chapter 28

Skin Cancer

Chapter Contents

Section 28.1

Facts about Skin Cancer

This section includes text excerpted from "Skin Cancer,"
Center for Disease Control and Prevention (CDC), April 23, 2018.

What Is Skin Cancer?

Skin cancer is the most common form of cancer in the United States. The two most common types of skin cancer—basal cell and squamous cell carcinomas—are highly curable, but can be disfiguring and costly to treat. Melanoma, the third most common skin cancer, is more dangerous and causes the most deaths. The majority of these three types of skin cancer are caused by overexposure to ultraviolet (UV) light.

Ultraviolet (UV) Light

Ultraviolet (UV) rays are an invisible kind of radiation that comes from the sun, tanning beds, and sunlamps. UV rays can penetrate and change skin cells.

The three types of UV rays are ultraviolet A (UVA), ultraviolet B (UVB), and ultraviolet C (UVC):

- More UVA rays reach the earth's surface than the other types of UV rays. UVA rays can reach deep into human skin, UVA rays can damaging connective tissue and the skin's deoxyribonucleic acid (DNA).

- Most UVB rays are absorbed by the ozone layer, so fewer of them reach the earth's surface compared to UVA rays. UVB rays, which help produce vitamin D in the skin, don't reach as far into the skin as UVA rays, but they can still cause sunburn and damage DNA.

- UVC rays are very dangerous, but they are absorbed completely by the ozone layer and do not reach the earth's surface.

In addition to causing sunburn, too much exposure to UV rays can change skin texture, cause the skin to age prematurely, and can lead to skin cancer. UV rays also have been linked to eye conditions such as cataracts.

The National Weather Service (NWS) and the U.S. Environmental Protection Agency (EPA) developed the UV Index to forecast the risk of overexposure to UV rays. It lets you know how much caution you should take when spending time outdoors.

The UV Index predicts exposure levels on a 0–15 scale; higher levels indicate a higher risk of overexposure. Calculated on a next-day basis for dozens of cities across the United States, the UV Index takes into account clouds and other local conditions that affect the amount of UV rays reaching the ground.

What Are the Risk Factors for Skin Cancer?

People with certain risk factors are more likely than others to develop skin cancer. Risk factors vary for different types of skin cancer, but some general risk factors are having:

- A lighter natural skin color
- Family history of skin cancer
- A personal history of skin cancer
- Exposure to the sun through work and play
- A history of sunburns, especially early in life
- A history of indoor tanning
- Skin that burns, freckles, reddens easily, or becomes painful in the sun
- Blue or green eyes
- Blond or red hair
- Certain types and a large number of moles

Tanning and Burning

Ultraviolet (UV) rays come from the sun or from indoor tanning (using a tanning bed, booth, or sunlamp to get tan). When UV rays reach the skin's inner layer, the skin makes more melanin. Melanin is the pigment that colors the skin. It moves toward the outer layers of the skin and becomes visible as a tan.

A tan does not indicate good health. A tan is a response to injury, because skin cells signal that they have been hurt by UV rays by producing more pigment.

People burn or tan depending on their skin type, the time of year, and how long they are exposed to UV rays. The six types of skin, based on how likely it is to tan or burn, are:

- Always burns, never tans

- Burns easily, tans minimally

- Burns moderately, tans gradually to light brown

- Burns minimally, always tans well to moderately brown

- Rarely burns, tans profusely to dark

- Never burns, deeply pigmented, least sensitive

Although everyone's skin can be damaged by UV exposure, people with skin types I and II are at the highest risk.

What Are the Symptoms of Skin Cancer?

A change in your skin is the most common sign of skin cancer. This could be a new growth, a sore that doesn't heal, or a change in a mole. Not all skin cancers look the same.

A simple way to remember the signs of melanoma is to remember the A-B-C-D-Es of melanoma:

- "A" stands for asymmetrical. Does the mole or spot have an irregular shape with two parts that look very different?

- "B" stands for border. Is the border irregular or jagged?

- "C" is for color. Is the color uneven?

- "D" is for diameter. Is the mole or spot larger than the size of a pea?

- "E" is for evolving. Has the mole or spot changed during the past few weeks or months?

Talk to your doctor if you notice changes in your skin such as a new growth, a sore that doesn't heal, a change in an old growth, or any of the A-B-C-D-Es of melanoma.

What Can I Do to Reduce My Risk of Skin Cancer?

Protection from ultraviolet (UV) radiation is important all year round, not just during the summer or at the beach. UV rays from the sun can reach you on cloudy and hazy days, as well as bright and sunny days. UV rays also reflect off of surfaces like water, cement, sand, and snow. Indoor tanning (using a tanning bed, booth, or sunlamp to get tan) exposes users to UV radiation.

The hours between 10 a.m. and 4 p.m. Daylight Saving Time (DST) (9 a.m. to 3 p.m. standard time) are the most hazardous for UV exposure outdoors in the continental United States. UV rays from sunlight are the greatest during the late spring and early summer in North America.

Center for Disease Prevention and Control (CDC) recommends easy options for protection from UV radiation:

- Stay in the shade, especially during midday hours.

- Wear clothing that covers your arms and legs.

- Wear a hat with a wide brim to shade your face, head, ears, and neck.

- Wear sunglasses that wrap around and block both UVA and UVB rays.

- Use sunscreen with a sun protection factor (SPF) of 15 or higher, and both UVA and UVB (broad spectrum) protection.

- Avoid indoor tanning.

Section 28.2

Diagnosing and Treating Melanoma

This section includes text excerpted from "Melanoma Treatment (PDQ®)—Patient Version," National Cancer Institute (NCI), March 12, 2018.

Melanoma is a disease in which malignant (cancer) cells form in melanocytes (cells that color the skin). The skin is the body's largest organ. It protects against heat, sunlight, injury, and infection. Skin also helps control body temperature and stores water, fat, and vitamin D. The skin has several layers, but the two main layers are the epidermis (upper or outer layer) and the dermis (lower or inner layer). Skin cancer begins in the epidermis, which is made up of three kinds of cells:

- **Squamous cells:** Thin, flat cells that form the top layer of the epidermis

- **Basal cells:** Round cells under the squamous cells

- **Melanocytes:** Cells that make melanin and are found in the lower part of the epidermis. Melanin is the pigment that gives skin its natural color. When skin is exposed to the sun or artificial light, melanocytes make more pigment and cause the skin to darken.

The number of new cases of melanoma has been increasing over the last 30 years. Melanoma is most common in adults, but it is sometimes found in children and adolescents.

Two Forms of Skin Cancer

There are two forms of skin cancer—melanoma and nonmelanoma. Melanoma is a rare form of skin cancer. It is more likely to invade nearby tissues and spread to other parts of the body than other types of skin cancer. When melanoma starts in the skin, it is called cutaneous melanoma. Melanoma may also occur in mucous membranes (thin, moist layers of tissue that cover surfaces such as the lips).

The most common types of skin cancer are basal cell carcinoma and squamous cell carcinoma. They are nonmelanoma skin cancers (NMSC). Nonmelanoma skin cancers rarely spread to other parts of the body. Melanoma can occur anywhere on the skin. In men, melanoma is often found on the trunk (the area from the shoulders to the hips) or the head and neck. In women, melanoma forms most often on the arms and legs. When melanoma occurs in the eye, it is called intraocular or ocular melanoma. Unusual moles, exposure to sunlight, and health history can affect the risk of melanoma.

Diagnosing Melanoma

If a mole or pigmented area of the skin changes or looks abnormal, the following tests and procedures can help find and diagnose melanoma:

Skin exam: A doctor or nurse checks the skin for moles, birthmarks, or other pigmented areas that look abnormal in color, size, shape, or texture.

Biopsy: A procedure to remove the abnormal tissue and a small amount of normal tissue around it. A pathologist looks at the tissue under a microscope to check for cancer cells. It can be hard to tell the difference between a colored mole and an early melanoma lesion. Patients may want to have the sample of tissue checked by a second pathologist. If the abnormal mole or lesion is cancer, the sample of tissue may also be tested for certain gene changes.

It is important that abnormal areas of the skin not be shaved off or cauterized (destroyed with a hot instrument, an electric current, or a caustic substance) because cancer cells that remain may grow and spread.

Treatment Option Overview

Different types of treatment are available for patients with melanoma. Some treatments are standard (the currently used treatment), and some are being tested in clinical trials. A treatment clinical trial is a research study meant to help improve current treatments or obtain information on new treatments for patients with cancer. When clinical trials show that a new treatment is better than the standard treatment, the new treatment may become the standard treatment. Patients may want to think about taking part in a clinical trial. Some clinical trials are open only to patients who have not started treatment.

Five types of standard treatment are used:

Surgery

Surgery to remove the tumor is the primary treatment of all stages of melanoma. A wide local excision is used to remove the melanoma and some of the normal tissue around it. Skin grafting (taking skin from another part of the body to replace the skin that is removed) may be done to cover the wound caused by surgery.

It is important to know whether cancer has spread to the lymph nodes. Lymph node mapping and sentinel lymph node biopsy are done to check for cancer in the sentinel lymph node (the first lymph node the cancer is likely to spread to from the tumor) during surgery. A radioactive substance and/or blue dye is injected near the tumor. The substance or dye flows through the lymph ducts to the lymph nodes. The first lymph node to receive the substance or dye is removed. A pathologist views the tissue under a microscope to look for cancer cells. If cancer cells are found, more lymph nodes will be removed and tissue samples will be checked for signs of cancer. This is called a lymphadenectomy.

Even if the doctor removes all the melanoma that can be seen at the time of surgery, some patients may be given chemotherapy after surgery to kill any cancer cells that are left. Chemotherapy given after surgery, to lower the risk that the cancer will come back, is called adjuvant therapy.

Surgery to remove cancer that has spread to the lymph nodes, lung, gastrointestinal (GI) tract, bone, or brain may be done to improve the patient's quality of life by controlling symptoms.

Chemotherapy

Chemotherapy is a cancer treatment that uses drugs to stop the growth of cancer cells, either by killing the cells or by stopping them from dividing. When chemotherapy is taken by mouth or injected into a vein or muscle, the drugs enter the bloodstream and can reach cancer cells throughout the body (systemic chemotherapy). When chemotherapy is placed directly into the cerebrospinal fluid, an organ, or a body cavity such as the abdomen, the drugs mainly affect cancer cells in those areas (regional chemotherapy).

One type of regional chemotherapy is hyperthermic isolated limb perfusion. With this method, anticancer drugs go directly to the arm or leg the cancer is in. The flow of blood to and from the limb is temporarily stopped with a tourniquet. A warm solution with the anticancer drug is put directly into the blood of the limb. This gives a high dose of drugs to the area where the cancer is.

The way the chemotherapy is given depends on the type and stage of the cancer being treated.

Radiation Therapy

Radiation therapy is a cancer treatment that uses high-energy X-rays or other types of radiation to kill cancer cells or keep them from growing. There are two types of radiation therapy:

External radiation therapy uses a machine outside the body to send radiation toward the cancer.

Internal radiation therapy uses a radioactive substance sealed in needles, seeds, wires, or catheters that are placed directly into or near the cancer.

The way the radiation therapy is given depends on the type and stage of the cancer being treated. External radiation therapy is used to treat melanoma, and may also be used as palliative therapy to relieve symptoms and improve quality of life.

Immunotherapy

Immunotherapy is a treatment that uses the patient's immune system to fight cancer. Substances made by the body or made in a laboratory are used to boost, direct, or restore the body's natural defenses against cancer. This type of cancer treatment is also called biotherapy or biologic therapy.

The following types of immunotherapy are being used in the treatment of melanoma:

- **Immune checkpoint inhibitor therapy:** Some types of immune cells, such as T cells, and some cancer cells have certain proteins, called checkpoint proteins, on their surface that keep immune responses in check. When cancer cells have large amounts of these proteins, they will not be attacked and killed by T cells. Immune checkpoint inhibitors block these proteins and the ability of T cells to kill cancer cells is increased. They are used to treat some patients with advanced melanoma or tumors that cannot be removed by surgery.

There are two types of immune checkpoint inhibitor therapy:

- **Anti-cytotoxic T lymphocyte antigen-4 (CTLA-4) inhibitor:** CTL4-A is a protein on the surface of T cells that helps keep the body's immune responses in check. When CTLA-4 attaches to another protein called B7 on a cancer cell, it stops the T cell from killing the cancer cell. CTLA-4 inhibitors attach to CTLA-4 and allow the T cells to kill cancer cells. Ipilimumab is a type of CTLA-4 inhibitor.

- **Programmed death 1 (PD-1) inhibitor:** PD-1 is a protein on the surface of T cells that helps keep the body's immune responses in check. When PD-1 attaches to another protein called PDL-1 on a cancer cell, it stops the T cell from killing the cancer cell. PD-1 inhibitors attach to PDL-1 and allow the T cells to kill cancer cells. Pembrolizumab and nivolumab are types of PD-1 inhibitors.

- **Interferon:** Interferon affects the division of cancer cells and can slow tumor growth.

343

- **Interleukin-2 (IL-2):** IL-2 boosts the growth and activity of many immune cells, especially lymphocytes (a type of white blood cell). Lymphocytes can attack and kill cancer cells.

- **Tumor necrosis factor (TNF) therapy:** TNF is a protein made by white blood cells in response to an antigen or infection. TNF is made in the laboratory and used as a treatment to kill cancer cells. It is being studied in the treatment of melanoma.

Targeted Therapy

Targeted therapy is a type of treatment that uses drugs or other substances to attack cancer cells. Targeted therapies usually cause less harm to normal cells than chemotherapy or radiation therapy do. The following types of targeted therapy are used or being studied in the treatment of melanoma:

- **Signal transduction inhibitor therapy:** Signal transduction inhibitors block signals that are passed from one molecule to another inside a cell. Blocking these signals may kill cancer cells.

  - Vemurafenib, dabrafenib, trametinib, and cobimetinib are signal transduction inhibitors used to treat some patients with advanced melanoma or tumors that cannot be removed by surgery. Vemurafenib and dabrafenib block the activity of proteins made by mutant *BRAF* genes. Trametinib and cobimetinib affect the growth and survival of cancer cells.

- **Oncolytic virus therapy:** A type of targeted therapy that is used in the treatment of melanoma. Oncolytic virus therapy uses a virus that infects and breaks down cancer cells but not normal cells. Radiation therapy or chemotherapy may be given after oncolytic virus therapy to kill more cancer cells.

- **Angiogenesis inhibitors:** A type of targeted therapy that is being studied in the treatment of melanoma. Angiogenesis inhibitors block the growth of new blood vessels. In cancer treatment, they may be given to prevent the growth of new blood vessels that tumors need to grow.

New targeted therapies and combinations of therapies are being studied in the treatment of melanoma.

Section 28.3

Diagnosing and Treating Nonmelanoma Skin Cancers

This section includes text excerpted from "Skin Cancer Treatment (PDQ®)—Patient Version," National Cancer Institute (NCI), August 28, 2017.

Skin cancer is a disease in which malignant (cancer) cells form in the tissues of the skin. The skin is the body's largest organ. It protects against heat, sunlight, injury, and infection. Skin also helps control body temperature and stores water, fat, and vitamin D. The skin has several layers, but the two main layers are the epidermis (upper or outer layer) and the dermis (lower or inner layer). Skin cancer begins in the epidermis, which is made up of three kinds of cells:

- **Squamous cells:** Thin, flat cells that form the top layer of the epidermis

- **Basal cells:** Round cells under the squamous cells

- **Melanocytes:** Cells that make melanin and are found in the lower part of the epidermis. Melanin is the pigment that gives skin its natural color. When skin is exposed to the sun, melanocytes make more pigment and cause the skin to darken

Skin cancer can occur anywhere on the body, but it is most common in skin that is often exposed to sunlight, such as the face, neck, hands, and arms.

Different Types of Cancer That Start in the Skin

There are different types of cancer that start in the skin. The most common types are basal cell carcinoma and squamous cell carcinoma, which are nonmelanoma skin cancers. Nonmelanoma skin cancers rarely spread to other parts of the body. Melanoma is a much rarer type of skin cancer. It is more likely to invade nearby tissues and spread to other parts of the body. Actinic keratosis is a skin condition that sometimes becomes squamous cell carcinoma. Skin color and being

345

exposed to sunlight can increase the risk of nonmelanoma skin cancer and actinic keratosis.

Diagnosing Nonmelanoma Skin Cancer

Tests or procedures that examine the skin are used to detect (find) and diagnose nonmelanoma skin cancer and actinic keratosis
The following procedures may be used:

- **Skin exam:** A doctor or nurse checks the skin for bumps or spots that look abnormal in color, size, shape, or texture.

- **Skin biopsy:** All or part of the abnormal-looking growth is cut from the skin and viewed under a microscope by a pathologist to check for signs of cancer. There are four main types of skin biopsies:

  - **Shave biopsy:** A sterile razor blade is used to "shave-off" the abnormal-looking growth.

  - **Punch biopsy:** A special instrument called a punch or a trephine is used to remove a circle of tissue from the abnormal-looking growth.

  - **Incisional biopsy:** A scalpel is used to remove part of a growth.

  - **Excisional biopsy:** A scalpel is used to remove the entire growth.

Treatment Options for Nonmelanoma Skin Cancers

Basal Cell Carcinoma

Treatment of basal cell carcinoma may include the following:

- Simple excision

- Mohs micrographic surgery

- Radiation therapy

- Electrodesiccation and curettage

- Cryosurgery

- Photodynamic therapy

- Topical chemotherapy

- Topical biologic therapy with imiquimod
- Laser surgery

Treatment of recurrent basal cell carcinoma is usually Mohs micrographic surgery. Treatment of basal cell carcinoma that is metastatic or cannot be treated with local therapy may include the following:

- Targeted therapy with a signal transduction inhibitor
- Chemotherapy
- A clinical trial of a new treatment

Squamous Cell Carcinoma

Treatment of squamous cell carcinoma may include the following:

- Simple excision
- Mohs micrographic surgery
- Radiation therapy
- Electrodesiccation and curettage
- Cryosurgery

Treatment of recurrent squamous cell carcinoma may include the following:

- Simple excision
- Mohs micrographic surgery
- Radiation therapy

Treatment of squamous cell carcinoma that is metastatic or cannot be treated with local therapy may include the following:

- Chemotherapy
- Retinoid therapy and biologic therapy with interferon
- A clinical trial of a new treatment

Chapter 29

Thyroid Cancer

Thyroid cancer is a disease in which malignant (cancer) cells form in the tissues of the thyroid gland. The thyroid is a gland at the base of the throat near the trachea (windpipe). It is shaped like a butterfly, with a right lobe and a left lobe. The isthmus, a thin piece of tissue, connects the two lobes. A healthy thyroid is a little larger than a quarter. It usually cannot be felt through the skin.

The thyroid uses iodine, a mineral found in some foods and in iodized salt, to help make several hormones. Thyroid hormones do the following:

- Control heart rate, body temperature, and how quickly food is changed into energy (metabolism)

- Control the amount of calcium in the blood

Thyroid nodules are common but usually are not cancer. Your doctor may find a lump (nodule) in your thyroid during a routine medical exam. A thyroid nodule is an abnormal growth of thyroid cells in the thyroid. Nodules may be solid or fluid-filled.

When a thyroid nodule is found, an ultrasound of the thyroid and a fine-needle aspiration biopsy are often done to check for signs of cancer. Blood tests to check thyroid hormone levels and for antithyroid antibodies in the blood may also be done to check for other types of thyroid disease.

This chapter includes text excerpted from "Thyroid Cancer Treatment (Adult) (PDQ®)—Patient Version," National Cancer Institute (NCI), March 30, 2018.

Thyroid nodules usually don't cause symptoms or need treatment. Sometimes the thyroid nodules become large enough that it is hard to swallow or breathe and more tests and treatment are needed. Only a small number of thyroid nodules are diagnosed as cancer.

Types of Thyroid Cancer

There are four main types of thyroid cancer:

1. Papillary thyroid cancer

2. Follicular thyroid cancer

3. Medullary thyroid cancer

4. Anaplastic thyroid cancer

Papillary and follicular thyroid cancer are sometimes called differentiated thyroid cancer. Medullary and anaplastic thyroid cancer are sometimes called poorly differentiated or undifferentiated thyroid cancer. Age, gender, and being exposed to radiation can affect the risk of thyroid cancer.

Risk Factors for Thyroid Cancer

Anything that increases your risk of getting a disease is called a risk factor. Having a risk factor does not mean that you will get cancer; not having risk factors doesn't mean that you will not get cancer. Talk with your doctor if you think you may be at risk.

Risk factors for thyroid cancer include the following:

- Being between 25 and 65 years old

- Being female

- Being exposed to radiation to the head and neck as an infant or child or being exposed to radiation from an atomic bomb. The cancer may occur as soon as 5 years after exposure

- Having a history of goiter (enlarged thyroid)

- Having a family history of thyroid disease or thyroid cancer

- Having certain genetic conditions such as familial medullary thyroid cancer (FMTC), multiple endocrine neoplasia type 2A syndrome (MEN2A), and multiple endocrine neoplasia type 2B syndrome (MEN2B)

- Being Asian

Medullary thyroid cancer is sometimes caused by a change in a gene that is passed from parent to child. The genes in cells carry hereditary information from parent to child. A certain change in the *RET* gene that is passed from parent to child (inherited) may cause medullary thyroid cancer. There is a genetic test that is used to check for the changed gene. The patient is tested first to see if he or she has the changed gene. If the patient has it, other family members may also be tested to find out if they are at increased risk for medullary thyroid cancer. Family members, including young children, who have the changed gene may have a thyroidectomy (surgery to remove the thyroid). This can decrease the chance of developing medullary thyroid cancer.

Signs of Thyroid Cancer

Signs of thyroid cancer include a swelling or lump in the neck. Thyroid cancer may not cause early signs or symptoms. It is sometimes found during a routine physical exam. Signs or symptoms may occur as the tumor gets bigger. Other conditions may cause the same signs or symptoms. Check with your doctor if you have any of the following:

- A lump (nodule) in the neck
- Trouble breathing
- Trouble swallowing
- Pain when swallowing
- Hoarseness

Diagnosing Thyroid Cancer

Tests that examine the thyroid, neck, and blood are used to detect (find) and diagnose thyroid cancer. The following tests and procedures may be used:

- **Physical exam and history:** An exam of the body to check general signs of health, including checking for signs of disease, such as lumps (nodules) or swelling in the neck, voice box, and lymph nodes, and anything else that seems unusual. A history of the patient's health habits and past illnesses and treatments will also be taken.

- **Laryngoscopy:** A procedure in which the doctor checks the larynx (voice box) with a mirror or with a laryngoscope.

351

A laryngoscope is a thin, tube-like instrument with a light and a lens for viewing. A thyroid tumor may press on vocal cords. The laryngoscopy is done to see if the vocal cords are moving normally.

- **Blood hormone studies:** A procedure in which a blood sample is checked to measure the amounts of certain hormones released into the blood by organs and tissues in the body. An unusual (higher or lower than normal) amount of a substance can be a sign of disease in the organ or tissue that makes it. The blood may be checked for abnormal levels of thyroid-stimulating hormone (TSH). TSH is made by the pituitary gland in the brain. It stimulates the release of thyroid hormone and controls how fast follicular thyroid cells grow. The blood may also be checked for high levels of the hormone calcitonin and antithyroid antibodies.

- **Blood chemistry studies:** A procedure in which a blood sample is checked to measure the amounts of certain substances, such as calcium, released into the blood by organs and tissues in the body. An unusual (higher or lower than normal) amount of a substance can be a sign of disease.

- **Ultrasound exam:** A procedure in which high-energy sound waves (ultrasound) are bounced off internal tissues or organs in the neck and make echoes. The echoes form a picture of body tissues called a sonogram. The picture can be printed to be looked at later. This procedure can show the size of a thyroid nodule and whether it is solid or a fluid-filled cyst. Ultrasound may be used to guide a fine-needle aspiration biopsy.

- **Computed tomography (CT) scan:** A procedure that makes a series of detailed pictures of areas inside the body, such as the neck, taken from different angles. The pictures are made by a computer linked to an X-ray machine. A dye may be injected into a vein or swallowed to help the organs or tissues show up more clearly. This procedure is also called computed tomography, computerized tomography, or computerized axial tomography.

- **Fine-needle aspiration biopsy of the thyroid:** The removal of thyroid tissue using a thin needle. The needle is inserted through the skin into the thyroid. Several tissue samples are removed from different parts of the thyroid. A pathologist views the tissue samples under a microscope to look for cancer cells.

Because the type of thyroid cancer can be hard to diagnose, patients should ask to have biopsy samples checked by a pathologist who has experience diagnosing thyroid cancer.

- **Surgical biopsy:** The removal of the thyroid nodule or one lobe of the thyroid during surgery so the cells and tissues can be viewed under a microscope by a pathologist to check for signs of cancer. Because the type of thyroid cancer can be hard to diagnose, patients should ask to have biopsy samples checked by a pathologist who has experience diagnosing thyroid cancer.

Stages of Thyroid Cancer

After thyroid cancer has been diagnosed, tests are done to find out if cancer cells have spread within the thyroid or to other parts of the body.

The process used to find out if cancer has spread within the thyroid or to other parts of the body is called staging. The information gathered from the staging process determines the stage of the disease. It is important to know the patient's age and the stage of the cancer in order to plan treatment.

The following tests and procedures may be used in the staging process:

- **CT scan:** A procedure that makes a series of detailed pictures of areas inside the body, such as the chest, abdomen, and brain, taken from different angles. The pictures are made by a computer linked to an X-ray machine. A dye may be injected into a vein or swallowed to help the organs or tissues show up more clearly. This procedure is also called computed tomography, computerized tomography, or computerized axial tomography.

- **Ultrasound exam:** A procedure in which high-energy sound waves (ultrasound) are bounced off internal tissues or organs and make echoes. The echoes form a picture of body tissues called a sonogram. The picture can be printed to be looked at later.

- **Chest X-ray:** An X-ray of the organs and bones inside the chest. An X-ray is a type of energy beam that can go through the body and onto film, making a picture of areas inside the body.

- **Bone scan:** A procedure to check if there are rapidly dividing cells, such as cancer cells, in the bone. A very small amount of radioactive material is injected into a vein and travels through the bloodstream. The radioactive material collects in the bones with cancer and is detected by a scanner.

- **Sentinel lymph node biopsy:** The removal of the sentinel lymph node during surgery. The sentinel lymph node is the first lymph node to receive lymphatic drainage from a tumor. It is the first lymph node the cancer is likely to spread to from the tumor. A radioactive substance and/or blue dye is injected near the tumor. The substance or dye flows through the lymph ducts to the lymph nodes. The first lymph node to receive the substance or dye is removed. A pathologist views the tissue under a microscope to look for cancer cells. If cancer cells are not found, it may not be necessary to remove more lymph nodes.

Stages are used to describe thyroid cancer based on the type of thyroid cancer and the age of the patient.

Papillary and follicular thyroid cancer in patients younger than 45 years:

- **Stage I:** In stage I papillary and follicular thyroid cancer, the tumor is any size and may have spread to nearby tissues and lymph nodes. Cancer has not spread to other parts of the body.

- **Stage II:** In stage II papillary and follicular thyroid cancer, the tumor is any size and cancer has spread from the thyroid to other parts of the body, such as the lungs or bone, and may have spread to lymph nodes.

Papillary and follicular thyroid cancer in patients 45 years and older:

- **Stage I:** In stage I papillary and follicular thyroid cancer, cancer is found only in the thyroid and the tumor is 2 centimeters or smaller.

- **Stage II:** In stage II papillary and follicular thyroid cancer, cancer is only in the thyroid and the tumor is larger than 2 centimeters but not larger than 4 centimeters.

- **Stage III:** In stage III papillary and follicular thyroid cancer, either of the following is found:

    - The tumor is larger than 4 centimeters and only in the thyroid or the tumor is any size and cancer has spread to tissues just outside the thyroid, but not to lymph nodes; or

- The tumor is any size and cancer may have spread to tissues just outside the thyroid. Cancer has spread to lymph nodes on one or both sides of the neck or between the lungs.

- **Stage IV:** Stage IV papillary and follicular thyroid cancer is divided into stages IVA, IVB, and IVC.

  In stage IVA, either of the following is found:

  - The tumor is any size and cancer has spread outside the thyroid to tissues under the skin, the trachea, the esophagus, the larynx (voice box), and/or the recurrent laryngeal nerve (a nerve that goes to the larynx); cancer may have spread to lymph nodes near the trachea or the larynx; or

  - The tumor is any size and cancer may have spread to tissues just outside the thyroid. Cancer has spread to lymph nodes on one or both sides of the neck or between the lungs.

  In stage IVB, cancer has spread to tissue in front of the spinal column or has surrounded the carotid artery or the blood vessels in the area between the lungs. Cancer may have spread to lymph nodes.

  In stage IVC, the tumor is any size and cancer has spread to other parts of the body, such as the lungs and bones, and may have spread to lymph nodes.

  Medullary thyroid cancer for all ages

- **Stage 0:** Stage 0 medullary thyroid cancer is found only with a special screening test. No tumor can be found in the thyroid.

- **Stage I:** Stage I medullary thyroid cancer is found only in the thyroid and is 2 centimeters or smaller.

- **Stage II:** In stage II medullary thyroid cancer, either of the following is found:

  - The tumor is larger than 2 centimeters and only in the thyroid; or

  - The tumor is any size and has spread to tissues just outside the thyroid, but not to lymph nodes.

- **Stage III:** In stage III medullary thyroid cancer, the tumor is any size, has spread to lymph nodes near the trachea and the larynx (voice box), and may have spread to tissues just outside the thyroid.

- **Stage IV:** Stage IV medullary thyroid cancer is divided into stages IVA, IVB, and IVC.

  In stage IVA, either of the following is found:

  - The tumor is any size and cancer has spread outside the thyroid to tissues under the skin, the trachea, the esophagus, the larynx (voice box), and/or the recurrent laryngeal nerve (a nerve that goes to the larynx); cancer may have spread to lymph nodes near the trachea or the larynx; or

  - The tumor is any size and cancer may have spread to tissues just outside the thyroid. Cancer has spread to lymph nodes on one or both sides of the neck or between the lungs.

  In stage IVB, cancer has spread to tissue in front of the spinal column or has surrounded the carotid artery or the blood vessels in the area between the lungs. Cancer may have spread to lymph nodes.

  In stage IVC, the tumor is any size and cancer has spread to other parts of the body, such as the lungs and bones, and may have spread to lymph nodes.

  Anaplastic thyroid cancer is considered stage IV thyroid cancer. It grows quickly and has usually spread within the neck when it is found. Stage IV anaplastic thyroid cancer is divided into stages IVA, IVB, and IVC.

- In stage IVA, cancer is found in the thyroid and may have spread to lymph nodes.

- In stage IVB, cancer has spread to tissue just outside the thyroid and may have spread to lymph nodes.

- In stage IVC, cancer has spread to other parts of the body, such as the lungs and bones, and may have spread to lymph nodes.

Treatment Options Overview for Thyroid Cancer

There are different types of treatment for patients with thyroid cancer. Different types of treatment are available for patients with thyroid cancer. Some treatments are standard (the currently used treatment), and some are being tested in clinical trials. A treatment clinical trial is a research study meant to help improve current treatments or obtain information on new treatments for patients with cancer. When clinical trials show that a new treatment is better than the standard treatment, the new treatment may become the standard treatment.

Patients may want to think about taking part in a clinical trial. Some clinical trials are open only to patients who have not started treatment.

Six types of standard treatment are used:

Surgery

Surgery is the most common treatment for thyroid cancer. One of the following procedures may be used:

- **Lobectomy:** Removal of the lobe in which thyroid cancer is found. Lymph nodes near the cancer may also be removed and checked under a microscope for signs of cancer.

- **Near-total thyroidectomy:** Removal of all but a very small part of the thyroid. Lymph nodes near the cancer may also be removed and checked under a microscope for signs of cancer.

- **Total thyroidectomy:** Removal of the whole thyroid. Lymph nodes near the cancer may also be removed and checked under a microscope for signs of cancer.

- **Tracheostomy:** Surgery to create an opening (stoma) into the windpipe to help you breathe. The opening itself may also be called a tracheostomy.

Radiation Therapy

Radiation therapy is a cancer treatment that uses high-energy X-rays or other types of radiation to kill cancer cells or keep them from growing. There are two types of radiation therapy:

- External radiation therapy uses a machine outside the body to send radiation toward the cancer. Sometimes the radiation is aimed directly at the tumor during surgery. This is called intraoperative radiation therapy.

- Internal radiation therapy uses a radioactive substance sealed in needles, seeds, wires, or catheters that are placed directly into or near the cancer.

Radiation therapy may be given after surgery to kill any thyroid cancer cells that were not removed. Follicular and papillary thyroid cancers are sometimes treated with radioactive iodine (RAI) therapy. RAI is taken by mouth and collects in any remaining thyroid tissue, including thyroid cancer cells that have spread to other places in the body. Since only thyroid tissue takes up iodine, the RAI destroys thyroid tissue and thyroid cancer cells without harming other tissue. Before a full treatment dose of RAI is given, a small test-dose is given to see if the tumor takes up the iodine.

The way the radiation therapy is given depends on the type and stage of the cancer being treated. External radiation therapy and radioactive iodine (RAI) therapy are used to treat thyroid cancer.

Chemotherapy

Chemotherapy is a cancer treatment that uses drugs to stop the growth of cancer cells, either by killing the cells or by stopping them from dividing. When chemotherapy is taken by mouth or injected into a vein or muscle, the drugs enter the bloodstream and can reach cancer cells throughout the body (systemic chemotherapy). When chemotherapy is placed directly into the cerebrospinal fluid, an organ, or a body cavity such as the abdomen, the drugs mainly affect cancer cells in those areas (regional chemotherapy).

The way the chemotherapy is given depends on the type and stage of the cancer being treated.

Thyroid Hormone Therapy

Hormone therapy is a cancer treatment that removes hormones or blocks their action and stops cancer cells from growing. Hormones are substances made by glands in the body and circulated in the bloodstream. In the treatment of thyroid cancer, drugs may be given to prevent the body from making thyroid-stimulating hormone (TSH), a hormone that can increase the chance that thyroid cancer will grow or recur.

Also, because thyroid cancer treatment kills thyroid cells, the thyroid is not able to make enough thyroid hormone. Patients are given thyroid hormone replacement pills.

Targeted Therapy

Targeted therapy is a type of treatment that uses drugs or other substances to identify and attack specific cancer cells without harming normal cells.

Tyrosine kinase inhibitor therapy is a type of targeted therapy that blocks signals needed for tumors to grow. Vandetanib and sorafenib are tyrosine kinase inhibitors that are used to treat certain types of thyroid cancer. New types of tyrosine kinase inhibitors (TKIs) are being studied to treat advanced thyroid cancer.

Watchful Waiting

Watchful waiting is closely monitoring a patient's condition without giving any treatment until signs or symptoms appear or change. New types of treatment are being tested in clinical trials. Treatment for thyroid cancer may cause side effects. Patients may want to think about taking part in a clinical trial. For some patients, taking part in a clinical trial may be the best treatment choice.

Part Five

Diagnosing and Treating Cancer

Chapter 30

How to Find a Doctor or Treatment Facility If You Have Cancer

If you have been diagnosed with cancer, finding a doctor and a treatment facility for your cancer care is an important step to getting the best treatment possible.

You will have many things to consider when choosing a doctor. It's important for you to feel comfortable with the specialist that you choose because you will be working closely with that person to make decisions about your cancer treatment.

Choosing a Doctor

When choosing a doctor for your cancer care, it may be helpful to know some of the terms used to describe a doctor's training and credentials. Most physicians who treat people with cancer are medical doctors (they have an M.D. degree) or osteopathic doctors (they have a D.O. degree). Standard training includes 4 years of study at a college or university, 4 years of medical school, and 3–7 years of postgraduate medical education through internships and residencies. Doctors must pass an exam to become licensed to practice medicine in their state.

This chapter includes text excerpted from "Finding Health Care Services," National Cancer Institute (NCI), August 25, 2017.

Specialists are doctors who have done their residency training in a specific field such as internal medicine. Independent specialty boards certify physicians after they have met needed requirements, including meeting certain education and training standards, being licensed to practice medicine, and passing an examination given by their specialty board. Once they have met these requirements, physicians are said to be "board certified."

Some specialists who treat cancer are:

- **Medical Oncologist:** Specializes in treating cancer

- **Hematologist:** Focuses on diseases of the blood and related tissues, including the bone marrow, spleen, and lymph nodes

- **Radiation oncologist:** Uses X-rays and other forms of radiation to diagnose and treat disease

- **Surgeon:** Performs operations on almost any area of the body and may specialize in a certain type of surgery

Finding a Doctor Who Specializes in Cancer Care

To find a doctor who specializes in cancer care, ask your primary care doctor to suggest someone. Or you may know of a specialist through the experience of a friend of family member. Also, your local hospital should be able to provide you with a list of specialists who practice there.

Another option for finding a doctor is your nearest National Cancer Institute (NCI)-designated cancer center. The Find a Cancer Center page (www.cancer.gov/research/nci-role/cancer-centers/find) provides contact information to help healthcare providers and cancer patients with referrals to all NCI-designated cancer centers in the United States.

The online directories listed below may also help you find a cancer care specialist.

- The American Board of Medical Specialists (ABMS), which creates and implements the standards for certifying and evaluating doctors, has a list of doctors that have met specific requirements and passed specialty exams.

- The American Medical Association (AMA) DoctorFinder (apps. ama-assn.org/doctorfinder) provides information on licensed doctors in the United States.

- The American Society of Clinical Oncology (ASCO) member database (www.cancer.net/find-cancer-doctor) has the names and affiliations of nearly 30,000 oncologists worldwide.

- The American College of Surgeons (ACS) lists member surgeons by region and specialty in their Find a Surgeon database (www. facs.org/search/find-a-surgeon). The ACS can also be reached at 800-621-4111.

- The American Osteopathic Association (AOA) Find a Doctor database (doctorsthatdo.org) provides an online list of practicing osteopathic physicians who are AOA members. The AOA can also be reached at 800-621-1773.

Local medical societies may also maintain lists of doctors in each specialty for you to check. Public and medical libraries may have print directories of doctors' names listed geographically by specialty. Depending on your health insurance plan, your choice may be limited to doctors who participate in your plan. Your insurance company can give you a list of doctors who take part in your plan. It's important to contact the office of the doctor you're considering to be sure that he or she is accepting new patients through your plan. It's also important to do this if you're using a federal or state health insurance program such as Medicare or Medicaid.

If you can change health insurance plans, you may want to decide which doctor you would like to use first and then choose the plan that includes your chosen physician. You also have the option of seeing a doctor outside your plan and paying more of the costs yourself.

To help make your decision when you're considering what doctor to choose, think about if the doctor:

- Has the education and training needed to meet your needs
- Has someone who covers for them if they are unavailable and who would have access to your medical records
- Has a helpful support staff
- Explains things clearly, listens to you, and treats you with respect
- Encourages you to ask questions
- Has office hours that meet your needs
- Is easy to get an appointment with

If you are choosing a surgeon, you will want to ask:

- Are they board certified?
- How often do they perform the type of surgery you need?
- How many of these procedures have they performed?
- At what hospital(s) do they practice?

It's important for you to feel good about the doctor you choose. You will be working with this person closely as you make decisions about your cancer treatment.

Getting a Second Opinion

After you talk to a doctor about the diagnosis and treatment plan for your cancer, you may want to get another doctor's opinion before you begin treatment. This is known as getting a second opinion. You can do this by asking another specialist to review all the materials related to your case. The doctor who gives the second opinion may agree with the treatment plan proposed by your first doctor, or they may suggest changes or another approach. Either way, getting a second opinion may:

- Give you more information

- Answer any questions you may have

- Give you a greater sense of control

- Help you feel more confident, knowing you have explored all your options

Getting a second opinion is very common. Yet some patients worry that their doctor will be offended if they ask for a second opinion. Usually, the opposite is true. Most doctors welcome a second opinion. And many health insurance companies pay for a second opinion or even require them, particularly if a doctor recommends surgery.

When talking with your doctor about getting a second opinion, it may be helpful to express that you're satisfied with your care but want to be certain you're as informed as possible about your treatment options. It's best to involve your doctor in the process of getting a second opinion, because he or she will need to make your medical records (such as your test results and X-rays) available to the doctor giving the second opinion. You may wish to bring a family member along for support when asking for a second opinion.

If your doctor can't suggest another specialist for a second opinion, many of the resources listed above for finding a doctor can help you find a specialist for a second opinion. You can also call NCI's Contact Center at 800-4-CANCER (800-422-6237) for guidance.

Choosing a Treatment Facility

As with choosing a doctor, your choice of facilities may be limited to those that take part in your health insurance plan. If you have already found a doctor for your cancer treatment, you may need to choose a treatment facility based on where your doctor practices. Or your doctor may be able to recommend a facility that provides quality care to meet your needs.

Some questions to ask when considering a treatment facility are:

- Does it have experience and success in treating my condition?

- Has it been rated by state, consumer, or other groups for its quality of care?

- How does it check on and work to improve its quality of care?

- Has it been approved by a nationally recognized accrediting body, such as the ACS Commission on Cancer (CoC) and/or The Joint Commission?

- Does it explain patients' rights and responsibilities? Are copies of this information available to patients?

- Does it offer support services, such as social workers and resources, to help me find financial assistance if I need it?

- Is it conveniently located?

If you belong to a health insurance plan, ask your insurance company if the facility you are choosing is approved by your plan. If you decide to pay for treatment yourself because you choose to go outside of your network or don't have insurance, discuss the possible costs with your doctor beforehand. You will want to talk to the hospital billing department as well. Nurses and social workers may also be able to give you more information about coverage, eligibility, and insurance issues.

The following resources may help you find a hospital or treatment facility for your care:

- NCI's Find a Cancer Center page (www.cancer.gov/research/nci-role/cancer-centers/find) provides contact information for NCI-designated cancer centers located throughout the country.

- The ACS's Commission on Cancer (CoC). The ACS website has a searchable database (www.facs.org/search/cancer-programs) of cancer care programs they have accredited. They can also be reached at 312-202-5085 or by e-mail at CoC@facs.org.

- The Joint Commission evaluates and accredits healthcare organizations and programs in the United States. It also provides guidance about choosing a treatment facility, and offers an online Quality Check® service (www.qualitycheck.org) that patients can use to check whether a specific facility has been accredited by the Joint Commission and to view its performance reports. They also can be reached at 630-792-5000.

For more information or assistance about finding a treatment facility, call NCI's Contact Center at 800-4-CANCER (800-422-6237).

Getting Treatment in the United States If You Are Not a U.S. Citizen

Some people who live outside the United States may wish to obtain a second opinion or have their cancer treatment in this country. Many facilities in the United States offer these services to international cancer patients. They may also provide support services, such as language interpretation or help with travel and finding lodging near the treatment facility.

If you live outside the United States and would like to get cancer treatment in this country, you should contact cancer treatment facilities directly to find out whether they have an international patient office. The NCI-Designated Cancer Centers Find a Cancer Center page offers contact information for NCI-designated cancer centers throughout the United States.

Citizens of other countries who are planning to travel to the United States for cancer treatment must first obtain a nonimmigrant visa for medical treatment from the U.S. Embassy or Consulate in their home country. Visa applicants must show that they:

• Want to come to the United States for medical treatment

• Plan to stay for a specific, limited period

• Have funds to cover expenses in the United States

• Have a residence and social and economic ties outside the United States

• Intend to return to their home country

To find out the fees and documents needed for the nonimmigrant visa and to learn more about the application process, contact the U.S. Embassy or Consulate in your home country. A list of links to the websites of U.S. Embassies and Consulates worldwide can be found on the U.S. Department of State's (DOS) website.

More information about nonimmigrant visa services is available on the U.S. State Department Visitor Visa page. If you are planning to travel to the United States, make sure to check the page for any possible updates or changes.

Finding a Treatment Facility outside the United States

Cancer information services are available in many countries to provide information and answer questions about cancer. They may also be able to help you find a cancer treatment facility close to where you live.

The International Cancer Information Service Group (ICISG), a worldwide network of more than 70 organizations that deliver cancer information, has a list of cancer information services on their website. Or you can email ICISG for questions or comments.

The Union for International Cancer Control (UICC) is another resource for people living outside the United States who want to find a cancer treatment facility. The UICC consists of international cancer-related organizations devoted to the worldwide fight against cancer. These organizations serve as resources for the public and may have helpful information about cancer and treatment facilities. To find a resource in or near your country, you may send the UICC an email or contact them at:

Union for International Cancer Control (UICC)
62 route de Frontenex
1207 Geneva
Switzerland
41-22-809-1811

Finding Health Insurance

The Affordable Care Act (ACA) changes how health insurance works in the United States, with implications for the prevention, screening, and treatment of cancer. Under this healthcare law, most Americans are required to have health insurance. If you do not have health insurance or want to look at new options, the online Health Insurance Marketplace lets you compare plans in your state based on price, benefits, quality, and other needs you may have. To learn about the Health Insurance Marketplace and your new coverage options, please go to Healthcare.gov or CuidadoDeSalud.gov or call toll-free at 800-318-2596 (TTY: 855-889-4325).

Home Care Services

Sometimes patients want to be cared for at home so they can be in familiar surroundings with family and friends. Home care services can help patients stay at home by using a team approach with doctors, nurses, social workers, physical therapists, and others.

If the patient qualifies for home care services, such services may include:

- Managing symptoms and monitoring care

- Delivery of medications

- Physical therapy

- Emotional and spiritual care

- Help with preparing meals and personal hygiene

- Providing medical equipment

For many patients and families, home care can be both rewarding and demanding. It can change relationships and require families to cope with all aspects of patient care. New issues may also arise that families need to address such as the logistics of having home care providers coming into the home at regular intervals. To prepare for these changes, patients and caregivers should ask questions and get as much information as possible from the home care team or organization. A doctor, nurse, or social worker can provide information about a patient's specific needs, the availability of services, and the local home care agencies.

Getting Financial Assistance for Home Care

Help with paying for home care services may be available from public or private sources. Private health insurance may cover some home care services, but benefits vary from plan to plan.

Some public resources to help pay for home care are:

- **Centers for Medicare & Medicaid Services (CMS):** A government agency responsible for the administration of several key federal healthcare programs. Two of these are:

    - **Medicare:** A government health insurance program for the elderly or disabled. For information, visit their website or call 800-MEDICARE (800-633-4227).

- **Medicaid:** A joint federal and state health insurance program for those who need help with medical expenses. Coverage varies by state.

Both Medicare and Medicaid may cover home care services for patients who qualify, but some rules apply. Talk to a social worker and other members of the healthcare team to find out more about home care providers and agencies. For more information contact the CMS online or call 877-267-2323.

- **Eldercare Locator:** Run by the U.S. Administration on Aging (AoA), it provides information about local Area Agencies on Aging and other assistance for older people. These agencies may provide funds for home care. Eldercare Locator can be reached at 800-677-1116 for more information.

- **U.S. Department of Veterans Affairs (VA):** Veterans who are disabled as a result of military service can receive home care services from the VA. However, only home care services provided by VA hospitals may be used. More information about these benefits can be found on their website or by calling 877-222-VETS (877-222-8387).

For other resources for home care, call the NCI Contact Center at 800-4-CANCER (800-422-6237) or visit cancer.gov.

Chapter 31

Diagnosing Cancer

Chapter Contents

Section 31.1

Commonly Used Diagnostic Tests and Procedures

This section contains text excerpted from the following sources: Text in this section begins with excerpts from "How Cancer Is Diagnosed," National Cancer Institute (NCI), March 9, 2015; Text under the heading "Questions to Ask Your Doctor about Your Diagnosis" is excerpted from "Questions to Ask Your Doctor about Your Diagnosis," National Cancer Institute (NCI), April 2, 2015.

If you have a symptom or your screening test result suggests cancer, the doctor must find out whether it is due to cancer or some other cause. The doctor may ask about your personal and family medical history and do a physical exam. The doctor also may order lab tests, scans, or other tests or procedures.

Lab Tests

High or low levels of certain substances in your body can be a sign of cancer. So, lab tests of the blood, urine, or other body fluids that measure these substances can help doctors make a diagnosis. However, abnormal lab results are not a sure sign of cancer. Lab tests are an important tool, but doctors cannot rely on them alone to diagnose cancer.

Imaging Procedures

Imaging procedures create pictures of areas inside your body that help the doctor see whether a tumor is present. These pictures can be made in several ways:

- **Computed tomography (CT) scan:** An X-ray machine linked to a computer takes a series of detailed pictures of your organs. You may receive a dye or other contrast material to highlight areas inside the body. Contrast material helps make these pictures easier to read.

- **Nuclear scan:** For this scan, you receive an injection of a small amount of radioactive material, which is sometimes called a tracer. It flows through your bloodstream and collects in certain bones or organs. A machine called a scanner detects and measures the radioactivity. The scanner creates pictures of bones or organs on a computer screen or on film. Your body gets rid of the radioactive substance quickly. This type of scan may also be called radionuclide scan.

- **Ultrasound:** An ultrasound device sends out sound waves that people cannot hear. The waves bounce off tissues inside your body like an echo. A computer uses these echoes to create a picture of areas inside your body. This picture is called a sonogram.

- **Magnetic resonance imaging (MRI):** A strong magnet linked to a computer is used to make detailed pictures of areas in your body. Your doctor can view these pictures on a monitor and print them on film.

- **Positron emission tomography (PET) scan:** For this scan, you receive an injection of a tracer. Then, a machine makes 3-D pictures that show where the tracer collects in the body. These scans show how organs and tissues are working.

- **X-rays:** X-rays use low doses of radiation to create pictures of the inside of your body.

Biopsy

In most cases, doctors need to do a biopsy to make a diagnosis of cancer. A biopsy is a procedure in which the doctor removes a sample of tissue. A pathologist then looks at the tissue under a microscope to see if it is cancer. The sample may be removed in several ways:

- **With a needle:** The doctor uses a needle to withdraw tissue or fluid.

- **With an endoscope:** The doctor looks at areas inside the body using a thin, lighted tube called an endoscope. The scope is inserted through a natural opening, such as the mouth. Then, the doctor uses a special tool to remove tissue or cells through the tube.

- **With surgery:** Surgery may be excisional or incisional.
  - In an excisional biopsy, the surgeon removes the entire tumor. Often some of the normal tissue around the tumor also is removed.

- In an incisional biopsy, the surgeon removes just part of the tumor.

Questions to Ask Your Doctor about Your Diagnosis

Learning that you have cancer can be a shock and you may feel overwhelmed at first. When you meet with your doctor, you will hear a lot of information. These questions may help you learn more about your cancer and what you can expect next.

- What type of cancer do I have?

- What is the stage of my cancer?

- Has it spread to other areas of my body?

- Will I need more tests before treatment begins? Which ones?

- Will I need a specialist(s) for my cancer treatment?

- Will you help me find a doctor to give me another opinion on the best treatment plan for me?

- How serious is my cancer?

- What are my chances of survival?

Section 31.2

Biopsy for Cancer

This section contains text excerpted from the following sources: Text in this section begins with the excerpts from "Biopsy," MedlinePlus, National Institutes of Health (NIH), May 2, 2017; Text under the heading "Role of Biopsy in Cancer Diagnosis" is excerpted from "Cancer Diagnosis," National Cancer Institute (NCI), February 1, 2002. Reviewed May 2018; Text under the heading "Types of Biopsies" is excerpted from "The Biopsy Report," National Cancer Institute (NCI), October 1, 2002. Reviewed May 2018; Text under the heading "Examination of Biopsy Specimen by Pathologist" is excerpted from "Pathology Reports," National Cancer Institute (NCI), September 23, 2010. Reviewed May 2018; Text under the heading "Sentinel Lymph Node Biopsy (SLNB)" is excerpted from "Sentinel Lymph Node Biopsy," National Cancer Institute (NCI), August 11, 2011. Reviewed May 2018.

A biopsy is a procedure that removes cells or tissue from your body. A doctor called a pathologist looks at the cells or tissue under a microscope to check for damage or disease. The pathologist may also do other tests on it. Biopsies can be done on all parts of the body. In most cases, a biopsy is the only test that can tell for sure if a suspicious area is cancer. But biopsies are performed for many other reasons too. There are different types of biopsies. A needle biopsy removes tissue with a needle passed through your skin to the site of the problem. Other kinds of biopsies may require surgery.

Role of Biopsy in Cancer Diagnosis

The diagnosis of cancer entails an attempt to accurately identify the anatomical site of origin of the malignancy and the type of cells involved. Cancer can arise in any organ or tissue in the body except fingernails, hair, and teeth.

The site refers to the location of the cancer within the body. The body part in which cancer first develops is known as the primary site. Cancer's primary site may determine how the tumor will behave; whether and where it may spread (metastasize) and what symptoms it is most likely to cause. The most common sites in which cancer develops include the skin, lungs, female breasts, colon and rectum, and corpus uteri.

The secondary site refers to the body part where metastasized cancer cells grow and form secondary tumors. A cancer is always described in terms of the primary site, even if it has spread to another part of the body. For instance, advanced breast cancer that has spread to the lymph nodes under the arm and to the bone and lungs is always considered breast cancer (and the spread to the lymph nodes, bones, and lungs describe the stage of the cancer).

A biopsy is preferred to establish, or rule out, a diagnosis of cancer. Tissue samples can be easily retrieved from a tumor near the body's surface. If the mass is inaccessible, an imaging exam that enables a tumor to be located precisely and visualized may be ordered before the biopsy is performed.

The histological type is determined by microscopic examination of suspected tissue that has been excised by biopsy or surgical resection. If the histological type is different from what is usually found in the tissue being examined, it can mean the cancer has spread to that area from some primary site. Metastasis can occur by direct extension, via the bloodstream or the lymphatic system, or by seeding or implantation of cancer cells.

A biopsy, together with advanced imaging technologies, may not only confirm the presence of cancer, but may also pinpoint the primary site and secondary site(s). In summary, a biopsy is the preferred method to confirm the diagnosis of cancer. Biopsies can provide information about histological type, classification, grade, potential aggressiveness and other information that may help determine the best treatment.

Types of Biopsies

The term biopsy refers to the removal and examination, gross and microscopic, of tissue or cells from the living body for the purpose of diagnosis. A variety of techniques exist for performing a biopsy of which the most common ones are:

- **Aspiration biopsy or bone marrow aspiration:** Biopsy of material (fluid, cells or tissue) obtained by suction through a needle attached to a syringe.

- **Bone marrow biopsy:** Examination of a piece of bone marrow by needle aspiration; can also be done as an open biopsy using a trephine (removing a circular disc of bone).

- **Curettage:** Removal of growths or other material by scraping with a curette.

- **Excisional biopsy (total):** The removal of a growth in its entirety by having a therapeutic as well as diagnostic purpose.

- **Incisional biopsy:** Incomplete removal of a growth for the purpose of diagnostic study.

- **Needle biopsy:** Same as aspiration biopsy.

- **Percutaneous biopsy:** A needle biopsy with the needle going through the skin.

- **Punch biopsy:** Biopsy of material obtained from the body tissue by a punch technique.

- **Sponge (gel foam) biopsy:** Removal of materials (cells, particles of tissue, and tissue juices) by rubbing a sponge over a lesion or over a mucous membrane for examination.

- **Surface biopsy:** Scraping of cells from surface epithelium, especially from the cervix, for microscopic examination.

- **Surgical biopsy:** Removal of tissue from the body by surgical excision for examination.

Examination of Biopsy Specimen by Pathologist

Tissue removed during a biopsy is sent to a pathology laboratory, where it is sliced into thin sections for viewing under a microscope. This is known as histologic (tissue) examination and is usually the best way to tell if cancer is present. The pathologist may also examine cytologic (cell) material. Cytologic material is present in urine, cerebrospinal fluid (the fluid around the brain and spinal cord), sputum (mucus from the lungs), peritoneal (abdominal cavity) fluid, pleural (chest cavity) fluid, cervical/vaginal smears, and in fluid removed during a biopsy.

Sentinel Lymph Node Biopsy (SLNB)

A sentinel lymph node is defined as the first lymph node to which cancer cells are most likely to spread from a primary tumor. Sometimes, there can be more than one sentinel lymph node. A sentinel lymph node biopsy (SLNB) is a procedure in which the sentinel lymph node is identified, removed, and examined to determine whether cancer cells are present. A negative SLNB result suggests that cancer has not developed the ability to spread to nearby lymph nodes or other organs. A positive SLNB result indicates that cancer is present in the sentinel lymph node and may be present in other nearby lymph nodes (called regional lymph nodes) and, possibly, other organs. This information can help a doctor determine the stage of the cancer (extent of the disease within the body) and develop an appropriate treatment plan.

What Happens during an SLNB?

A surgeon injects a radioactive substance, a blue dye, or both near the tumor to locate the position of the sentinel lymph node. The surgeon then uses a device that detects radioactivity to find the sentinel node or looks for lymph nodes that are stained with the blue dye. Once the sentinel lymph node is located, the surgeon makes a small incision (about 1/2 inch) in the overlying skin and removes the node.

The sentinel node is then checked for the presence of cancer cells by a pathologist. If cancer is found, the surgeon may remove additional lymph nodes, either during the same biopsy procedure or during a follow-up surgical procedure. SLNBs may be done on an outpatient basis or may require a short stay in the hospital.

SLNB is usually done at the same time the primary tumor is removed. However, the procedure can also be done either before or after removal of the tumor.

What Are the Benefits of SLNB?

In addition to helping doctors stage cancers and estimate the risk that tumor cells have developed the ability to spread to other parts of the body, SLNB may help some patients avoid more extensive lymph node surgery. Removing additional nearby lymph nodes to look for cancer cells may not be necessary if the sentinel node is negative for cancer. All lymph node surgery can have adverse effects, and some of these effects may be reduced or avoided if fewer lymph nodes are removed.

Section 31.3

Pelvic Examination

This section contains text excerpted from the following sources:
Text in this section begins with excerpts from "Screening Pelvic
Examinations in Asymptomatic Average Risk Adult Women," U.S.
Department of Veterans Affairs (VA), September 2013. Reviewed
May 2018; Text under the heading "Procedure" is excerpted from
"Pelvic Exam," National Cancer Institute (NCI), March 4, 2013.
Reviewed May 2018; Text beginning with the heading "Colposcopy" is
excerpted from "Understanding Cervical Changes—A Health Guide
for Women," National Cancer Institute (NCI), May 2017; Text under
the heading "The Effectiveness of PE as a Screening Tool for Non-
Cervical Cancers" is excerpted from "Evidence Is Lacking to Support
Pelvic Examinations as a Screening Tool for Non-Cervical Cancers
or Other Conditions," U.S. National Library of Medicine (NLM),
February 1, 2016.

The routine pelvic examination (PE) has been a usual part of preventive care for women for many decades. Many women and providers
believe that the routine pelvic exam should be included in an annual
comprehensive well-woman visit. The exam consists of inspection of
the external genitalia, speculum examination of the vagina and cervix,
bimanual examination, and sometimes rectal or rectovaginal examination. Traditionally, the examination in the asymptomatic average-risk
women has been used to screen for pathology through palpation, visualization, and specimen collection.

Pathology potentially detectable on the pelvic examination
includes malignancies (e.g., cervical, ovarian, uterine, bladder, vaginal, or vulvar); infections (e.g., chlamydia, gonorrhea, warts, candi-
diasis, and bacterial vaginosis); pelvic inflammatory disease (PID);
or other pathology (e.g., atrophic vaginitis, cervical polyps, uterine
prolapse, and fibroids). In addition, pelvic examinations are often
performed prior to the provision of hormonal contraception. The
term "pelvic examination" includes any of the following components,
alone or in combination: assessment of the external genitalia, internal speculum examination, bimanual palpation, and rectovaginal
examination.

The Procedure

A doctor or nurse inserts one or two lubricated, gloved fingers of one hand into the vagina and presses on the lower abdomen with the other hand. This is done to feel the size, shape, and position of the uterus and ovaries. The vagina, cervix, fallopian tubes, and rectum are also checked.

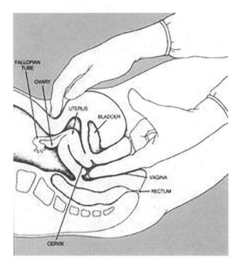

Figure 31.1. *Pelvic Exam* (Source: "Pelvic Exam Illustration," National Cancer Institute (NCI).)

Figure 31.1 shows a side view of the female reproductive anatomy during a pelvic exam. The uterus, left fallopian tube, left ovary, cervix, vagina, bladder, and rectum are shown. Two gloved fingers are shown inserted into the vagina, while the other hand is shown pressing on the lower abdomen.

Colposcopy

Your healthcare provider will examine your cervix using a colposcope and perform a biopsy if required. A colposcopy is a procedure to examine your cervix. During this procedure, your doctor inserts a speculum to gently open the vagina and see the cervix. Diluted white vinegar is put on the cervix, causing abnormal areas to turn white. Your doctor then places an instrument called a colposcope close to the vagina. It has a bright light and a magnifying lens and allows your doctor to look closely at your cervix. A colposcopy usually includes a biopsy. A biopsy is done so that the cells or tissues can be checked under a microscope for signs of disease. In addition to removing a sample for further testing, some types of biopsies may be used as treatment, to remove abnormal cervical tissue or lesions.

Pelvic Exam and Cervical Cancer Screening

Cervical cancer screening tests are usually done during a pelvic exam. During this exam, you lie on your back on an exam table, bend your knees, and put your feet into stirrups. The healthcare provider gently opens your vagina with a speculum to see the cervix. A soft, narrow brush or spatula is used to collect a small sample of cells from your cervix.

The sample of cervical cells is sent to the lab and checked for any abnormal cervical cells. The same sample can also be checked for human papillomavirus (HPV), with an HPV test. When both a Pap (Papanicolaou) test and an HPV test are done, this is called cotesting. A pelvic exam includes more than just taking samples for a Pap and/or HPV test. Your healthcare provider will also check the size, shape, and position of the uterus and ovaries and feel for any lumps or cysts. The rectum may also be checked for lumps or abnormal areas. Most healthcare providers will tell you what to expect at each step of the exam, so you will be at ease. When you talk with your healthcare provider, you may also ask to be tested for sexually transmitted infections (STIs).

The Effectiveness of PE as a Screening Tool for Noncervical Cancers

A systematic review by the Division of Cancer Prevention and Control (DCPC), Centers for Disease Control and Prevention (CDC), identified very little evidence for the effectiveness of PE screening for prevention of noncervical cancer or any benign conditions. The harms identified, however, were real, documented and not without significance. Women who feel pain and discomfort are less likely to return for a preventive care visit consisting of other evidence-based screening or care. PEs were also a barrier among obese women: a group of women that may benefit from chronic disease screenings or counseling.

Unfortunately, this review was not able to differentiate between the benefits and harms of the individual examination components (speculum, external genital examination and bimanual). The bimanual examination (BME) is often the component that is associated with the most embarrassment, pain or discomfort and may benefit from a more focused review. Cervical cancer was not examined as an outcome because of the assumption that the speculum examination is necessary for cytology collection, and cytology has been shown to be an effective screening test for cervical cancer. Combining the speculum examination with the cytology for cervical cancer screening resulted in an unhelpful category that included two very different components of screening that are used for different reasons: the speculum examination is the method used to obtain the sample, while cytology is the test conducted on the sample.

This review was accompanied by a statement from a well-respected body of U.S. internal medicine specialists that recommended against performing screening PE. In a recent survey, a third of internists still used the PE routinely to screen for ovarian cancer, compared to 55 percent of family medicine physicians and 98 percent of obstetricians and gynecologists. In 2010, the most common reason for a visit to the U.S. office-based obstetrics and gynecology practice was for preventive care, and American College of Obstetricians and Gynecologists (ACOG) continues to recommend annual PE among most adult women despite the lack of evidence of its effectiveness.

Section 31.4

Loop Electrosurgical Excision Procedure (LEEP)

"Loop Electrosurgical Excision Procedure (LEEP),"
© 2018 Omnigraphics. Reviewed May 2018.

The loop electrosurgical excision procedure (LEEP) is one of the most commonly used interventions to treat cervical intraepithelial neoplasia, also called cervical dysplasia, which refers to abnormal cells on the surface of the cervix discovered during a pelvic examination or on the basis of a Papanicolaou (Pap) smear test. In addition to being an effective, low-cost, and the least invasive method to treat precancerous lesions in the cervix, LEEP is also used as a diagnostic tool for cancers of the cervix and vagina.

The procedure can be performed in an outpatient setting and usually under regional anesthesia—although sometimes it may require sedation with general anesthesia if the patient's condition deems it necessary. As the name suggests, a low voltage electric current is applied through a fine wire loop to excise the abnormal cells, cauterize the lesion, and make way for regrowth of normal cells. Loops of varying sizes and shapes can be used depending on the orientation of the lesion and the cervical transformation zone, an area of constantly changing cells in the cervical canal that is most prone to abnormalities. Sometimes, a part of the abnormal tissue is excised during LEEP to obtain an endocervical specimen for evaluation.

The Procedure

LEEP is generally done when there is no menstrual discharge so as to monitor postprocedural bleeding. It is also not usually scheduled during pregnancy as it may carry a small risk of spontaneous abortion or preterm labor. The physician should be informed of any medication, such as blood thinners or herbal supplements, being used as the patient may be required to discontinue this use prior to LEEP.

The preparation for LEEP requires no fasting and is more or less the same as for a pelvic exam. The patient is asked to empty her bladder and is positioned on the examination table with both legs supported by a pair of obstetric stirrups, or foot stirrups, as is done for a pelvic exam. The physician then inserts a speculum in the vagina to dilate the walls of the vagina and access the cervix. A colposcope, an instrument with a luminous source and a magnifying lens, is then positioned at the vaginal opening for visual inspection of the vulva, vagina, and cervix, and identification of abnormal areas. The cervix is first soaked with a 3–5 percent acetic acid solution, which turns abnormal areas white and allows greater visualization of the dysplastic area. After this, the cervix is anesthetized to numb the area, and a tenaculum (a type of forceps with two opposing ends) is typically used to stabilize the cervix for the procedure. The LEEP wire is then inserted through the speculum to the site of abnormal tissue. Thermal energy is then generated in the wire and a radio frequency current passes through it and is transferred to the target tissue. The rapid buildup of heat causes spontaneous vaporization of the intracellular water, which in turn leads to disintegration and, finally, death of the precancerous tissue.

Typically, ectocervical LEEP sampling removes only a thin layer of the peripheral tissue (6–8 mm in depth). In patients requiring further exploration, a second endocervical sample of around 5 mm depth may be obtained using a smaller loop.

Medication

Preoperative nonsteroidal anti-inflammatory drugs (NSAIDs) may be administered to help with pain and cramping associated with the procedure, and anxiolytic agents and other relaxation techniques are also widely used to treat anxiety and ensure that the patient remains still during the procedure. Vasoconstricting solutions, such as epinephrine or vasopressin, may also be administered to enable hemostasis.

Postoperative Instruction

Mild to moderate cramping and bleeding comparable to a light menstrual discharge are commonly experienced after a LEEP procedure. Patients are advised against lifting more than 20 pounds of weight or engaging in strenuous exercise or competitive sports for 3 to 4 weeks following the procedure. Patients are usually instructed to avoid sexual intercourse, using tampons, or douching to lower the risk of bleeding and infection. Straining during bowel movements is also to be avoided and over-the-counter (OTC) laxatives may be prescribed to prevent constipation.

Complications

Intra- and postoperative bleeding, although rare, is a possible complication arising from the procedure, particularly with deeper endocervical sampling. While most cases of hemorrhage can be successfully managed with conservative treatment (electrocautery or medication), a few may require surgical ligature with absorbable sutures to achieve hemostasis (stoppage of bleeding).

Generally, the procedure carries a very low risk of infection, and prophylactic antibiotics are rarely indicated. However, if a patient develops abdominal pain, fever, or malodorous vaginal discharge, antibiotics may be prescribed to treat the infection.

Cervical stenosis, or blocking of the cervical canal, is one of the possible complications of a LEEP procedure. While scarring is a natural healing process following the procedure, a small percentage of patients go on to develop cervical stenosis as a result of robust scarring. The larger the amount of tissue cauterized, the greater the likelihood of scar formation and obstruction of the cervical canal.

Stenosis can be either anatomic or complete. Anatomic stenosis does not restrict menstrual flow and needs no corrective intervention. A complete stenosis, which is associated with loss of both anatomic and functional opening of the cervix, may compromise cervical competence and complicate fertility, particularly in cases in which substantial tissue has been removed. Such cases are usually resolved by simple endocervical dilation about six weeks after the LEEP procedure or the placement of a stent or intrauterine device. The scar tissue may also be opened up just prior to fertility treatments such as insemination and embryo transfer.

Prognosis

LEEP is an effective method of intervention for low-grade cervical dysplasia, and is usually associated with few long-term adverse events. Most of the cases resolve and no residual disease is indicated in subsequent colposcopies or Pap smears. However, if follow-up Pap smears indicate persistent dysplasia or recurrent high-grade lesions, then a hysterectomy may be necessary. One of the major drawbacks arising from this "see-and-treat" procedure—as LEEP is popularly referred to—is the inherent risk of overutilization, particularly for low-grade dysplasia, which is usually associated with a high potential for spontaneous regression.

References

1. "The Fight against Cervical Cancer," Military Health System (MHS), n.d.

2. "Loop Electrosurgical Excision Procedure (LEEP)," Johns Hopkins Medicine, n.d.

3. "Instructions for Care after a Loop Electrical Excision Procedure (LEEP)," U.S. Department of Veterans Affairs (VA), May 2005.

Section 31.5

Tumor Markers

This section includes text excerpted from "Diagnosis and Staging—Tumor Markers," National Cancer Institute (NCI), November 4, 2015.

What Are Tumor Markers?

Tumor markers are substances that are produced by cancer or by other cells of the body in response to cancer or certain benign (non-cancerous) conditions. Most tumor markers are made by normal cells as well as by cancer cells; however, they are produced at much higher levels in cancerous conditions. These substances can be found in the blood, urine, stool, tumor tissue, or other tissues or bodily fluids of some patients with cancer. Most tumor markers are proteins. However, more recently, patterns of gene expression and changes to deoxyribonucleic acid (DNA) have also begun to be used as tumor markers.

Many different tumor markers have been characterized and are in clinical use. Some are associated with only one type of cancer, whereas others are associated with two or more cancer types. No "universal" tumor marker that can detect any type of cancer has been found. There are some limitations to the use of tumor markers. Sometimes, non-cancerous conditions can cause the levels of certain tumor markers to increase. In addition, not everyone with a particular type of cancer will have a higher level of a tumor marker associated with that cancer. Moreover, tumor markers have not been identified for every type of cancer.

How Are Tumor Markers Used in Cancer Care?

Tumor markers are used to help detect, diagnose, and manage some types of cancer. Although an elevated level of a tumor marker may suggest the presence of cancer, this alone is not enough to diagnose cancer. Therefore, measurements of tumor markers are usually combined with other tests, such as biopsies, to diagnose cancer.

Tumor marker levels may be measured before treatment to help doctors plan the appropriate therapy. In some types of cancer, the level of a tumor marker reflects the stage (extent) of the disease and/or the patient's prognosis (likely outcome or course of disease). Tumor markers may also be measured periodically during cancer therapy. A decrease in the level of a tumor marker or a return to the marker's normal level may indicate that the cancer is responding to treatment, whereas no change or an increase may indicate that the cancer is not responding. Tumor markers may also be measured after treatment has ended to check for recurrence (the return of cancer).

How Are Tumor Markers Measured?

A doctor takes a sample of tumor tissue or bodily fluid and sends it to a laboratory, where various methods are used to measure the level of the tumor marker. If the tumor marker is being used to determine whether treatment is working or whether there is a recurrence, the marker's level will be measured in multiple samples taken over time. Usually, these "serial measurements," which show whether the level of a marker is increasing, staying the same, or decreasing, are more meaningful than a single measurement.

What Tumor Markers Are Currently Being Used, and for Which Cancer Types?

A number of tumor markers are currently being used for a wide range of cancer types. Although most of these can be tested in laboratories that meet standards set by the Clinical Laboratory Improvement Amendments, some cannot be and may, therefore, be considered experimental. Tumor markers that are currently in common use are listed below.

ALK Gene Rearrangements and Overexpression

- Cancer types: Nonsmall cell lung cancer and anaplastic large cell lymphoma

- Tissue analyzed: Tumor

- How used: To help determine treatment and prognosis

Alpha-Fetoprotein (AFP)

- Cancer types: Liver cancer and germ cell tumors

- Tissue analyzed: Blood

- How used: To help diagnose liver cancer and follow response to treatment; to assess stage, prognosis, and response to treatment of germ cell tumors

Beta-2-Microglobulin (B2M)

- Cancer types: Multiple myeloma, chronic lymphocytic leukemia, and some lymphomas
- Tissue analyzed: Blood, urine, or cerebrospinal fluid
- How used: To determine prognosis and follow response to treatment

Beta-human Chorionic Gonadotropin (Beta-hCG)

- Cancer types: Choriocarcinoma and germ cell tumors
- Tissue analyzed: Urine or blood
- How used: To assess stage, prognosis, and response to treatment

BRCA1 *and* **BRCA2** *Gene Mutations*

- Cancer type: Ovarian cancer
- Tissue analyzed: Blood
- How used: To determine whether treatment with a particular type of targeted therapy is appropriate

BCR-ABL Fusion Gene (Philadelphia Chromosome)

- Cancer type: Chronic myeloid leukemia (CML), acute lymphoblastic leukemia (ALL), and acute myelogenous leukemia (AML)
- Tissue analyzed: Blood and/or bone marrow
- How used: To confirm diagnosis, predict response to targeted therapy, and monitor disease status

BRAF V600 Mutations

- Cancer types: Cutaneous melanoma and colorectal cancer
- Tissue analyzed: Tumor
- How used: To select patients who are most likely to benefit from treatment with certain targeted therapies

C-Kit / CD117

- Cancer types: Gastrointestinal stromal tumor (GIST) and mucosal melanoma
- Tissue analyzed: Tumor
- How used: To help in diagnosing and determining treatment

CA15-3 / CA27.29

- Cancer type: Breast cancer
- Tissue analyzed: Blood
- How used: To assess whether treatment is working or disease has recurred

CA 19-9 (Cancer Antigen 19-9)

- Cancer types: Pancreatic cancer, gallbladder cancer, bile duct cancer, and gastric cancer
- Tissue analyzed: Blood
- How used: To assess whether treatment is working

CA 125 (Cancer Antigen 125)

- Cancer type: Ovarian cancer
- Tissue analyzed: Blood
- How used: To help in diagnosis, assessment of response to treatment, and evaluation of recurrence

Calcitonin

- Cancer type: Medullary thyroid cancer (MTC)
- Tissue analyzed: Blood
- How used: To aid in diagnosis, check whether treatment is working, and assess recurrence

Carcinoembryonic Antigen (CEA)

- Cancer types: Colorectal cancer and some other cancers
- Tissue analyzed: Blood

- How used: To keep track of how well cancer treatments are working or check if cancer has come back

CD20

- Cancer type: Non-Hodgkin lymphoma (NHL)
- Tissue analyzed: Blood
- How used: To determine whether treatment with a targeted therapy is appropriate

Chromogranin A (CgA)

- Cancer type: Neuroendocrine tumors
- Tissue analyzed: Blood
- How used: To help in diagnosis, assessment of treatment response, and evaluation of recurrence

Chromosomes 3, 7, 17, and 9p21

- Cancer type: Bladder cancer
- Tissue analyzed: Urine
- How used: To help in monitoring for tumor recurrence

Circulating Tumor Cells of Epithelial Origin (CELLSEARCH®)

- Cancer types: Metastatic breast and colorectal cancers
- Tissue analyzed: Blood
- How used: To inform clinical decision making, and to assess prognosis

Cytokeratin Fragment 21-1

- Cancer type: Lung cancer
- Tissue analyzed: Blood
- How used: To help in monitoring for recurrence

Epidermal Growth Factor Receptor (EGFR) Gene Mutation Analysis

- Cancer type: Nonsmall cell lung cancer

- Tissue analyzed: Tumor
- How used: To help determine treatment and prognosis

Estrogen Receptor (ER)/Progesterone Receptor (PR)

- Cancer type: Breast cancer
- Tissue analyzed: Tumor
- How used: To determine whether treatment with hormone therapy and some targeted therapies is appropriate

Fibrin/Fibrinogen

- Cancer type: Bladder cancer
- Tissue analyzed: Urine
- How used: To monitor progression and response to treatment

Human Epididymis Protein 4 (HE4)

- Cancer type: Ovarian cancer
- Tissue analyzed: Blood
- How used: To plan cancer treatment, assess disease progression, and monitor for recurrence

HER2/Neu Gene Amplification or Protein Overexpression

- Cancer types: Breast cancer, gastric cancer, and gastroesophageal junction adenocarcinoma
- Tissue analyzed: Tumor
- How used: To determine whether treatment with certain targeted therapies is appropriate

Immunoglobulins

- Cancer types: Multiple myeloma and Waldenström macroglobulinemia (WM)
- Tissue analyzed: Blood and urine
- How used: To help diagnose disease, assess response to treatment, and look for recurrence

KRAS Gene Mutation Analysis

- Cancer types: Colorectal cancer and nonsmall cell lung cancer
- Tissue analyzed: Tumor
- How used: To determine whether treatment with a particular type of targeted therapy is appropriate

Lactate Dehydrogenase

- Cancer types: Germ cell tumors, lymphoma, leukemia, melanoma, and neuroblastoma
- Tissue analyzed: Blood
- How used: To assess stage, prognosis, and response to treatment

Neuron-Specific Enolase (NSE)

- Cancer types: Small cell lung cancer and neuroblastoma
- Tissue analyzed: Blood
- How used: To help in diagnosis and to assess response to treatment

Nuclear Matrix Protein 22

- Cancer type: Bladder cancer
- Tissue analyzed: Urine
- How used: To monitor response to treatment

Programmed Death Ligand 1 (PD-L1)

- Cancer type: Nonsmall cell lung cancer
- Tissue analyzed: Tumor
- How used: To determine whether treatment with a particular type of targeted therapy is appropriate

Thyroglobulin

- Cancer type: Thyroid cancer
- Tissue analyzed: Blood
- How used: To evaluate response to treatment and look for recurrence

Urokinase Plasminogen Activator (uPA) and Plasminogen Activator Inhibitor (PAI-1)

- Cancer type: Breast cancer
- Tissue analyzed: Tumor
- How used: To determine aggressiveness of cancer and guide treatment

5-Protein Signature (OVA1®)

- Cancer type: Ovarian cancer
- Tissue analyzed: Blood
- How used: To preoperatively assess pelvic mass for suspected ovarian cancer

21-Gene Signature (Oncotype DX®)

- Cancer type: Breast cancer
- Tissue analyzed: Tumor
- How used: To evaluate risk of recurrence

70-Gene Signature (Mammaprint®)

- Cancer type: Breast cancer
- Tissue analyzed: Tumor
- How used: To evaluate risk of recurrence

Can Tumor Markers Be Used in Cancer Screening?

Because tumor markers can be used to assess the response of a tumor to treatment and for prognosis, researchers have hoped that they might also be useful in screening tests that aim to detect cancer early, before there are any symptoms. For a screening test to be useful, it should have very high sensitivity (ability to correctly identify people who have the disease) and specificity (ability to correctly identify people who do not have the disease). If a test is highly sensitive, it will identify most people with the disease—that is, it will result in very few false-negative results. If a test is highly specific, only a small number of people will test positive for the disease who do not have it—in other words, it will result in very few false-positive results.

Although tumor markers are extremely useful in determining whether a tumor is responding to treatment or assessing whether it has recurred, no tumor marker identified to date is sufficiently sensitive or specific to be used on its own to screen for cancer.

Similarly, results from the PLCO trial showed that CA-125, a tumor marker that is sometimes elevated in the blood of women with ovarian cancer but can also be elevated in women with benign conditions, is not sufficiently sensitive or specific to be used together with transvaginal ultrasound to screen for ovarian cancer in women at average risk of the disease. An analysis of 28 potential markers for ovarian cancer in blood from women who later went on to develop ovarian cancer found that none of these markers performed even as well as CA-125 at detecting the disease in women at average risk.

What Kind of Research Is Underway to Develop More Accurate Tumor Markers?

Cancer researchers are turning to proteomics (the study of protein structure, function, and patterns of expression) in hopes of developing new biomarkers that can be used to identify disease in its early stages, to predict the effectiveness of treatment, or to predict the chance of cancer recurrence after treatment has ended. Scientists are also evaluating patterns of gene expression for their ability to help determine a patient's prognosis or response to therapy. For example, results of the National Cancer Institute (NCI)-sponsored Trial Assigning Individua Lized Options for Treatment (Rx), or TAILORx, showed that for women recently diagnosed with lymph node-negative, hormone receptor-positive, HER2-negative breast cancer who had undergone surgery, those with the lowest 21-gene (Oncotype Dx®) recurrence scores had very low recurrence rates when given hormone therapy alone and thus can be spared chemotherapy. The trial is ongoing to see whether women at intermediate risk of recurrence, based on the 21-gene test, do better with chemotherapy in addition to hormone therapy than with hormone therapy alone.

Chapter 32

What Do Your Cancer Test Results Mean?

Chapter Contents

Section 32.1

Understanding a Pathology Report

This section includes text excerpted from "Pathology Reports,"
National Cancer Institute (NCI), September 23, 2010.
Reviewed May 2018.

What Is a Pathology Report?

A pathology report is a document that contains the diagnosis determined by examining cells and tissues under a microscope. The report may also contain information about the size, shape, and appearance of a specimen as it looks to the naked eye. This information is known as the gross description. A pathologist is a doctor who does this examination and writes the pathology report. Pathology reports play an important role in cancer diagnosis and staging (describing the extent of cancer within the body, especially whether it has spread), which helps determine treatment options.

How Is Tissue Processed after a Biopsy or Surgery? What Is a Frozen Section?

The tissue removed during a biopsy or surgery must be cut into thin sections, placed on slides, and stained with dyes before it can be examined under a microscope. Two methods are used to make the tissue firm enough to cut into thin sections: frozen sections and paraffin-embedded (permanent) sections. All tissue samples are prepared as permanent sections, but sometimes frozen sections are also prepared.

Permanent sections are prepared by placing the tissue in fixative (usually formalin) to preserve the tissue, processing it through additional solutions, and then placing it in paraffin wax. After the wax has hardened, the tissue is cut into very thin slices, which are placed on slides and stained. The process normally takes several days. A permanent section provides the best quality for examination by the pathologist and produces more accurate results than a frozen section.

Frozen sections are prepared by freezing and slicing the tissue sample. They can be done in about 15–20 minutes while the patient is in the operating room. Frozen sections are done when an immediate answer is needed; for example, to determine whether the tissue is cancerous so as to guide the surgeon during the course of an operation.

How Long after the Tissue Sample Is Taken Will the Pathology Report Be Ready?

The pathologist sends a pathology report to the doctor within 10 days after the biopsy or surgery is performed. Pathology reports are written in technical medical language. Patients may want to ask their doctors to give them a copy of the pathology report and to explain the report to them. Patients also may wish to keep a copy of their pathology report in their own records.

What Information Does a Pathology Report Usually Include?

The pathology report may include the following information:

- **Patient information:** Name, birth date, biopsy date
- **Gross description:** Color, weight, and size of tissue as seen by the naked eye
- **Microscopic description:** How the sample looks under the microscope and how it compares with normal cells
- **Diagnosis:** Type of tumor/cancer and grade (how abnormal the cells look under the microscope and how quickly the tumor is likely to grow and spread)
- **Tumor size:** Measured in centimeters
- **Tumor margins:** There are three possible findings when the biopsy sample is the entire tumor:
  - Positive margins mean that cancer cells are found at the edge of the material removed
  - Negative, not involved, clear, or free margins mean that no cancer cells are found at the outer edge
  - Close margins are neither negative nor positive
- **Other information:** Usually, notes about samples that have been sent for other tests or a second opinion
  - Pathologist's signature and name and address of the laboratory

What Might the Pathology Report Say about the Physical and Chemical Characteristics of the Tissue?

After identifying the tissue as cancerous, the pathologist may perform additional tests to get more information about the tumor that cannot be determined by looking at the tissue with routine stains, such as hematoxylin and eosin (also known as H&E), under a microscope. The pathology report will include the results of these tests. For example, the pathology report may include information obtained from immunochemical stains (IHC). IHC uses antibodies to identify specific antigens on the surface of cancer cells. IHC can often be used to:

- Determine where the cancer started

- Distinguish among different cancer types, such as carcinoma, melanoma, and lymphoma

- Help diagnose and classify leukemias and lymphomas

The pathology report may also include the results of flow cytometry. Flow cytometry is a method of measuring properties of cells in a sample, including the number of cells, percentage of live cells, cell size and shape, and presence of tumor markers on the cell surface. Tumor markers are substances produced by tumor cells or by other cells in the body in response to cancer or certain noncancerous conditions.) Flow cytometry can be used in the diagnosis, classification, and management of cancers such as acute leukemia, chronic lymphoproliferative disorders, and non-Hodgkin lymphoma (NHL).

Finally, the pathology report may include the results of molecular diagnostic and cytogenetic studies. Such studies investigate the presence or absence of malignant cells, and genetic or molecular abnormalities in specimens.

What Information about the Genetics of the Cells Might Be Included in the Pathology Report?

Cytogenetics uses tissue culture and specialized techniques to provide genetic information about cells, particularly genetic alterations. Some genetic alterations are markers or indicators of a specific cancer. For example, the Philadelphia chromosome is associated with chronic myelogenous leukemia (CML). Some alterations can provide information about prognosis, which helps the doctor make treatment recommendations. Some tests that might be performed on a tissue sample include:

- **Fluorescence in situ hybridization (FISH).** Determines the positions of particular genes. It can be used to identify chromosomal abnormalities and to map genes.

- **Polymerase chain reaction (PCR).** A method of making many copies of particular deoxyribonucleic acid (DNA) sequences of relevance to the diagnosis.

- **Real-time PCR or quantitative PCR.** A method of measuring how many copies of a particular DNA sequence are present.

- **Reverse-transcriptase polymerase chain reaction (RT-PCR).** A method of making many copies of a specific ribonucleic acid (RNA) sequence.

- **Southern blot hybridization.** Detects specific DNA fragments.

- **Western blot hybridization.** Identifies and analyzes proteins or peptides.

Can Individuals Get a Second Opinion about Their Pathology Results?

Although most cancers can be easily diagnosed, sometimes patients or their doctors may want to get a second opinion about the pathology results. Patients interested in getting a second opinion should talk with their doctor. They will need to obtain the slides and/or paraffin block from the pathologist who examined the sample or from the hospital where the biopsy or surgery was done.

Many institutions provide second opinions on pathology specimens. National Cancer Institute (NCI)-designated cancer centers or academic institutions are reasonable places to consider. Patients should contact the facility in advance to determine if this service is available, the cost, and shipping instructions.

Section 32.2

Questions and Answers about Cancer Staging

This section includes text excerpted from "Cancer Staging,"
National Cancer Institute (NCI), March 9, 2015.

Stage refers to the extent of your cancer, such as how large the tumor is, and if it has spread. Knowing the stage of your cancer helps your doctor:

- Understand how serious your cancer is and your chances of survival

- Plan the best treatment for you

- Identify clinical trials that may be treatment options for you

A cancer is always referred to by the stage it was given at diagnosis, even if it gets worse or spreads. New information about how a cancer has changed over time gets added on to the original stage. So, the stage doesn't change, even though the cancer might.

How Stage Is Determined

To learn the stage of your disease, your doctor may order X-rays, lab tests, and other tests or procedures.

Systems That Describe Stage

There are many staging systems. Some, such as the TNM (T—size of primary tumor; N—regional lymph nodes; M—distant metastasis) staging system, are used for many types of cancer. Others are specific to a particular type of cancer. Most staging systems include information about:

- Where the tumor is located in the body

- The cell type (such as, adenocarcinoma or squamous cell carcinoma)

- The size of the tumor

- Whether the cancer has spread to nearby lymph nodes

- Whether the cancer has spread to a different part of the body

- Tumor grade, which refers to how abnormal the cancer cells look and how likely the tumor is to grow and spread

The TNM Staging System

The TNM system is the most widely used cancer staging system. Most hospitals and medical centers use the TNM system as their main method for cancer reporting. You are likely to see your cancer described by this staging system in your pathology report, unless you have a cancer for which a different staging system is used. Examples of cancers with different staging systems include brain and spinal cord tumors and blood cancers.

In the TNM system:

- The T refers to the size and extent of the main tumor. The main tumor is usually called the primary tumor.

- The N refers to the number of nearby lymph nodes that have cancer.

- The M refers to whether the cancer has metastasized. This means that the cancer has spread from the primary tumor to other parts of the body.

When your cancer is described by the TNM system, there will be numbers after each letter that give more details about the cancer—for example, T1N0MX or T3N1M0. The following explains what the letters and numbers mean:

Primary tumor (T)

- TX: Main tumor cannot be measured.

- T0: Main tumor cannot be found.

- T1, T2, T3, T4: Refers to the size and/or extent of the main tumor. The higher the number after the T, the larger the tumor or the more it has grown into nearby tissues. T's may be further divided to provide more detail, such as T3a and T3b.

Regional lymph nodes (N)

- NX: Cancer in nearby lymph nodes cannot be measured.

- N0: There is no cancer in nearby lymph nodes.

- N1, N2, N3: Refers to the number and location of lymph nodes that contain cancer. The higher the number after the N, the more lymph nodes that contain cancer.

Distant metastasis (M)

- MX: Metastasis cannot be measured.

- M0: Cancer has not spread to other parts of the body.

- M1: Cancer has spread to other parts of the body.

Other Ways to Describe Stage

The TNM system helps describe cancer in great detail. But, for many cancers, the TNM combinations are grouped into five less-detailed stages. When talking about your cancer, your doctor or nurse may describe it as one of these stages:

Table 32.1. Cancer Staging

Stage	What It Means
Stage 0	Abnormal cells are present but have not spread to nearby tissue. Also called carcinoma in situ, or CIS. CIS is not cancer, but it may become cancer.
Stage I, Stage II, and Stage III	Cancer is present. The higher the number, the larger the cancer tumor and the more it has spread into nearby tissues.
Stage IV	The cancer has spread to distant parts of the body.

Another staging system that is used for all types of cancer groups the cancer into one of five main categories. This staging system is more often used by cancer registries than by doctors. But, you may still hear your doctor or nurse describe your cancer in one of the following ways:

- **In situ**: Abnormal cells are present but have not spread to nearby tissue

- **Localized**: Cancer is limited to the place where it started, with no sign that it has spread

- **Regional**: Cancer has spread to nearby lymph nodes, tissues, or organs

- **Distant**: Cancer has spread to distant parts of the body

- **Unknown**: There is not enough information to figure out the stage

Section 32.3

Questions and Answers about Tumor Grades

This section includes text excerpted from "Tumor Grade Fact Sheet Tumor Grade," National Cancer Institute (NCI), May 3, 2013. Reviewed May 2018.

What Is Tumor Grade?

Tumor grade is the description of a tumor based on how abnormal the tumor cells and the tumor tissue look under a microscope. It is an indicator of how quickly a tumor is likely to grow and spread. If the cells of the tumor and the organization of the tumors tissue are close to those of normal cells and tissue, the tumor is called "well-differentiated." These tumors tend to grow and spread at a slower rate than tumors that are "undifferentiated" or "poorly differentiated," which have abnormal-looking cells and may lack normal tissue structures. Based on these and other differences in microscopic appearance, doctors assign a numerical "grade" to most cancers. The factors used to determine tumor grade can vary between different types of cancer.

Tumor grade is not the same as the stage of a cancer. Cancer stage refers to the size and/or extent (reach) of the original (primary) tumor and whether or not cancer cells have spread in the body. Cancer stage is based on factors such as the location of the primary tumor, tumor size, regional lymph node involvement (the spread of cancer to nearby lymph nodes), and the number of tumors present.

How Is Tumor Grade Determined?

If a tumor is suspected to be malignant, a doctor removes all or part of it during a procedure called a biopsy. A pathologist (a doctor who identifies diseases by studying cells and tissues under a microscope) then examines the biopsied tissue to determine whether the tumor is benign or malignant. The pathologist also determines the tumor's grade and identifies other characteristics of the tumor. The National Cancer Institute (NCI) Pathology Reports describes the type

405

of information that can be found in a pathologist's report about the visual and microscopic examination of tissue removed during a biopsy or other surgery.

How Are Tumor Grades Classified?

Grading systems differ depending on the type of cancer. In general, tumors are graded as 1, 2, 3, or 4, depending on the amount of abnormality. In Grade 1 tumors, the tumor cells and the organization of the tumor tissue appear close to normal. These tumors tend to grow and spread slowly. In contrast, the cells and tissue of Grade 3 and Grade 4 tumors do not look like normal cells and tissue. Grade 3 and Grade 4 tumors tend to grow rapidly and spread faster than tumors with a lower grade.

If a grading system for a tumor type is not specified, the following system is generally used:

- GX: Grade cannot be assessed (undetermined grade)
- G1: Well differentiated (low grade)
- G2: Moderately differentiated (intermediate grade)
- G3: Poorly differentiated (high grade)
- G4: Undifferentiated (high grade)

What Is Breast Cancer's Grading System?

Doctors most often use the Nottingham grading system (also called the Elston-Ellis modification of the Scarff-Bloom-Richardson grading system) for breast cancer. This system grades breast tumors based on the following features:

- Tubule formation: How much of the tumor tissue has normal breast (milk) duct structures
- Nuclear grade: An evaluation of the size and shape of the nucleus in the tumor cells
- Mitotic rate: How many dividing cells are present, which is a measure of how fast the tumor cells are growing and dividing

Each of the categories gets a score between 1 and 3; a score of "1" means the cells and tumor tissue look the most like normal cells and tissue, and a score of "3" means the cells and tissue look the most abnormal. The scores for the three categories are then added, yielding a total score of 3–9. Three grades are possible:

- Total score = 3–5: G1 (Low grade or well differentiated)

- Total score = 6–7: G2 (Intermediate grade or moderately differentiated)

- Total score = 8–9: G3 (High grade or poorly differentiated)

How Does Tumor Grade Affect a Patient's Treatment Options?

Doctors use tumor grade and other factors, such as cancer stage and a patient's age and general health, to develop a treatment plan and to determine a patient's prognosis (the likely outcome or course of a disease; the chance of recovery or recurrence). Generally, a lower grade indicates a better prognosis. A higher-grade cancer may grow and spread more quickly and may require immediate or more aggressive treatment. The importance of tumor grade in planning treatment and determining a patient's prognosis is greater for certain types of cancer, such as soft tissue sarcoma, primary brain tumors, and breast cancer. Patients should talk with their doctor for more information about tumor grade and how it relates to their treatment and prognosis.

Chapter 33

Getting a Second Opinion before Surgery

What Is a Second Opinion?

A second opinion is when another doctor (in addition to your regular doctor) gives his or her view about your health problem and how it should be treated. Getting a second opinion can help you make a more informed decision about your care.

Medicare Part B (Medical Insurance) helps pay for a second opinion before surgery. When your doctor says you have a health problem that needs surgery, you have the right to:

- Know and understand your treatment choices

- Have another doctor look at those choices with you (second opinion)

- Participate in treatment decisions by making your wishes known

When Should I Get a Second Opinion?

If your doctor says you need surgery to diagnose or treat a health problem that isn't an emergency, consider getting a second opinion. It's up to you to decide when and if you'll have surgery.

This chapter includes text excerpted from "Getting a Second Opinion before Surgery," Centers for Medicare & Medicaid Services (CMS), April 2018.

Medicare doesn't pay for surgeries or procedures that aren't medically necessary, like cosmetic surgery. This means that Medicare also won't pay for second opinions for surgeries or procedures that aren't medically necessary.

Don't wait for a second opinion if you need emergency surgery. Some types of emergencies may require surgery right away, like:

- Acute appendicitis

- Blood clot or aneurysm

- Accidental injuries

How Do I Find a Doctor for a Second Opinion?

Make sure the doctor giving the second opinion accepts Medicare. To find a doctor for a second opinion:

- Visit Medicare.gov/physiciancompare to find doctors who accept Medicare.

- Call 800-MEDICARE (800-633-4227). TTY users can call 877-486-2048. Ask for information about doctors who accept Medicare.

- Ask your doctor for the name of another doctor to see for a second opinion. Don't hesitate to ask—most doctors want you to get a second opinion. You can also ask another doctor you trust to recommend a doctor.

What Should I Do before Getting a Second Opinion?

Before you visit the second doctor:

- Ask the first doctor to send your medical records to the doctor giving the second opinion. That way, you may not have to repeat the tests you already had.

- Call the second doctor's office and make sure they have your records.

- Write down a list of questions to take with you to the appointment.

- Ask a family member or friend to go to the appointment with you.

During the visit with the second doctor:

- Tell the doctor what surgery you're thinking about having.

- Tell the doctor what tests you already had.

- Ask the questions you have on your list and encourage your friend or loved one to ask any questions that he or she may have.

The second doctor may ask you to have additional tests performed as a result of the visit. Medicare will help pay for these tests just as it helps pay for other services that are medically necessary.

What If the First and Second Opinions Are Different?

If the second doctor doesn't agree with the first, you may feel confused about what to do. In that case, you may want to:

- Talk more about your condition with your first doctor.

- Talk to a third doctor. Medicare helps pay for a third opinion, if the first and second opinions are different.

Getting a second or third opinion doesn't mean you have to change doctors. You decide which doctor you want to do your surgery.

How Much Does Medicare Pay for a Second Opinion?

Medicare Part B helps pay for a second (or third) opinion and related tests just as it helps pay for other services that are medically necessary. If you have Part B and Original Medicare:

- Medicare pays 80 percent of the Medicare-approved amount.

- Your share is usually 20 percent of the Medicare-approved amount after you pay your yearly Part B deductible.

Do Medicare Advantage Plans Cover Second Opinions?

If you're in a Medicare Advantage Plan (like an health maintenance organization (HMO) or preferred provider organization (PPO)), you have the right to get a second opinion. If the first two opinions are different, your plan will help pay for a third opinion.

Even though you have the right to get a second opinion, keep these things in mind:

- Some plans will only help pay for a second opinion if you have a referral (a written OK) from your primary care doctor.

- Some plans will only help pay for a second opinion from a doctor who's in your plan's provider network.

Call your Medicare Advantage Plan for more information.

If you have Medicaid, it might also pay for second surgical opinions. To find out, call your Medicaid office. You can get the phone number by:

- Visiting Medicare.gov/contacts.

- Calling 800-MEDICARE (800-633-4227). TTY users can call 877-486-2048.

You have the right to get Medicare information in an accessible format, like large print, Braille, or audio. You also have the right to file a complaint if you feel you've been discriminated against. Visit Medicare.gov/aboutus/nondiscrimination/accessibility-nondiscrimination.html, or call 800-MEDICARE for more information.

Chapter 34

Commonly Used Surgical Procedures for Women with Cancer

Chapter Contents

Section 34.1

Hysterectomy

This section includes text excerpted from "Hysterectomy,"
Office on Women's Health (OWH), U.S. Department of
Health and Human Services (HHS), February 15, 2018.

A hysterectomy is a surgery to remove a woman's uterus (also known as the womb). The uterus is where a baby grows when a woman is pregnant. During the surgery, the whole uterus is usually removed. Your doctor may also remove your fallopian tubes and ovaries. After a hysterectomy, you no longer have menstrual periods and cannot become pregnant.

What Happens during a Hysterectomy?

Hysterectomy is a surgery to remove a woman's uterus (her womb). The whole uterus is usually removed. Your doctor also may remove your fallopian tubes and ovaries. Talk to your doctor before your surgery to discuss your options. For example, if both ovaries are removed, you will have symptoms of menopause. Ask your doctor about the risks and benefits of removing your ovaries. You may also be able to try an alternative to hysterectomy, such as medicine or another type of treatment, first.

Why Would I Need a Hysterectomy?

You may need a hysterectomy if you have one of the following:

- **Uterine fibroids.** Uterine fibroids are noncancerous growths in the wall of the uterus. In some women, they cause pain or heavy bleeding.

- **Heavy or unusual vaginal bleeding.** Changes in hormone levels, infection, cancer, or fibroids can cause heavy, prolonged bleeding.

- **Uterine prolapse.** This is when the uterus slips from its usual place down into the vagina. This is more common in women who had several vaginal births, but it can also happen after menopause or because of obesity. Prolapse can lead to urinary and bowel problems and pelvic pressure.

- **Endometriosis.** Endometriosis happens when the tissue that normally lines the uterus grows outside of the uterus on the ovaries where it doesn't belong. This can cause severe pain and bleeding between periods.

- **Adenomyosis.** In this condition, the tissue that lines the uterus grows inside the walls of the uterus where it doesn't belong. The uterine walls thicken and cause severe pain and heavy bleeding.

- **Cancer** (or precancer) of the uterus, ovary, cervix, or endometrium (the lining of the uterus). Hysterectomy may be the best option if you have cancer in one of these areas. Other treatment options may include chemotherapy and radiation. Your doctor will talk with you about the type of cancer you have and how advanced it is.

Keep in mind that there may be alternative ways to treat your health problem without having a hysterectomy. Hysterectomy is a major surgery. Talk with your doctor about all of your treatment options.

What Are Some Alternatives to Hysterectomy?

Hysterectomy is major surgery. Sometimes a hysterectomy may be medically necessary, such as with prolonged heavy bleeding or certain types of cancer. But sometimes you can try other treatments first. These include:

- **Watchful waiting.** You and your doctor may wish to wait if you have uterine fibroids, which tend to shrink after menopause.

- **Exercises.** For uterine prolapse, you can try Kegel exercises (squeezing the pelvic floor muscles). Kegel exercises help restore tone to the muscles holding the uterus in place.

- **Medicine.** Your doctor may give you medicine to help with endometriosis. Over-the-counter (OTC) pain medicines taken during your period also may help with pain and bleeding. Hormonal birth control, such as the pill, shot, or vaginal ring, or a hormonal intrauterine device (IUD) may help with

415

irregular or heavy vaginal bleeding or periods that last longer than usual.

- **Vaginal pessary (for uterine prolapse).** A pessary is a rubber or plastic donut-shaped object, similar to a diaphragm used for birth control. The pessary is inserted into the vagina to hold the uterus in place. Uterine prolapse happens when the uterus drops or "falls out" because it loses support after childbirth or pelvic surgery.

- **Surgery.** You and your doctor may choose to try a surgery that involves smaller or fewer cuts than hysterectomy. The smaller cuts may help you heal faster with less scarring. Depending on your symptoms, these options may include:

  - **Surgery to treat endometriosis.** Laparoscopic surgery uses a thin, lighted tube with a small camera. The doctor puts the camera and surgery tools into your pelvic area through very small cuts. This surgery can remove scar tissue or growths from endometriosis without harming the surrounding healthy organs such as ovaries. You may still get pregnant after this surgery.

  - **Surgery to help stop heavy or long-term vaginal bleeding.**

    - Dilation and curettage (D&C) removes the lining of the uterus that builds up every month before your period. Often, a hysteroscopy is done at the same time. Your doctor inserts the hysteroscope (a thin telescope) into your uterus to see the inside of the uterine cavity. D&C may also remove noncancerous growths or polyps from the uterus. After the D&C, a new uterine lining will build up during your next menstrual cycle as usual. You may still get pregnant after this surgery.

    - Endometrial ablation destroys the lining of the uterus permanently. Depending on the size and condition of your uterus, your doctor may use tools that freeze, heat, or use microwave energy to destroy the uterine lining. This surgery should not be used if you still want to become pregnant or if you have gone through menopause.

  - **Surgery to remove uterine fibroids without removing the uterus.** This is called a myomectomy. Depending on the location of your fibroids, the myomectomy can be done through the pelvic area or through the vagina and cervix. You may be able to get pregnant after this surgery. If your doctor recommends this surgery, ask your doctor if a power morcellator will be used. The U.S. Food and Drug Administration (FDA) has warned against the use of power morcellators for most women.

- **Surgery to shrink fibroids without removing the uterus.** This is called myolysis. The surgeon heats the fibroids, which causes them to shrink and die. Myolysis may be done laparoscopically (through very small cuts in the pelvic area). You may still get pregnant after myolysis.

- **Treatments to shrink fibroids without surgery.** These treatments include uterine artery embolization (UAE) and magnetic resonance (MR)-guided focused ultrasound (MR(f)US). UAE puts tiny plastic or gel particles into the vessels supplying blood to the fibroid. Once the blood supply is blocked, the fibroid shrinks and dies. MR(f)US sends ultrasound waves to the fibroids that heat and shrink the fibroids. After UAE or MR(f)US, you will not be able to get pregnant.

How Common Are Hysterectomies?

Each year in the United States, nearly 500,000 women get hysterectomies. A hysterectomy is the second most common surgery among women in the United States. The most common surgery in women is childbirth by cesarean delivery (C-section).

What Are the Different Types of Hysterectomies?

- A total hysterectomy removes all of the uterus, including the cervix. The ovaries and the fallopian tubes may or may not be removed. This is the most common type of hysterectomy.

- A partial, also called subtotal or supracervical, hysterectomy removes just the upper part of the uterus. The cervix is left in place. The ovaries may or may not be removed.

- A radical hysterectomy removes all of the uterus, cervix, the tissue on both sides of the cervix, and the upper part of the vagina. A radical hysterectomy is most often used to treat certain types of cancer, such as cervical cancer. The fallopian tubes and the ovaries may or may not be removed.

Will the Doctor Remove My Ovaries during the Hysterectomy?

Whether your ovaries are removed during the hysterectomy may depend on the reason for your hysterectomy. Ovaries may be removed during hysterectomy to lower the risk for ovarian cancer. However, women who have not yet gone through menopause also lose the protection of estrogen, which helps protect women from conditions such as heart disease and osteoporosis. Recent studies suggest that removing only the fallopian tubes but keeping the ovaries may help lower the risk for the most common type of ovarian cancer, which is believed to start in the fallopian tubes. The decision to keep or remove your ovaries is one you can make after talking about the risks and benefits with your doctor.

Will the Hysterectomy Cause Me to Enter Menopause?

All women who have a hysterectomy will stop getting their period. Whether you will have other symptoms of menopause after a hysterectomy depends on whether your doctor removes your ovaries during the surgery. If you keep your ovaries during the hysterectomy, you should not have other menopausal symptoms right away. But you may have symptoms a few years younger than the average age for menopause (52 years).

Because your uterus is removed, you no longer have periods and cannot get pregnant. But your ovaries might still make hormones, so you might not have other signs of menopause. You may have hot flashes, a symptom of menopause, because the surgery may have blocked blood flow to the ovaries. This can prevent the ovaries from releasing estrogen. If both ovaries are removed during the hysterectomy, you will no longer have periods and you may have other menopausal symptoms right away. Because your hormone levels drop quickly without ovaries, your symptoms may be stronger than with natural menopause. Ask your doctor about ways to manage your symptoms.

How Is a Hysterectomy Performed?

A hysterectomy can be done in several different ways. It will depend on your health history and the reason for your surgery.

Talk to your doctor about the different options:

- **Abdominal hysterectomy.** Your doctor makes a cut, usually in your lower abdomen.

- **Vaginal hysterectomy.** This is done through a small cut in the vagina.

- **Laparoscopic hysterectomy.** A laparoscope is an instrument with a thin, lighted tube and a small camera that allows your doctor to see your pelvic organs. Laparoscopic surgery is when the doctor makes very small cuts to put the laparoscope and surgical tools inside of you. During a laparoscopic hysterectomy the uterus is removed through the small cuts made in either your abdomen or your vagina.

- **Robotic surgery.** Your doctor guides a robotic arm to do the surgery through small cuts in your lower abdomen, like a laparoscopic hysterectomy.

How Long Does It Take to Recover from a Hysterectomy?

Recovering from a hysterectomy takes time. Most women stay in the hospital one to two days after surgery. Some doctors may send you home the same day of your surgery. Some women stay in the hospital longer, often when the hysterectomy is done because of cancer.

Your doctor will likely have you get up and move around as soon as possible after your hysterectomy. This includes going to the bathroom on your own. However, you may have to pee through a thin tube called a catheter for one or two days after your surgery.

The time it takes for you to return to normal activities depends on the type of surgery:

- Abdominal surgery can take from four to six weeks to recover.

- Vaginal, laparoscopic, or robotic surgery can take from three to four weeks to recover.

You should get plenty of rest and not lift heavy objects for four to six weeks after surgery. At that time, you should be able to take tub baths and resume sexual intercourse. How long it takes for you to recover will depend on your surgery and your health before the surgery. Talk to your doctor.

What Changes Can I Expect after a Hysterectomy?

Hysterectomy is a major surgery, so recovery can take a few weeks. But for most women, the biggest change is a better quality of life. You should have relief from the symptoms that made the surgery necessary.

Other changes that you may experience after a hysterectomy include:

- **Menopause.** You will no longer have periods. If your ovaries are removed during the hysterectomy, you may have other menopause symptoms.

- **Change in sexual feelings.** Some women have vaginal dryness or less interest in sex after a hysterectomy, especially if the ovaries are removed.

- **Increased risk for other health problems.** If both ovaries are removed, this may put you at higher risk for certain conditions such as: bone loss, heart disease, and urinary incontinence (leaking of urine). Talk to your doctor about how to prevent these problems.

- **Sense of loss.** Some women may feel grief or depression over the loss of fertility or the change in their bodies. Talk to your doctor if you have symptoms of depression, including feelings of sadness, a loss of interest in food or things you once enjoyed, or less energy, that last longer than a few weeks after your surgery.

Will My Sex Life Change after a Hysterectomy?

It might. If you had a good sex life before your hysterectomy, you should be able to return to it without any problems after recovery. Many women report a better sex life after hysterectomy because of relief from pain or heavy vaginal bleeding. If your hysterectomy causes you to have symptoms of menopause, you may experience vaginal dryness or a lack of interest in sex. Using a water-based lubricant can help with dryness. Talk to your partner and try to allow more time to get aroused during sex.

I've Had a Hysterectomy. Do I Still Need to Have Pap (Papanicolaou) Tests?

Maybe. You will still need regular Pap tests (or Pap smear) to screen for cervical cancer if you:

- Did not have your cervix removed

- Had a hysterectomy because of cancer or precancer

Ask your doctor what is best for you and how often you should have Pap tests.

Section 34.2

Surgery Choices for Women with DCIS or Breast Cancer

This section includes text excerpted from "Surgery Choices for Women with DCIS or Breast Cancer," National Cancer Institute (NCI), November 2012. Reviewed May 2018.

Talk with Surgeons

Talk with a breast cancer surgeon about your choices. Find out what happens during surgery, the types of problems that sometimes occur, and any treatment you might need after surgery. Ask a lot of questions and learn as much as you can. You may also wish to talk with family members, friends, or others who have had breast cancer surgery.

After talking with a surgeon, think about getting a second opinion. A second opinion means getting the advice of another surgeon. This surgeon might tell you about other treatment options. Or, he or she may agree with the advice you got from the first doctor. Some people worry about hurting their surgeon's feelings if they get a second opinion. But, it is very common and good surgeons don't mind. Also, some insurance companies require it. It is better to get a second opinion than worry that you made the wrong choice.

If you think you might have a mastectomy, this is also a good time to learn about breast reconstruction. Think about meeting with a reconstructive plastic surgeon to learn about this surgery and if it seems like a good option for you.

Learn the Facts about DCIS and Breast Cancer

Ductal Carcinoma in Situ (DCIS)

- If you have DCIS, this means that abnormal cells were found in the lining of the breast duct, but they have not spread outside the duct to the breast tissue. These abnormal cells are not invasive cancer, but they may become cancer. DCIS is also called Stage 0 or noninvasive cancer.

- Because doctors do not know which cases of DCIS will turn into invasive cancer and which ones will not, DCIS is treated with surgery the same as invasive cancer. Surgery choices for DCIS are based on how much of the breast has abnormal cells in it and where they are in the breast.

Breast Cancer

- When you find out you have breast cancer, your doctor will do tests to find out what stage it is. Stage describes how big the tumor is, if it has spread, and where it has spread. Surgery can be used to treat some, but not all, stages of breast cancer. This resource has information for women whose cancer can be removed with surgery. If your cancer cannot be removed with surgery, this resource does not have the information you need. Ask your doctor or nurse if you are not sure if surgery is right for you.

Learn about Your Surgery Choices

Most women who have DCIS or breast cancer that can be treated with surgery have three surgery choices. They are:

1. Breast-sparing surgery, followed by radiation therapy

2. Mastectomy

3. Mastectomy with breast reconstruction surgery

Breast-Sparing Surgery

Breast-sparing surgery means the surgeon removes only the DCIS or cancer and some normal tissue around it. If you have cancer, the surgeon will also remove one or more lymph nodes from under your arm. Breast-sparing surgery usually keeps your breast looking much like it did before surgery.

Other words for breast-sparing surgery include:

- Lumpectomy
- Partial mastectomy
- Breast-conserving surgery
- Segmental mastectomy

After breast-sparing surgery, most women also receive radiation therapy. The main goal of this treatment is to keep cancer from coming back in the same breast. Some women will also need chemotherapy, hormone therapy, and/or targeted therapy.

Mastectomy

With a mastectomy, the surgeon removes the whole breast that contains the DCIS or cancer. There are two main types of mastectomy. They are:

- **Total (simple) mastectomy.** The surgeon removes your whole breast. Sometimes, the surgeon also takes out one or more of the lymph nodes under your arm.

- **Modified radical mastectomy.** The surgeon removes your whole breast, many of the lymph nodes under your arm, and the lining over your chest muscles.

Some women will also need radiation therapy, chemotherapy, hormone therapy, and/or targeted therapy.

If you have a mastectomy, you may choose to wear a prosthesis (breast-like form) in your bra or have breast reconstruction surgery.

Breast Reconstruction Surgery

You can have breast reconstruction surgery at the same time as the mastectomy, or anytime after. This type of surgery is done by a plastic surgeon with special training in reconstruction surgery. The surgeon uses an implant or tissue from another part of your body to create a breast-like shape that replaces the breast that was removed. The surgeon may also make the form of a nipple and add a tattoo that looks like the areola (the dark area around your nipple). There are two main types of breast reconstruction surgery:

Breast implant. Breast reconstruction with an implant is often done in steps. The first step is called tissue expansion. In this step, the

423

plastic surgeon places a balloon expander under the chest muscle. Over weeks or months, saline (salt water) will be added to the expander to stretch the chest muscle and the skin on top of it. This process makes a pocket for the implant.

Once the pocket is the correct size, the surgeon will remove the expander and place an implant (filled with saline or silicone gel) into the pocket. This creates a new breast-like shape. Although it looks like a breast, you will not have the same feeling in it because nerves were cut during your mastectomy.

Breast implants do not last a lifetime. If you choose to have an implant, chances are you will need more surgery later on to remove or replace it. Implants can cause problems such as breast hardness, pain, and infection. An implant may also break, move, or shift. These problems can happen soon after surgery or years later.

Tissue flap. In tissue flap surgery, a reconstructive plastic surgeon builds a new breast-like shape from muscle, fat, and skin taken from other parts of your body (usually your belly or back). This new breast-like shape should last the rest of your life. Women who are very thin or obese, who smoke, or who have serious health problems often cannot have tissue flap surgery.

Healing after tissue flap surgery often takes longer than healing after breast implant surgery. You may have other problems, as well. For example, if you have a muscle removed, you might lose strength in the area from which it was taken. Or, you may get an infection or have trouble healing. Tissue flap surgery is best done by a reconstructive plastic surgeon who has special training in this type of surgery and has done it many times before.

Think about What Is Important to You

After you have talked with a breast cancer surgeon and learned the facts, you may also want to talk with your spouse or partner, family, friends, or other women who have had breast cancer surgery.

Then, think about what is important to you. Thinking about these questions and talking them over with others might help.

Surgery Choices

- If I have breast-sparing surgery, am I willing and able to have radiation therapy 5 days a week for 5–8 weeks?

- If I have a mastectomy, do I also want breast reconstruction surgery?

- If I have breast reconstruction surgery, do I want it at the same time as my mastectomy?

- What treatment does my insurance cover? What do I have to pay for?

Life after Surgery

- How important is it to me how my breast looks after cancer surgery?

- How important is it to me how my breast feels after cancer surgery?

- If I have a mastectomy and do not have reconstruction, will my insurance cover prosthesis and special bras?

- Where can I find a breast prosthesis and special bras?

Section 34.3

Oophorectomy

"Oophorectomy," © 2018 Omnigraphics
Reviewed May 2018.

The surgical removal of one or both ovaries, the primary female reproductive organs that produce ova (eggs) and reproductive hormones (estrogen and progesterone), is called an oophorectomy. This procedure is usually indicated for treatment of ovarian abnormalities that have failed to respond to conservative therapy. The surgery involving removal of both ovaries is called bilateral oophorectomy; while the procedure involving removal of only one ovary is called unilateral oophorectomy. A partial oophorectomy (or ovariotomy) is the surgery involving the removal of ovarian cysts, or resection (removal of tissue) from the ovaries.

An oophorectomy may sometimes be combined with a salpingectomy (surgery to remove the fallopian tubes), particularly in those with an increased risk of ovarian cancer. In such cases, the surgical procedure is then called a salpingo-oophorectomy. Although a relatively safe procedure, oophorectomy may carry certain risks inherent in surgeries, including bleeding, infection, or damage to nearby organs.

Indications

The decision to perform an oophorectomy depends largely on the patient's age, medical history, and future pregnancy plans. Indications for oophorectomies generally include malignancy, benign cysts or tumors in the ovary or the fallopian tube, endometriosis, pelvic inflammatory disease, and ectopic pregnancy. Sometimes, an emergency oophorectomy becomes necessary when the ligament supporting the ovary twists or forms a knot obstructing blood and nerve supply to the ovary. Called ovarian torsion, this is an uncommon diagnosis, but requires immediate attention and corrective surgery to prevent loss of the ovary. However, if reduced blood flow over a prolonged period has resulted in necrosis (tissue death), an oophorectomy is performed to remove the nonviable ovary.

An oophorectomy is also commonly performed as a risk-reducing procedure to prevent ovarian cancer in those with an elevated genetic risk of developing breast and/or ovarian cancer. Bilateral oophorectomies may sometimes be performed concurrently with a hysterectomy, although they are not usually recommended for premenopausal women unless the benefits far outweigh the long-term adverse effects associated with the surgery.

Preparation

The preoperative protocol for oophorectomy is same as any other surgery. Routine hematological and urine analyses in conjunction with imaging tests, such as ultrasound and computerized tomography (CT), help the surgeon plan for the procedure. Specific tests may also be carried out for any preexisting health conditions. An intravenous (IV) catheter is inserted in the arm for administering medicines and fluids.

Techniques

An oophorectomy is generally performed under general anesthesia and may involve one of the following procedures:

Open Abdominal Surgery (Laparotomy)

An incision is made in the lower abdomen to access the ovary. Blood vessels are removed and tied before separating the ovary from the surrounding tissue and removing it. The abdomen is then closed in layers with staples or stitches after sealing all bleeding points. Open surgeries are usually preferred when adhesions, or bands of scar tissue that bind the tissues or organs together, have formed as a consequence of prior abdominal surgery. A laparotomy is associated with a longer recovery period and carries a higher risk of bleeding and infection as compared to minimally invasive laparoscopic procedures.

Minimally Invasive Surgery

Also called laparoscopic surgery, it is performed under general or local anesthesia and is usually associated with less bleeding, lower risk of infection, and a faster recovery when compared to traditional open surgeries. A tubular instrument known as a trochar is inserted in the abdomen through one or more small incisions called ports. A laparoscope, an instrument fitted with a light source and camera, is passed into the abdomen or the pelvis through the trochar. The laparoscope relays images of the insides of the pelvis and abdomen to a high-resolution external monitor and allows the surgeon to visualize the pelvic organs. Specialized surgical instruments are then inserted through the trochar and the ovary or its parts are removed through one of the abdominal incisions.

Robot-assisted laparoscopic oophorectomy is being increasingly used as surgical intervention for benign conditions, or early-stage ovarian cancer. In this procedure, the surgeon uses a computer to control the surgical instruments, thus allowing better visualization of the organs (ovaries and ureters) and blood vessels. This procedure has been proven to allow better maneuverability with surgical tools than conventional laparoscopic surgery, and the technique continues to be researched for improvement. Intraoperative complications and surgical outcomes associated with the technique, by and large, depend on the surgeon's experience in robotic technology.

Postoperative Care

Most oophorectomies take only a few hours, and the expected hospital stay usually ranges from 2 to 4 days, depending on the specific indication for the surgery. The healthcare provider prescribes pain medication and provides instructions on postoperative care. An IV catheter may be placed in the urethra to drain urine for a few days. A temporary drain may also be placed in the incision to drain blood and fluid.

Open abdominal incisions are usually kept clean and dry for a few weeks. Any sign of infection, including abdominal pain, redness, swelling, vaginal discharge, opening of the incision, or fever should be reported to the medical team. Staples, if any, will be removed during the postoperative visit, which usually takes place approximately 1 to 2 weeks following the surgery. Wound closure strips are then placed on the sutures. Caution must be exercised to avoid constipation during this time, and this is usually achieved through diet modification, laxatives, and increased fluid intake. The medical team may also recommend simple exercises and will advise patients on when normal activities can be resumed.

Long-Term Effects

While serious complications stemming directly from the intra-abdominal surgery are rare, oophorectomy is generally associated with a number of adverse outcomes, particularly in premenopausal women. For this reason, elective oophorectomy, once a routine part of hysterectomy, is being increasingly replaced by ovarian conservation. Some of the potential negative outcomes of oophorectomy include increased risks of cardiovascular disease and osteoporosis. Small-scale clinical trials have also established the association between oophorectomy and cognitive impairment, and the risk is seen to increase significantly with oophorectomy at a younger age. Similar studies also report an increased likelihood of developing Parkinson disease following an oophorectomy.

Loss of ovarian function before natural menopause can also negatively impact psychological well-being and sexual function. Oophorectomized women generally suffer from anxiety and depression and also experience symptoms of "surgical menopause," including hot flashes, dyspareunia, and poor sexual satisfaction. While unilateral oophorectomies do not diminish the ability for natural conception, a bilateral oophorectomy will lead to infertility and require assisted reproductive techniques to achieve pregnancy. While some adverse effects from oophorectomy may be treated with hormone replacement therapy, loss of ovarian function unarguably impacts a patient's quality of life and increases the risk of many chronic conditions associated with aging.

References

1. "Prophylactic Oophorectomy in Pre-Menopausal Women and Long Term Health—A Review," National Center for Biotechnology Information (NCBI), January 1, 2009.

2. "Oophorectomy: The Debate between Ovarian Conservation and Elective Oophorectomy," National Center for Biotechnology Information (NCBI), January 1, 2014.

3. "Oophorectomy (Ovary Removal Surgery)," Mayo Clinic, n.d.

Section 34.4

Minimally Invasive Surgery (Laparoscopic Surgery)

This section contains text excerpted from the following sources: Text in this section begins with excerpts from "NCI Dictionary of Cancer Terms," National Cancer Institute (NCI), September 5, 2013. Reviewed May 2018; Text under the heading "Scope of Laparoscopic Surgery" is excerpted from "SBIR Phase II: Enhanced Dexterity Minimally Invasive Surgical Platform," National Science Foundation (NSF), November 19, 2014. Reviewed May 2018; Text under the heading "Diagnostic Laparoscopy" is excerpted from "Diagnostic Laparoscopy," U.S. National Library of Medicine (NLM), April 30, 2018; Text under the heading "Robotic and Minimally Invasive Surgery" is excerpted from "Robotic Surgery: Risks versus Rewards," Agency for Healthcare Research and Quality (AHRQ), U.S. Department of Health and Human Services (HHS), February 2016; Text under the heading "Instructions for Care after Outpatient Laparoscopic Surgery" is excerpted from "Instructions for Care after Outpatient Laparoscopic Surgery (Gynecology)," U.S. Department of Veterans Affairs (VA), May 2005. Reviewed May 2018.

Surgery that is done using small incisions (cuts) and few stitches. During minimally invasive surgery, one or more small incisions may be made in the body. A laparoscope (thin, tube-like instrument with a light and a lens for viewing) is inserted through one opening to guide the surgery. Tiny surgical instruments are inserted through other openings to do the surgery. Minimally invasive surgery may cause less pain, scarring, and damage to healthy tissue, and the patient may have a faster recovery than with traditional surgery.

Scope of Laparoscopic Surgery

In addition to patient benefits of less postsurgical pain, less scarring, and quicker recovery, minimally invasive surgery also reduces healthcare cost due to shorter hospital stays and lower risk of postoperative complications. Minimally invasive surgery impacts all surgical specialties, including gynecology, general, bariatric, urologic, and cardiothoracic. Although more than 1.5 million such procedures are performed in the United States each year, wider adoption is limited by the high cost of current surgical robots, training burden of traditional hand-held instruments, and complexity of certain minimally invasive procedures.

Diagnostic Laparoscopy

Diagnostic laparoscopy is a procedure that allows a doctor to look directly at the contents of the abdomen or pelvis.

How the Test Is Performed

The procedure is usually done in the hospital or outpatient surgical center under general anesthesia (while you are asleep and pain-free). The procedure is performed in the following way:

- The surgeon makes a small cut (incision) below the belly button.

- A needle or tube is inserted into the incision. Carbon dioxide gas is passed into the abdomen through the needle or tube. The gas helps expand the area, giving the surgeon more room to work, and helps the surgeon see the organs more clearly.

- A tube is placed through the cut in your abdomen. A tiny video camera (laparoscope) goes through this tube and is used to see the inside of your pelvis and abdomen. More small cuts may be made if other instruments are needed to get a better view of certain organs.

- If you are having gynecologic laparoscopy, dye may be injected into your cervix area so the surgeon can view the fallopian tubes.

- After the exam, the gas, laparoscope, and instruments are removed, and the cuts are closed. You will have bandages over those areas.

Robotic and Minimally Invasive Surgery

Robotic-assisted surgery (RAS) is a derivative of standard laparoscopic surgery and was developed to overcome the limitations of standard laparoscopy. Like traditional laparoscopy, RAS uses small incisions and insufflation of the anatomical operative space with carbon dioxide. The robotic camera and various instruments are placed through the ports into the body and can be manipulated by the surgeon performing the operation. In the case of RAS, though, the surgeon, seated at a computer console in the operating room, uses robot assistance to utilize the tools (instead of doing it himself or herself directly at the bedside). In RAS, a bedside assistant exchanges the instruments and performs manual tasks like retraction and suction.

The use of robotic assistance in surgery has expanded exponentially since it was first approved in 2000. Robotic-assisted surgery (RAS) has found its way into almost every surgical subspecialty and now has approved uses in urology, gynecology, cardiothoracic surgery, general surgery, and otolaryngology. RAS is most commonly used in urology and gynecology; more than 75 percent of robotic procedures performed are within these two specialties. Robotic surgical systems have the potential to improve surgical technique and outcomes, but they also create a unique set of risks and patient safety concerns.

RAS Outcomes

The outcomes in RAS seem to correlate with individual surgeon experience. For example, in cancer surgery, surgeons with more experience are more likely to have clean margins. Other studies have documented lower complication rates with an increasing number of procedures. These findings of practice makes perfect are not specific to robotic surgery; such findings have been seen in many procedures. There are varying reports of exactly how many cases are required to master the robotic learning curve, and the number varies by surgical procedure.

Notwithstanding the concerns, RAS has been accepted as generally safe. Multiple risk factors can increase the possibility of complications and errors: patient factors (i.e., obesity or underlying comorbidities), surgeon factors (training and experience), and robotic factors (i.e., mechanical malfunction).

431

Instructions for Care after Outpatient Laparoscopic Surgery

You have just had laparoscopic surgery in the outpatient surgery unit. Self-care will be important for healing. You will want to understand and follow these directions:

1. You may well feel the effects of the anesthesia for the first 24 hours after surgery. You can return to your regular diet if you feel up to it. If you feel nauseated (sick to your stomach) gradually work your way back to your regular diet over the next 24—48 hours.

2. Do not drive for 24 hours after your surgery.

3. You will be given pain medicine. Be sure you know how often you can take it before you go home.

4. You can return to your regular activities after 48 hours, unless your doctor tells you something else. Avoid douches, tampons, and sexual intercourse for one week after surgery

5. You may remove the dressing (band-aid) after 48 hours. You need to keep the wound clean and dry. If your clothes will rub your wound or if you might get dirt or dust on it at work, put on a clean band-aid.

6. You may shower 24 hours after surgery. Remove the band-aid first. When drying the area, pat dry or dry with a hair dryer. Do not rub the wound with the towel or washcloth. Do not leave a wet band-aid on the wound.

7. Check your wound at least once a day for these signs of infection:

    *   Increased pain

    *   Increased swelling

    *   Increased redness or warmth

    *   Any drainage (oozing)

    *   Fever (a temperature higher than 100.4o) or chills

8. If you have any bleeding that soaks through the band-aid from the skin edges, put pressure on the wound for five minutes, then put on the wound for 15 minutes out of every hour for eight hours.

If you have been given medicine or ointment, be sure you understand the instructions you were given before you leave. Follow all instructions carefully. If you have stitches that must be removed, you will be given an appointment to return in five to seven days to have them removed. At this time, the doctor will also see how well you are healing. Self-dissolving stitches are usually used to close the incision (cut). If you have self-dissolving stitches, you will be scheduled for a follow-up appointment about two weeks after your surgery.

Section 34.5

Cryosurgery

This section includes text excerpted from "Cryosurgery in Cancer Treatment," National Cancer Institute (NCI), September 10, 2003. Reviewed May 2018.

What Is Cryosurgery?

Cryosurgery (also called cryotherapy) is the use of extreme cold produced by liquid nitrogen (or argon gas) to destroy abnormal tissue. Cryosurgery is used to treat external tumors, such as those on the skin. For external tumors, liquid nitrogen is applied directly to the cancer cells with a cotton swab or spraying device.

Cryosurgery is also used to treat tumors inside the body (internal tumors and tumors in the bone). For internal tumors, liquid nitrogen or argon gas is circulated through a hollow instrument called a cryoprobe, which is placed in contact with the tumor. The doctor uses ultrasound or magnetic resonance imaging (MRI) to guide the cryoprobe and monitor the freezing of the cells, thus limiting damage to nearby healthy tissue. (In ultrasound, sound waves are bounced off organs and other tissues to create a picture called a sonogram.) A ball of ice crystals forms around the probe, freezing nearby cells. Sometimes more than one probe is used to deliver the liquid nitrogen to various parts of the tumor. The probes may be put into the tumor during surgery or through the skin (percutaneously). After cryosurgery, the frozen tissue thaws and is either naturally absorbed by the body (for internal tumors), or it dissolves and forms a scab (for external tumors).

What Types of Cancer Can Be Treated with Cryosurgery?

Cryosurgery is used to treat several types of cancer, and some precancerous or noncancerous conditions. In addition to liver tumor, cryosurgery can be an effective treatment for the following:

- Retinoblastoma (a childhood cancer that affects the retina of the eye). Doctors have found that cryosurgery is most effective when the tumor is small and only in certain parts of the retina

- Early-stage skin cancers (both basal cell and squamous cell carcinomas)

- Precancerous skin growths known as actinic keratosis

- Precancerous conditions of the cervix known as cervical intraepithelial neoplasia (CIN) (abnormal cell changes in the cervix that can develop into cervical cancer)

Cryosurgery is also used to treat some types of low-grade cancerous and noncancerous tumors of the bone. It may reduce the risk of joint damage when compared with more extensive surgery, and help lessen the need for amputation. The treatment is also used to treat acquired immunodeficiency syndrome (AIDS)-related Kaposi sarcoma when the skin lesions are small and localized.

Researchers are evaluating cryosurgery as a treatment for a number of cancers, including breast, colon, and kidney cancer. They are also exploring cryotherapy in combination with other cancer treatments, such as hormone therapy, chemotherapy, radiation therapy, or surgery.

Can Cryosurgery Be Used to Treat Primary Liver Cancer or Liver Metastases (Cancer That Has Spread to the Liver from Another Part of the Body)? What Are the Side Effects?

Cryosurgery may be used to treat primary liver cancer that has not spread. It is used especially if surgery is not possible due to factors such as other medical conditions. The treatment also may be used for cancer that has spread to the liver from another site (such as the colon or rectum). In some cases, chemotherapy and/or radiation therapy may be given before or after cryosurgery. Cryosurgery in the liver may cause damage to the bile ducts and/or major blood vessels, which can lead to hemorrhage (heavy bleeding) or infection.

Does Cryosurgery Have Any Complications or Side Effects?

Cryosurgery does have side effects, although they may be less severe than those associated with surgery or radiation therapy. The effects depend on the location of the tumor. Cryosurgery for cervical intraepithelial neoplasia has not been shown to affect a woman's fertility, but it can cause cramping, pain, or bleeding. When used to treat skin cancer (including Kaposi sarcoma), cryosurgery may cause scarring and swelling; if nerves are damaged, loss of sensation may occur, and, rarely, it may cause a loss of pigmentation and loss of hair in the treated area. When used to treat tumors of the bone, cryosurgery may lead to the destruction of nearby bone tissue and result in fractures, but these effects may not be seen for some time after the initial treatment and can often be delayed with other treatments. In rare cases, cryosurgery may interact badly with certain types of chemotherapy. Although the side effects of cryosurgery may be less severe than those associated with conventional surgery or radiation, more studies are needed to determine the long-term effects.

What Are the Advantages of Cryosurgery?

Cryosurgery offers advantages over other methods of cancer treatment. It is less invasive than surgery, involving only a small incision or insertion of the cryoprobe through the skin. Consequently, pain, bleeding, and other complications of surgery are minimized. Cryosurgery is less expensive than other treatments and requires shorter recovery time and a shorter hospital stay, or no hospital stay at all. Sometimes cryosurgery can be done using only local anesthesia.

Because physicians can focus cryosurgical treatment on a limited area, they can avoid the destruction of nearby healthy tissue. The treatment can be safely repeated and may be used along with standard treatments such as surgery, chemotherapy, hormone therapy, and radiation. Cryosurgery may offer an option for treating cancers that are considered inoperable or that do not respond to standard treatments. Furthermore, it can be used for patients who are not good candidates for conventional surgery because of their age or other medical conditions.

What Are the Disadvantages of Cryosurgery?

The major disadvantage of cryosurgery is the uncertainty surrounding its long-term effectiveness. While cryosurgery may be effective in treating tumors the physician can see by using imaging tests (tests that produce pictures of areas inside the body), it can miss microscopic cancer spread. Furthermore, because the effectiveness of the technique is still being assessed, insurance coverage issues may arise.

What Does the Future Hold for Cryosurgery?

Additional studies are needed to determine the effectiveness of cryosurgery in controlling cancer and improving survival. Data from these studies will allow physicians to compare cryosurgery with standard treatment options such as surgery, chemotherapy, and radiation. Moreover, physicians continue to examine the possibility of using cryosurgery in combination with other treatments.

Where Is Cryosurgery Available?

Cryosurgery is widely available in gynecologists' offices for the treatment of cervical neoplasias. A limited number of hospitals and cancer centers throughout the country currently have skilled doctors and the necessary technology to perform cryosurgery for other noncancerous, precancerous, and cancerous conditions. Individuals can consult with their doctors or contact hospitals and cancer centers in their area to find out where cryosurgery is being used.

Chapter 35

Chemotherapy

Chemotherapy (also called chemo) is a type of cancer treatment that uses drugs to kill cancer cells.

How Chemotherapy Works against Cancer

Chemotherapy works by stopping or slowing the growth of cancer cells, which grow and divide quickly. Chemotherapy is used to:

- **Treat cancer:** Chemotherapy can be used to cure cancer, lessen the chance it will return, or stop or slow its growth.

- **Ease cancer symptoms:** Chemotherapy can be used to shrink tumors that are causing pain and other problems.

Who Receives Chemotherapy

Chemotherapy is used to treat many types of cancer. For some people, chemotherapy may be the only treatment you receive. But most often, you will have chemotherapy and other cancer treatments. The types of treatment that you need depends on the type of cancer you have, if it has spread and where, and if you have other health problems.

This chapter contains text excerpted from "Types of Cancer Treatment—Chemotherapy to Treat Cancer," National Cancer Institute (NCI), April 29, 2015.

How Chemotherapy Is Used with Other Cancer Treatments

When used with other treatments, chemotherapy can:

- Make a tumor smaller before surgery or radiation therapy. This is called neoadjuvant chemotherapy.

- Destroy cancer cells that may remain after treatment with surgery or radiation therapy. This is called adjuvant chemotherapy.

- Help other treatments work better

- Kill cancer cells that have returned or spread to other parts of your body

Chemotherapy Can Cause Side Effects

Chemotherapy not only kills fast-growing cancer cells, but also kills or slows the growth of healthy cells that grow and divide quickly. Examples are cells that line your mouth and intestines and those that cause your hair to grow. Damage to healthy cells may cause side effects, such as mouth sores, nausea, and hair loss. Side effects often get better or go away after you have finished chemotherapy.

The most common side effect is fatigue, which is feeling exhausted and worn out. You can prepare for fatigue by:

- Asking someone to drive you to and from chemotherapy

- Planning time to rest on the day of and day after chemotherapy

- Asking for help with meals and child care on the day of and at least one day after chemotherapy

There are many ways you can help manage chemotherapy side effects.

How Much Chemotherapy Costs

The cost of chemotherapy depends on:

- The types and doses of chemotherapy used

- How long and how often chemotherapy is given

- Whether you get chemotherapy at home, in a clinic or office, or during a hospital stay

- The part of the country where you live

Talk with your health insurance company about what services it will pay for. Most insurance plans pay for chemotherapy. To learn more, talk with the business office where you go for treatment.

What to Expect When Receiving Chemotherapy

How Chemotherapy Is Given

Chemotherapy may be given in many ways. Some common ways include:

- **Oral:** The chemotherapy comes in pills, capsules, or liquids that you swallow

- **Intravenous (IV):** The chemotherapy goes directly into a vein

- **Injection:** The chemotherapy is given by a shot in a muscle in your arm, thigh, or hip, or right under the skin in the fatty part of your arm, leg, or belly

- **Intrathecal:** The chemotherapy is injected into the space between the layers of tissue that cover the brain and spinal cord

- **Intraperitoneal (IP):** The chemotherapy goes directly into the peritoneal cavity, which is the area in your body that contains organs such as your intestines, stomach, and liver

- **Intra-arterial (IA):** The chemotherapy is injected directly into the artery that leads to the cancer

- **Topical:** The chemotherapy comes in a cream that you rub onto your skin

Chemotherapy is often given through a thin needle that is placed in a vein on your hand or lower arm. Your nurse will put the needle in at the start of each treatment and remove it when treatment is over. Intravenous (IV) chemotherapy may also be given through catheters or ports, sometimes with the help of a pump.

- **Catheter.** A catheter is a thin, soft tube. A doctor or nurse places one end of the catheter in a large vein, often in your chest area. The other end of the catheter stays outside your body. Most catheters stay in place until you have finished your chemotherapy treatments. Catheters can also be used to give you other drugs and to draw blood. Be sure to watch for signs of infection around your catheter. See the section about infection for more information.

- **Port.** A port is a small, round disc that is placed under your skin during minor surgery. A surgeon puts it in place before you begin your course of treatment, and it remains there until you have finished. A catheter connects the port to a large vein, most often in your chest. Your nurse can insert a needle into your port to give you chemotherapy or draw blood. This needle can be left in place for chemotherapy treatments that are given for longer than one day. Be sure to watch for signs of infection around your port.

- **Pump.** Pumps are often attached to catheters or ports. They control how much and how fast chemotherapy goes into a catheter or port, allowing you to receive your chemotherapy outside of the hospital. Pumps can be internal or external. External pumps remain outside your body. Internal pumps are placed under your skin during surgery.

How Your Doctor Decides Which Chemotherapy Drugs to Give You

There are many different chemotherapy drugs. Which ones are included in your treatment plan depends mostly on:

- The type of cancer you have and how advanced it is
- Whether you have had chemotherapy before
- Whether you have other health problems, such as diabetes or heart disease

Where You Go for Chemotherapy

You may receive chemotherapy during a hospital stay, at home, or as an outpatient at a doctor's office, clinic, or hospital. Outpatient means you do not stay overnight. No matter where you go for chemotherapy, your doctor and nurse will watch for side effects and help you manage them.

How Often You Receive Chemotherapy

Treatment schedules for chemotherapy vary widely. How often and how long you get chemotherapy depends on:

- Your type of cancer and how advanced it is

- Whether chemotherapy is used to:
  - Cure your cancer
  - Control its growth
  - Ease symptoms
- The type of chemotherapy you are getting
- How your body responds to the chemotherapy

You may receive chemotherapy in cycles. A cycle is a period of chemotherapy treatment followed by a period of rest. For instance, you might receive chemotherapy every day for 1 week followed by 3 weeks with no chemotherapy. These 4 weeks make up one cycle. The rest period gives your body a chance to recover and build new healthy cells.

Missing a Chemotherapy Treatment

It is best not to skip a chemotherapy treatment. But, sometimes your doctor may change your chemotherapy schedule if you are having certain side effects. If this happens, your doctor or nurse will explain what to do and when to start treatment again.

How Chemotherapy May Affect You

Chemotherapy affects people in different ways. How you feel depends on:

- The type of chemotherapy you are getting
- The dose of chemotherapy you are getting
- Your type of cancer
- How advanced your cancer is
- How healthy you are before treatment

Since everyone is different and people respond to chemotherapy in different ways, your doctor and nurses cannot know for sure how you will feel during chemotherapy.

How Will I Know If My Chemotherapy Is Working?

You will see your doctor often. During these visits, she will ask you how you feel, do a physical exam, and order medical tests and scans.

Tests might include blood tests. Scans might include magnetic resonance imaging (MRI), computed tomography (CT), or positron emission tomography (PET) scans. You cannot tell if chemotherapy is working based on its side effects. Some people think that severe side effects mean that chemotherapy is working well, or that no side effects mean that chemotherapy is not working. The truth is that side effects have nothing to do with how well chemotherapy is fighting your cancer.

Special Diet Needs

Chemotherapy can damage the healthy cells that line your mouth and intestines and cause eating problems. Tell your doctor or nurse if you have trouble eating while you are receiving chemotherapy. You might also find it helpful to speak with a dietitian.

Working during Chemotherapy

Many people can work during chemotherapy, as long as they match their work schedule to how they feel. Whether or not you can work may depend on what kind of job you have. If your job allows, you may want to see if you can work part-time or from home on days you do not feel well. Many employers are required by law to change your work schedule to meet your needs during cancer treatment. Talk with your employer about ways to adjust your work during chemotherapy.

Chapter 36

Radiation Therapy

What Is Radiation Therapy?

Radiation therapy uses high-energy radiation to shrink tumors and kill cancer cells. X-rays, gamma rays, and charged particles are types of radiation used for cancer treatment. The radiation may be delivered by a machine outside the body (external-beam radiation therapy), or it may come from radioactive material placed in the body near cancer cells (internal radiation therapy, also called brachytherapy). Systemic radiation therapy uses radioactive substances, such as radioactive iodine, that travel in the blood to kill cancer cells. About half of all cancer patients receive some type of radiation therapy sometime during the course of their treatment.

How Does Radiation Therapy Kill Cancer Cells?

Radiation therapy kills cancer cells by damaging their deoxyribonucleic acid or DNA (the molecules inside cells that carry genetic information and pass it from one generation to the next). Radiation therapy can either damage DNA directly or create charged particles (free radicals) within the cells that can in turn damage the DNA.

Cancer cells whose DNA is damaged beyond repair stop dividing or die. When the damaged cells die, they are broken down and eliminated by the body's natural processes.

This chapter contains text excerpted from "Radiation Therapy for Cancer," National Cancer Institute (NCI), June 30, 2010. Reviewed May 2018.

Does Radiation Therapy Kill Only Cancer Cells?

No, radiation therapy can also damage normal cells, leading to side effects. Doctors take potential damage to normal cells into account when planning a course of radiation therapy. The amount of radiation that normal tissue can safely receive is known for all parts of the body. Doctors use this information to help them decide where to aim radiation during treatment.

Why Do Patients Receive Radiation Therapy?

Radiation therapy is sometimes given with curative intent (that is, with the hope that the treatment will cure a cancer, either by eliminating a tumor, preventing cancer recurrence, or both). In such cases, radiation therapy may be used alone or in combination with surgery, chemotherapy, or both. Radiation therapy may also be given with palliative intent. Palliative treatments are not intended to cure. Instead, they relieve symptoms and reduce the suffering caused by cancer.

Some examples of palliative radiation therapy are:

- Radiation given to the brain to shrink tumors formed from cancer cells that have spread to the brain from another part of the body (metastases)

- Radiation given to shrink a tumor that is pressing on the spine or growing within a bone, which can cause pain

- Radiation given to shrink a tumor near the esophagus, which can interfere with a patient's ability to eat and drink

How Is Radiation Therapy Planned for an Individual Patient?

A radiation oncologist develops a patient's treatment plan through a process called treatment planning, which begins with simulation.

During simulation, detailed imaging scans show the location of a patient's tumor and the normal areas around it. These scans are usually computed tomography (CT) scans, but they can also include magnetic resonance imaging (MRI), positron emission tomography (PET), and ultrasound scans.

CT scans are often used in treatment planning for radiation therapy. During CT scanning, pictures of the inside of the body are created by a computer linked to an X-ray machine.

During simulation and daily treatments, it is necessary to ensure that the patient will be in exactly the same position every day relative to the machine delivering the treatment or doing the imaging. Body molds, head masks, or other devices may be constructed for an individual patient to make it easier for a patient to stay still. Temporary skin marks and even tattoos are used to help with precise patient positioning.

Patients getting radiation to the head may need a mask. The mask helps keep the head from moving so that the patient is in the exact same position for each treatment.

After simulation, the radiation oncologist then determines the exact area that will be treated, the total radiation dose that will be delivered to the tumor, how much dose will be allowed for the normal tissues around the tumor, and the safest angles (paths) for radiation delivery.

The staff working with the radiation oncologist (including physicists and dosimetrists) use sophisticated computers to design the details of the exact radiation plan that will be used. After approving the plan, the radiation oncologist authorizes the start of treatment. On the first day of treatment, and usually at least weekly after that, many checks are made to ensure that the treatments are being delivered exactly the way they were planned.

Radiation doses for cancer treatment are measured in a unit called a gray (Gy), which is a measure of the amount of radiation energy absorbed by 1 kilogram (Kg) of human tissue. Different doses of radiation are needed to kill different types of cancer cells.

Radiation can damage some types of normal tissue more easily than others. For example, the reproductive organs (testicles and ovaries) are more sensitive to radiation than bones. The radiation oncologist takes all of this information into account during treatment planning.

If an area of the body has previously been treated with radiation therapy, a patient may not be able to have radiation therapy to that area a second time, depending on how much radiation was given during the initial treatment. If one area of the body has already received the maximum safe lifetime dose of radiation, another area might still be treated with radiation therapy if the distance between the two areas is large enough.

The area selected for treatment usually includes the whole tumor plus a small amount of normal tissue surrounding the tumor. The normal tissue is treated for two main reasons:

- To take into account body movement from breathing and normal movement of the organs within the body, which can change the location of a tumor between treatments

- To reduce the likelihood of tumor recurrence from cancer cells that have spread to the normal tissue next to the tumor (called microscopic local spread)

How Is Radiation Therapy Given to Patients?

Radiation can come from a machine outside the body (external-beam radiation therapy (EBRT)) or from radioactive material placed in the body near cancer cells (internal radiation therapy, more commonly called brachytherapy). Systemic radiation therapy uses a radioactive substance, given by mouth or into a vein, that travels in the blood to tissues throughout the body.

The type of radiation therapy prescribed by a radiation oncologist depends on many factors, including:

- The type of cancer

- The size of the cancer

- The cancer's location in the body

- How close the cancer is to normal tissues that are sensitive to radiation

- How far into the body the radiation needs to travel

- The patient's general health and medical history

- Whether the patient will have other types of cancer treatment

- Other factors, such as the patient's age and other medical conditions

External-Beam Radiation Therapy (EBRT)

External-beam radiation therapy (EBRT) is most often delivered in the form of photon beams (either X-rays or gamma rays). A photon is the basic unit of light and other forms of electromagnetic radiation. It can be thought of as a bundle of energy. The amount of energy in a photon can vary. For example, the photons in gamma rays have the highest energy, followed by the photons in X-rays.

Many types of EBRT are delivered using a machine called a linear accelerator (also called a LINAC). A LINAC uses electricity to form a stream of fast-moving subatomic particles. This creates high-energy radiation that may be used to treat cancer.

Patients usually receive EBRT in daily treatment sessions over the course of several weeks. The number of treatment sessions depends on many factors, including the total radiation dose that will be given.

One of the most common types of EBRT is called 3-dimensional conformal radiation therapy (3D-CRT). 3D-CRT uses very sophisticated computer software and advanced treatment machines to deliver radiation to very precisely shaped target areas.

Many other methods of EBRT are currently being tested and used in cancer treatment. These methods include:

- **Intensity-modulated radiation therapy (IMRT).** IMRT uses hundreds of tiny radiation beam-shaping devices, called collimators, to deliver a single dose of radiation. The collimators can be stationary or can move during treatment, allowing the intensity of the radiation beams to change during treatment sessions. This kind of dose modulation allows different areas of a tumor or nearby tissues to receive different doses of radiation.

Unlike other types of radiation therapy, IMRT is planned in reverse (called inverse treatment planning). In inverse treatment planning, the radiation oncologist chooses the radiation doses to different areas of the tumor and surrounding tissue, and then a high-powered computer program calculates the required number of beams and angles of the radiation treatment. In contrast, during traditional (forward) treatment planning, the radiation oncologist chooses the number and angles of the radiation beams in advance and computers calculate how much dose will be delivered from each of the planned beams.

The goal of IMRT is to increase the radiation dose to the areas that need it and reduce radiation exposure to specific sensitive areas of surrounding normal tissue. Compared with 3D-CRT, IMRT can reduce the risk of some side effects, such as damage to the salivary glands (which can cause dry mouth, or xerostomia), when the head and neck are treated with radiation therapy. However, with IMRT, a larger volume of normal tissue overall is exposed to radiation. Whether IMRT leads to improved control of tumor growth and better survival compared with 3D-CRT is not yet known.

- **Image-guided radiation therapy (IGRT).** In IGRT, repeated imaging scans (CT, MRI, or PET) are performed during treatment. These imaging scans are processed by computers to identify changes in a tumor's size and location due to treatment and to allow the position of the patient or the planned radiation dose to be adjusted during treatment as needed. Repeated imaging can increase the accuracy of radiation treatment and may allow reductions in the planned volume of tissue to be treated, thereby decreasing the total radiation dose to normal tissue.

- **Tomotherapy.** Tomotherapy is a type of image-guided IMRT. A tomotherapy machine is a hybrid between a CT imaging scanner and an EBRT machine. The part of the tomotherapy machine that delivers radiation for both imaging and treatment can rotate completely around the patient in the same manner as a normal CT scanner.

Tomotherapy machines can capture CT images of the patient's tumor immediately before treatment sessions, to allow for very precise tumor targeting and sparing of normal tissue.

Like standard IMRT, tomotherapy may be better than 3D-CRT at sparing normal tissue from high radiation doses. However, clinical trials comparing 3D-CRT with tomotherapy have not been conducted.

- **Stereotactic radiosurgery (SRS).** SRS can deliver one or more high doses of radiation to a small tumor. SRS uses extremely accurate image-guided tumor targeting and patient positioning. Therefore, a high dose of radiation can be given without excess damage to normal tissue.

SRS can be used to treat only small tumors with well-defined edges. It is most commonly used in the treatment of brain or spinal tumors and brain metastases from other cancer types. For the treatment of some brain metastases, patients may receive radiation therapy to the entire brain (called whole-brain radiation therapy) in addition to SRS.

SRS requires the use of a head frame or other device to immobilize the patient during treatment to ensure that the high dose of radiation is delivered accurately.

- **Stereotactic body radiation therapy (SBRT).** SBRT delivers radiation therapy in fewer sessions, using smaller radiation fields and higher doses than 3D-CRT in most cases. By definition, SBRT treats tumors that lie outside the brain and spinal cord. Because these tumors are more likely to move with the normal motion of the body, and therefore, cannot be targeted as accurately as tumors within the brain or spine, SBRT is usually given in more than one dose. SBRT can be used to treat only small, isolated tumors, including cancers in the lung and liver.

Many doctors refer to SBRT systems by their brand names, such as the CyberKnife®.

- **Proton therapy.** EBRT can be delivered by proton beams as well as the photon beams described above. Protons are a type of charged particle.

Proton beams differ from photon beams mainly in the way they deposit energy in living tissue. Whereas photons deposit energy in small packets all along their path through tissue, protons deposit much of their energy at the end of their path (called the Bragg peak) and deposit less energy along the way.

In theory, use of protons should reduce the exposure of normal tissue to radiation, possibly allowing the delivery of higher doses of radiation to a tumor. Proton therapy has not yet been compared with standard EBRT in clinical trials.

Other charged particle beams. Electron beams are used to irradiate superficial tumors, such as skin cancer or tumors near the surface of the body, but they cannot travel very far through tissue. Therefore, they cannot treat tumors deep within the body.

Patients can discuss these different methods of radiation therapy with their doctors to see if any is appropriate for their type of cancer and if it is available in their community or through a clinical trial.

Internal Radiation Therapy

Internal radiation therapy (brachytherapy) is radiation delivered from radiation sources (radioactive materials) placed inside or on the body. Several brachytherapy techniques are used in cancer treatment. Interstitial brachytherapy uses a radiation source placed within tumor tissue. Intracavitary brachytherapy uses a source placed within a surgical cavity or a body cavity, such as the chest cavity, near a tumor. Episcleral brachytherapy, which is used to treat melanoma inside the eye, uses a source that is attached to the eye.

In brachytherapy, radioactive isotopes are sealed in tiny pellets or "seeds." These seeds are placed in patients using delivery devices, such as needles, catheters, or some other type of carrier. As the isotopes decay naturally, they give off radiation that damages nearby cancer cells.

If left in place, after a few weeks or months, the isotopes decay completely and no longer give off radiation. The seeds will not cause harm if they are left in the body.

Brachytherapy may be able to deliver higher doses of radiation to some cancers than EBRT while causing less damage to normal tissue.

Brachytherapy can be given as a low-dose-rate or a high-dose-rate treatment:

- In low-dose-rate treatment, cancer cells receive continuous low-dose radiation from the source over a period of several days.

- In high-dose-rate treatment, a robotic machine attached to delivery tubes placed inside the body guides one or more radioactive sources into or near a tumor, and then removes the sources at the end of each treatment session. High-dose-rate treatment can be given in one or more treatment sessions.

- An example of a high-dose-rate treatment is the MammoSite® system, which is being studied to treat patients with breast cancer who have undergone breast-conserving surgery.

The placement of brachytherapy sources can be temporary or permanent:

- For permanent brachytherapy, the sources are surgically sealed within the body and left there, even after all of the radiation has been given off. The remaining material (in which the radioactive isotopes were sealed) does not cause any discomfort or harm to the patient. Permanent brachytherapy is a type of low-dose-rate brachytherapy.

- For temporary brachytherapy, tubes (catheters) or other carriers are used to deliver the radiation sources, and both the carriers and the radiation sources are removed after treatment. Temporary brachytherapy can be either low-dose-rate or high-dose-rate treatment.

Doctors can use brachytherapy alone or in addition to EBRT to provide a "boost" of radiation to a tumor while sparing surrounding normal tissue.

Systemic Radiation Therapy

In systemic radiation therapy, a patient swallows or receives an injection of a radioactive substance, such as radioactive iodine or a radioactive substance bound to a monoclonal antibody.

Radioactive iodine (I-131) is a type of systemic radiation therapy commonly used to help treat some types of thyroid cancer. Thyroid cells naturally take up radioactive iodine.

For systemic radiation therapy for some other types of cancer, a monoclonal antibody helps target the radioactive substance to the right place. The antibody joined to the radioactive substance travels through the blood, locating and killing tumor cells. For example:

- The drug ibritumomab tiuxetan (Zevalin®) has been approved by the U.S. Food and Drug Administration (FDA) for the treatment of certain types of B-cell non-Hodgkin lymphoma (NHL). The antibody part of this drug recognizes and binds to a protein found on the surface of B lymphocytes.

- The combination drug regimen of tositumomab and iodine (I-131) tositumomab (Bexxar®) has been approved for the treatment of certain types of NHL. In this regimen, nonradioactive tositumomab antibodies are given to patients first, followed by treatment with tositumomab antibodies that have (I-131) attached. Tositumomab recognizes and binds to the same protein on B lymphocytes as ibritumomab. The nonradioactive form of the antibody helps protect normal B lymphocytes from being damaged by radiation from (I-131).

Many other systemic radiation therapy drugs are in clinical trials for different cancer types. Some systemic radiation therapy drugs relieve pain from cancer that has spread to the bone (bone metastases). This is a type of palliative radiation therapy. The radioactive drugs samarium-153-lexidronam (Quadramet®) and strontium-89 chloride (Metastron®) are examples of radiopharmaceuticals used to treat pain from bone metastases.

Why Are Some Types of Radiation Therapy Given in Many Small Doses?

Patients who receive most types of external-beam radiation therapy usually have to travel to the hospital or an outpatient facility up to 5 days a week for several weeks. One dose (a single fraction) of the total planned dose of radiation is given each day. Occasionally, two treatments a day are given.

Most types of external-beam radiation therapy are given in once-daily fractions. There are two main reasons for once-daily treatment:

- To minimize the damage to normal tissue

- To increase the likelihood that cancer cells are exposed to radiation at the points in the cell cycle when they are most vulnerable to DNA damage

451

In recent decades, doctors have tested whether other fractionation schedules are helpful, including:

- **Accelerated fractionation:** Treatment given in larger daily or weekly doses to reduce the number of weeks of treatment

- **Hyperfractionation:** Smaller doses of radiation given more than once a day

- **Hypofractionation:** Larger doses given once a day or less often to reduce the number of treatments

Researchers hope that different types of treatment fractionation may either be more effective than traditional fractionation or be as effective but more convenient.

When Will a Patient Get Radiation Therapy?

A patient may receive radiation therapy before, during, or after surgery. Some patients may receive radiation therapy alone, without surgery or other treatments. Some patients may receive radiation therapy and chemotherapy at the same time. The timing of radiation therapy depends on the type of cancer being treated and the goal of treatment (cure or palliation).

Radiation therapy given before surgery is called preoperative or neoadjuvant radiation. Neoadjuvant radiation may be given to shrink a tumor so it can be removed by surgery and be less likely to return after surgery. Radiation therapy given during surgery is called intraoperative radiation therapy (IORT). IORT can be external-beam radiation therapy (with photons or electrons) or brachytherapy. When radiation is given during surgery, nearby normal tissues can be physically shielded from radiation exposure. IORT is sometimes used when normal structures are too close to a tumor to allow the use of external-beam radiation therapy.

Radiation therapy given after surgery is called postoperative or adjuvant radiation therapy.

Radiation therapy given after some types of complicated surgery (especially in the abdomen or pelvis) may produce too many side effects; therefore, it may be safer if given before surgery in these cases.

The combination of chemotherapy and radiation therapy given at the same time is sometimes called chemoradiation or radiochemotherapy. For some types of cancer, the combination of chemotherapy and radiation therapy may kill more cancer cells (increasing the likelihood of a cure), but it can also cause more side effects. After cancer treatment, patients receive regular follow-up care from their oncologists to monitor their health and to check for possible cancer recurrence.

Does Radiation Therapy Make a Patient Radioactive?

External-beam radiation does not make a patient radioactive. During temporary brachytherapy treatments, while the radioactive material is inside the body, the patient is radioactive; however, as soon as the material is removed, the patient is no longer radioactive. For temporary brachytherapy, the patient will usually stay in the hospital in a special room that shields other people from the radiation.

During permanent brachytherapy, the implanted material will be radioactive for several days, weeks, or months after the radiation source is put in place. During this time, the patient is radioactive. However, the amount of radiation reaching the surface of the skin is usually very low. Nonetheless, this radiation can be detected by radiation monitors and contact with pregnant woman and young children may be restricted for a few days or weeks.

Some types of systemic radiation therapy may temporarily make a patient's bodily fluids (such as saliva, urine, sweat, or stool) emit a low level of radiation. Patients receiving systemic radiation therapy may need to limit their contact with other people during this time, and especially avoid contact with children younger than 18 and pregnant women. A patient's doctor or nurse will provide more information to family members and caretakers if any of these special precautions are needed. Over time (usually days or weeks), the radioactive material retained within the body will break down so that no radiation can be measured outside the patient's body.

What Are the Potential Side Effects of Radiation Therapy?

Radiation therapy can cause both early (acute) and late (chronic) side effects. Acute side effects occur during treatment, and chronic side effects occur months or even years after treatment ends. The side effects that develop depend on the area of the body being treated, the dose given per day, the total dose given, the patient's general medical condition, and other treatments given at the same time.

Acute radiation side effects are caused by damage to rapidly dividing normal cells in the area being treated. These effects include skin irritation or damage at regions exposed to the radiation beams. Examples include damage to the salivary glands or hair loss when the head or neck area is treated, or urinary problems when the lower abdomen is treated.

Most acute effects disappear after treatment ends, though some (like salivary gland damage) can be permanent. The drug amifostine (Ethyol®) can help protect the salivary glands from radiation damage if it is given during treatment. Amifostine is the only drug approved by the FDA to protect normal tissues from radiation during treatment. This type of drug is called a radioprotector. Other potential radioprotectors are being tested in clinical trials.

Fatigue is a common side effect of radiation therapy regardless of which part of the body is treated. Nausea with or without vomiting is common when the abdomen is treated and occurs sometimes when the brain is treated. Medications are available to help prevent or treat nausea and vomiting during treatment.

Late side effects of radiation therapy may or may not occur. Depending on the area of the body treated, late side effects can include:

- Fibrosis (the replacement of normal tissue with scar tissue, leading to restricted movement of the affected area)

- Damage to the bowels, causing diarrhea and bleeding

- Memory loss

- Infertility (inability to have a child)

- Rarely, a second cancer caused by radiation exposure

Second cancers that develop after radiation therapy depend on the part of the body that was treated. For example, girls treated with radiation to the chest for Hodgkin lymphoma have an increased risk of developing breast cancer later in life. In general, the lifetime risk of a second cancer is highest in people treated for cancer as children or adolescents.

Whether or not a patient experiences late side effects depends on other aspects of their cancer treatment in addition to radiation therapy, as well as their individual risk factors. Some chemotherapy drugs, genetic risk factors, and lifestyle factors (such as smoking) can also increase the risk of late side effects.

When suggesting radiation therapy as part of a patient's cancer treatment, the radiation oncologist will carefully weigh the known risks of treatment against the potential benefits for each patient (including relief of symptoms, shrinking a tumor, or potential cure). The results of hundreds of clinical trials and doctors' individual experiences help radiation oncologists decide which patients are likely to benefit from radiation therapy.

What Research Is Being Done to Improve Radiation Therapy?

Doctors and other scientists are conducting research studies called clinical trials to learn how to use radiation therapy to treat cancer more safely and effectively. Clinical trials allow researchers to examine the effectiveness of the treatments in comparison with standard ones, as well as to compare the side effects of the treatments.

Researchers are working on improving image-guided radiation so that it provides real-time imaging of the tumor target during treatment. Real-time imaging could help compensate for normal movement of the internal organs from breathing and for changes in tumor size during treatment.

Researchers are also studying radiosensitizers and radioprotectors, chemicals that modify a cell's response to radiation:

- Radiosensitizers are drugs that make cancer cells more sensitive to the effects of radiation therapy. Several agents are under study as radiosensitizers. In addition, some anticancer drugs, such as 5-fluorouracil and cisplatin, make cancer cells more sensitive to radiation therapy.

- Radioprotectors (also called radioprotectants) are drugs that protect normal cells from damage caused by radiation therapy. These drugs promote the repair of normal cells exposed to radiation. Many agents are currently being studied as potential radioprotectors.

The use of carbon ion beams in radiation therapy is being investigated by researchers, but, at this time, the use of these beams remains experimental. Carbon ion beams are available at only a few medical centers around the world. They are not currently available in the United States. Researchers hope that carbon ion beams may be effective in treating some tumors that are resistant to traditional radiation therapy. People with cancer who are interested in taking part in a clinical trial should talk with their doctor.

Chapter 37

Bone Marrow and Peripheral Blood Stem Cell Transplantation

Stem cell transplants are procedures that restore blood-forming stem cells in people who have had theirs destroyed by the very high doses of chemotherapy or radiation therapy that are used to treat certain cancers.

Blood-forming stem cells are important because they grow into different types of blood cells. The main types of blood cells are:

- White blood cells (WBCs), which are part of your immune system and help your body fight infection

- Red blood cells (RBCs), which carry oxygen throughout your body

- Platelets, which help the blood clot

You need all three types of blood cells to be healthy.

This chapter contains text excerpted from the following sources: Text in this chapter begins with excerpts from "Stem Cell Transplants in Cancer Treatment," National Cancer Institute (NCI), April 29, 2015; Text beginning with the heading "What Are Bone Marrow and Hematopoietic Stem Cells?" is excerpted from "Blood-Forming Stem Cell Transplants," National Cancer Institute (NCI), August 12, 2013. Reviewed May 2018.

Types of Stem Cell Transplants

In a stem cell transplant, you receive healthy blood-forming stem cells through a needle in your vein. Once they enter your bloodstream, the stem cells travel to the bone marrow, where they take the place of the cells that were destroyed by treatment. The blood-forming stem cells that are used in transplants can come from the bone marrow, bloodstream, or umbilical cord. Transplants can be:

- Autologous, which means the stem cells come from you, the patient

- Allogeneic, which means the stem cells come from someone else. The donor may be a blood relative but can also be someone who is not related.

- Syngeneic, which means the stem cells come from your identical twin, if you have one

To reduce possible side effects and improve the chances that an allogeneic transplant will work, the donor's blood-forming stem cells must match yours in certain ways.

How Stem Cell Transplants Work against Cancer

Stem cell transplants do not usually work against cancer directly. Instead, they help you recover your ability to produce stem cells after treatment with very high doses of radiation therapy, chemotherapy, or both. However, in multiple myeloma and some types of leukemia, the stem cell transplant may work against cancer directly. This happens because of an effect called graft-versus-tumor that can occur after allogeneic transplants. Graft-versus-tumor (GvT) occurs when white blood cells from your donor (the graft) attack any cancer cells that remain in your body (the tumor) after high-dose treatments. This effect improves the success of the treatments.

Who Receives Stem Cell Transplants

Stem cell transplants are most often used to help people with leukemia and lymphoma. They may also be used for neuroblastoma and multiple myeloma. Stem cell transplants for other types of cancer are being studied in clinical trials, which are research studies involving people.

Side Effects of Stem Cell Transplants

The high doses of cancer treatment that you have before a stem cell transplant can cause problems such as bleeding and an increased risk of infection. Talk with your doctor or nurse about other side effects that you might have and how serious they might be.

If you have an allogeneic transplant, you might develop a serious problem called graft-versus-host disease (GVHD). GVHD can occur when white blood cells from your donor (the graft) recognize cells in your body (the host) as foreign and attack them. This problem can cause damage to your skin, liver, intestines, and many other organs. It can occur a few weeks after the transplant or much later. GVHD can be treated with steroids or other drugs that suppress your immune system. The closer your donor's blood-forming stem cells match yours, the less likely you are to have GVHD. Your doctor may also try to prevent it by giving you drugs to suppress your immune system.

Cost of Stem Cell Transplants

Stem cells transplants are complicated procedures that are very expensive. Most insurance plans cover some of the costs of transplants for certain types of cancer. Talk with your health plan about which services it will pay for. Talking with the business office where you go for treatment may help you understand all the costs involved.

What to Expect When Receiving a Stem Cell Transplant

Where You Go for a Stem Cell Transplant

When you need an allogeneic stem cell transplant, you will need to go to a hospital that has a specialized transplant center. The National Marrow Donor Program® (NMDP) maintains a list of transplant centers in the United States that can help you find a transplant center.

Unless you live near a transplant center, you may need to travel from home for your treatment. You might need to stay in the hospital during your transplant, you may be able to have it as an outpatient, or you may need to be in the hospital only part of the time. When you are not in the hospital, you will need to stay in a hotel or apartment nearby. Many transplant centers can assist with finding nearby housing.

How Long It Takes to Have a Stem Cell Transplant

A stem cell transplant can take a few months to complete. The process begins with treatment of high doses of chemotherapy, radiation therapy, or a combination of the two. This treatment goes on for a week or two. Once you have finished, you will have a few days to rest.

Next, you will receive the blood-forming stem cells. The stem cells will be given to you through an intravenous (IV) catheter. This process is like receiving a blood transfusion. It takes 1–5 hours to receive all the stem cells.

After receiving the stem cells, you begin the recovery phase. During this time, you wait for the blood cells you received to start making new blood cells.

Even after your blood counts return to normal, it takes much longer for your immune system to fully recover—several months for autologous transplants and 1–2 years for allogeneic or syngeneic transplants.

How Stem Cell Transplants May Affect You

Stem cell transplants affect people in different ways. How you feel depends on:

- The type of transplant that you have
- The doses of treatment you had before the transplant
- How you respond to the high-dose treatments
- Your type of cancer
- How advanced your cancer is
- How healthy you were before the transplant

Since people respond to stem cell transplants in different ways, your doctor or nurses cannot know for sure how the procedure will make you feel.

How to Tell If Your Stem Cell Transplant Worked

Doctors will follow the progress of the new blood cells by checking your blood counts often. As the newly transplanted stem cells produce blood cells, your blood counts will go up.

Special Diet Needs

The high-dose treatments that you have before a stem cell transplant can cause side effects that make it hard to eat, such as mouth sores and nausea. Tell your doctor or nurse if you have trouble eating while you are receiving treatment. You might also find it helpful to speak with a dietitian.

Working during Your Stem Cell Transplant

Whether or not you can work during a stem cell transplant may depend on the type of job you have. The process of a stem cell transplant, with the high-dose treatments, the transplant, and recovery, can take weeks or months. You will be in and out of the hospital during this time. Even when you are not in the hospital, sometimes you will need to stay near it, rather than staying in your own home. So, if your job allows, you may want to arrange to work remotely part-time. Many employers are required by law to change your work schedule to meet your needs during cancer treatment. Talk with your employer about ways to adjust your work during treatment. You can learn more about these laws by talking with a social worker.

What Are Bone Marrow and Hematopoietic Stem Cells?

Bone marrow is the soft, sponge-like material found inside bones. It contains immature cells known as hematopoietic or blood-forming stem cells. (Hematopoietic stem cells are different from embryonic stem cells. Embryonic stem cells can develop into every type of cell in the body.) Hematopoietic stem cells divide to form more blood-forming stem cells, or they mature into one of three types of blood cells: white blood cells, which fight infection; red blood cells, which carry oxygen; and platelets, which help the blood to clot. Most hematopoietic stem cells are found in the bone marrow, but some cells, called peripheral blood stem cells (PBSCs), are found in the bloodstream. Blood in the umbilical cord also contains hematopoietic stem cells. Cells from any of these sources can be used in transplants.

What Are Bone Marrow Transplantation and Peripheral Blood Stem Cell Transplantation?

Bone marrow transplantation (BMT) and peripheral blood stem cell transplantation (PBSCT) are procedures that restore stem cells that have been destroyed by high doses of chemotherapy and/or radiation therapy. There are three types of transplants:

- In autologous transplants, patients receive their own stem cells.

- In syngeneic transplants, patients receive stem cells from their identical twin.

- In allogeneic transplants, patients receive stem cells from their brother, sister, or parent. A person who is not related to the patient (an unrelated donor) also may be used.

Why Are BMT and PBSCT Used in Cancer Treatment?

One reason BMT and PBSCT are used in cancer treatment is to make it possible for patients to receive very high doses of chemotherapy and/or radiation therapy. To understand more about why BMT and PBSCT are used, it is helpful to understand how chemotherapy and radiation therapy work. Chemotherapy and radiation therapy generally affect cells that divide rapidly. They are used to treat cancer because cancer cells divide more often than most healthy cells. However, because bone marrow cells also divide frequently, high-dose treatments can severely damage or destroy the patient's bone marrow. Without healthy bone marrow, the patient is no longer able to make the blood cells needed to carry oxygen, fight infection, and prevent bleeding. BMT and PBSCT replace stem cells destroyed by treatment. The healthy, transplanted stem cells can restore the bone marrow's ability to produce the blood cells the patient needs. In some types of leukemia, the graft-versus-tumor (GVT) effect that occurs after allogeneic BMT and PBSCT is crucial to the effectiveness of the treatment. GVT occurs when white blood cells from the donor (the graft) identify the cancer cells that remain in the patient's body after the chemotherapy and/or radiation therapy (the tumor) as foreign and attack them.

What Types of Cancer Are Treated with BMT and PBSCT?

BMT and PBSCT are most commonly used in the treatment of leukemia and lymphoma. They are most effective when the leukemia or lymphoma is in remission (the signs and symptoms of cancer have disappeared). BMT and PBSCT are also used to treat other cancers such as neuroblastoma (cancer that arises in immature nerve cells and affects mostly infants and children) and multiple myeloma. Researchers are evaluating BMT and PBSCT in clinical trials (research studies) for the treatment of various types of cancer.

How Are the Donor's Stem Cells Matched to the Patient's Stem Cells in Allogeneic or Syngeneic Transplantation?

To minimize potential side effects, doctors most often use transplanted stem cells that match the patient's own stem cells as closely as possible. People have different sets of proteins, called human leukocyte-associated (HLA) antigens, on the surface of their cells. The set of proteins, called the HLA type, is identified by a special blood test.

In most cases, the success of allogeneic transplantation depends in part on how well the HLA antigens of the donor's stem cells match those of the recipient's stem cells. The higher the number of matching HLA antigens, the greater the chance that the patient's body will accept the donor's stem cells. In general, patients are less likely to develop a complication known as graft-versus-host disease (GVHD) if the stem cells of the donor and patient are closely matched.

Close relatives, especially brothers and sisters, are more likely than unrelated people to be HLA-matched. However, only 25–35 percent of patients have an HLA-matched sibling. The chances of obtaining HLA-matched stem cells from an unrelated donor are slightly better, approximately 50 percent. Among unrelated donors, HLA matching is greatly improved when the donor and recipient have the same ethnic and racial background. Although the number of donors is increasing overall, individuals from certain ethnic and racial groups still have a lower chance of finding a matching donor. Large volunteer donor registries can assist in finding an appropriate unrelated donor.

Because identical twins have the same genes, they have the same set of HLA antigens. As a result, the patient's body will accept a transplant from an identical twin. However, identical twins represent a small number of all births, so syngeneic transplantation is rare.

How Is Bone Marrow Obtained for Transplantation?

The stem cells used in BMT come from the liquid center of the bone, called the marrow. In general, the procedure for obtaining bone marrow, which is called "harvesting," is similar for all three types of BMTs (autologous, syngeneic, and allogeneic). The donor is given either general anesthesia, which puts the person to sleep during the procedure, or regional anesthesia, which causes loss of feeling below the waist. Needles are inserted through the skin over the pelvic (hip) bone or, in rare cases, the sternum (breastbone), and into the bone marrow to draw the marrow out of the bone. Harvesting the marrow takes about an hour.

The harvested bone marrow is then processed to remove blood and bone fragments. Harvested bone marrow can be combined with a preservative and frozen to keep the stem cells alive until they are needed. This technique is known as cryopreservation. Stem cells can be cryopreserved for many years.

How Are PBSCs Obtained for Transplantation?

The stem cells used in PBSCT come from the bloodstream. A process called apheresis or leukapheresis is used to obtain PBSCs for transplantation. For 4 or 5 days before apheresis, the donor may be given a medication to increase the number of stem cells released into the bloodstream. In apheresis, blood is removed through a large vein in the arm or a central venous catheter (a flexible tube that is placed in a large vein in the neck, chest, or groin area). The blood goes through a machine that removes the stem cells. The blood is then returned to the donor and the collected cells are stored. Apheresis typically takes 4–6 hours. The stem cells are then frozen until they are given to the recipient.

How Are Umbilical Cord Stem Cells Obtained for Transplantation?

Stem cells also may be retrieved from umbilical cord blood. For this to occur, the mother must contact a cord blood bank before the baby's birth. The cord blood bank may request that she complete a questionnaire and give a small blood sample. Cord blood banks may be public or commercial. Public cord blood banks accept donations of cord blood and may provide the donated stem cells to another matched individual in their network. In contrast, commercial cord blood banks will store the cord blood for the family, in case it is needed later for the child or another family member.

After the baby is born and the umbilical cord has been cut, blood is retrieved from the umbilical cord and placenta. This process poses minimal health risk to the mother or the child. If the mother agrees, the umbilical cord blood is processed and frozen for storage by the cord blood bank. Only a small amount of blood can be retrieved from the umbilical cord and placenta, so the collected stem cells are typically used for children or small adults.

Are Any Risks Associated with Donating Bone Marrow?

Because only a small amount of bone marrow is removed, donating usually does not pose any significant problems for the donor. The most serious risk associated with donating bone marrow involves the use of anesthesia during the procedure. The area where the bone marrow was taken out may feel stiff or sore for a few days, and the donor may feel tired. Within a few weeks, the donor's body replaces the donated marrow; however, the time required for a donor to recover varies. Some people are back to their usual routine within 2 or 3 days, while others may take up to 3–4 weeks to fully recover their strength.

Are Any Risks Associated with Donating PBSCs?

Apheresis usually causes minimal discomfort. During apheresis, the person may feel lightheadedness, chills, numbness around the lips, and cramping in the hands. Unlike bone marrow donation, PBSC donation does not require anesthesia. The medication that is given to stimulate the mobilization (release) of stem cells from the marrow into the bloodstream may cause bone and muscle aches, headaches, fatigue, nausea, vomiting, and/or difficulty sleeping. These side effects generally stop within 2–3 days of the last dose of the medication.

How Does the Patient Receive the Stem Cells during the Transplant?

After being treated with high-dose anticancer drugs and/or radiation, the patient receives the stem cells through an intravenous (IV) line just like a blood transfusion. This part of the transplant takes 1–5 hours.

Are Any Special Measures Taken When the Cancer Patient Is Also the Donor (Autologous Transplant)?

The stem cells used for autologous transplantation must be relatively free of cancer cells. The harvested cells can sometimes be treated before transplantation in a process known as "purging" to get rid of cancer cells. This process can remove some cancer cells from the harvested cells and minimize the chance that cancer will come back. Because purging may damage some healthy stem cells, more cells are obtained from the patient before the transplant so that enough healthy stem cells will remain after purging.

What Happens after the Stem Cells Have Been Transplanted to the Patient?

After entering the bloodstream, the stem cells travel to the bone marrow, where they begin to produce new white blood cells, red blood cells, and platelets in a process known as "engraftment." Engraftment usually occurs within about 2–4 weeks after transplantation. Doctors monitor it by checking blood counts on a frequent basis. Complete recovery of immune function takes much longer, however—up to several months for autologous transplant recipients and 1–2 years for patients receiving allogeneic or syngeneic transplants. Doctors evaluate the results of various blood tests to confirm that new blood cells are being produced and that the cancer has not returned. Bone marrow aspiration (the removal of a small sample of bone marrow through a needle for examination under a microscope) can also help doctors determine how well the new marrow is working.

What Are the Possible Side Effects of BMT and PBSCT?

The major risk of both treatments is an increased susceptibility to infection and bleeding as a result of the high-dose cancer treatment. Doctors may give the patient antibiotics to prevent or treat infection. They may also give the patient transfusions of platelets to prevent bleeding and red blood cells to treat anemia. Patients who undergo BMT and PBSCT may experience short-term side effects such as nausea, vomiting, fatigue, loss of appetite, mouth sores, hair loss, and skin reactions.

Potential long-term risks include complications of the pretransplant chemotherapy and radiation therapy, such as infertility (the inability to produce children); cataracts (clouding of the lens of the eye, which causes loss of vision); secondary (new) cancers; and damage to the liver, kidneys, lungs, and/or heart.

With allogeneic transplants, GVHD sometimes develops when white blood cells from the donor (the graft) identify cells in the patient's body (the host) as foreign and attack them. The most commonly damaged organs are the skin, liver, and intestines. This complication can develop within a few weeks of the transplant (acute GVHD) or much later (chronic GVHD). To prevent this complication, the patient may receive medications that suppress the immune system. Additionally, the donated stem cells can be treated to remove the white blood cells that cause GVHD in a process called "T-cell depletion." If GVHD develops, it can be very serious and is treated with steroids or other immunosuppressive agents. GVHD can be difficult to treat, but some studies suggest that patients with leukemia who develop GVHD are less likely to have the cancer come back. Clinical trials are being conducted to find ways to prevent and treat GVHD. The likelihood and severity of complications are specific to the patient's treatment and should be discussed with the patient's doctor.

What Is a "Mini-Transplant"?

A "mini-transplant" (also called a nonmyeloablative or reduced-intensity transplant) is a type of allogeneic transplant. This approach is being studied in clinical trials for the treatment of several types of cancer, including leukemia, lymphoma, multiple myeloma, and other cancers of the blood.

A mini-transplant uses lower, less toxic doses of chemotherapy and/or radiation to prepare the patient for an allogeneic transplant. The use of lower doses of anticancer drugs and radiation eliminates some, but not all, of the patient's bone marrow. It also reduces the number of cancer cells and suppresses the patient's immune system to prevent rejection of the transplant.

Unlike traditional BMT or PBSCT, cells from both the donor and the patient may exist in the patient's body for some time after a mini-transplant. Once the cells from the donor begin to engraft, they may cause the GVT effect and work to destroy the cancer cells that were not eliminated by the anticancer drugs and/or radiation. To boost the GVT effect, the patient may be given an injection of the donor's white blood cells. This procedure is called a "donor lymphocyte infusion."

What Is a "Tandem Transplant"?

A "tandem transplant" is a type of autologous transplant. This method is being studied in clinical trials for the treatment of several types of cancer, including multiple myeloma and germ cell cancer. During a tandem transplant, a patient receives two sequential courses of high-dose chemotherapy with stem cell transplant. Typically, the two courses are given several weeks to several months apart. Researchers hope that this method can prevent the cancer from recurring (coming back) at a later time.

467

How Do Patients Cover the Cost of BMT or PBSCT?

Advances in treatment methods, including the use of PBSCT, have reduced the amount of time many patients must spend in the hospital by speeding recovery. This shorter recovery time has brought about a reduction in cost. However, because BMT and PBSCT are complicated technical procedures, they are very expensive. Many health insurance companies cover some of the costs of transplantation for certain types of cancer. Insurers may also cover a portion of the costs if special care is required when the patient returns home.

There are options for relieving the financial burden associated with BMT and PBSCT. A hospital social worker is a valuable resource in planning for these financial needs. Federal government programs and local service organizations may also be able to help. National Cancer Institute's (NCI) Cancer Information Service (CIS) can provide patients and their families with additional information about sources of financial assistance at 800-4-CANCER (800-422-6237). NCI is part of the National Institutes of Health (NIH).

What Are the Costs of Donating Bone Marrow, PBSCs, or Umbilical Cord Blood?

All medical costs for the donation procedure are covered by Be The Match®, or by the patient's medical insurance, as are travel expenses and other nonmedical costs. The only costs to the donor might be time taken off from work. A woman can donate her baby's umbilical cord blood to public cord blood banks at no charge. However, commercial blood banks do charge varying fees to store umbilical cord blood for the private use of the patient or his or her family.

Chapter 38

Biological Therapies for Cancer

What Is Biological Therapy?

Biological therapy involves the use of living organisms, substances derived from living organisms, or laboratory-produced versions of such substances to treat disease. Some biological therapies for cancer use vaccines or bacteria to stimulate the body's immune system to act against cancer cells. These types of biological therapy, which are sometimes referred to collectively as "immunotherapy" or "biological response modifier therapy," do not target cancer cells directly. Other biological therapies, such as antibodies or segments of genetic material (ribonucleic acid (RNA) or deoxyribonucleic acid (DNA)), do target cancer cells directly. Biological therapies that interfere with specific molecules involved in tumor growth and progression are also referred to as targeted therapies. For patients with cancer, biological therapies may be used to treat the cancer itself or the side effects of other cancer treatments. Although many forms of biological therapy have been approved by the U.S. Food and Drug Administration (FDA), others remain experimental and are available to cancer patients principally through participation in clinical trials (research studies involving people).

This chapter includes text excerpted from "Biological Therapies for Cancer," National Cancer Institute (NCI), June 12, 2013. Reviewed May 2018.

What Is the Immune System and What Role Does It Play in Biological Therapy for Cancer?

The immune system is a complex network of organs, tissues, and specialized cells. It recognizes and destroys foreign invaders, such as bacteria or viruses, as well as some damaged, diseased, or abnormal cells in the body, including cancer cells. An immune response is triggered when the immune system encounters a substance, called an antigen, it recognizes as "foreign."

White blood cells (WBCs) are the primary players in immune system responses. Some white blood cells, including macrophages and natural killer cells, patrol the body, seeking out foreign invaders and diseased, damaged, or dead cells. These white blood cells provide a general—or nonspecific—level of immune protection.

Other white blood cells, including cytotoxic T cells and B cells, act against specific targets. Cytotoxic T cells release chemicals that can directly destroy microbes or abnormal cells. B cells make antibodies that latch onto foreign intruders or abnormal cells and tag them for destruction by another component of the immune system. Still, other white blood cells, including dendritic cells, play supporting roles to ensure that cytotoxic T cells and B cells do their jobs effectively.

It is generally believed that the immune system's natural capacity to detect and destroy abnormal cells prevents the development of many cancers. Nevertheless, some cancer cells are able to evade detection by using one or more strategies. For example, cancer cells can undergo genetic changes that lead to the loss of cancer-associated antigens, making them less "visible" to the immune system. They may also use several different mechanisms to suppress immune responses or to avoid being killed by cytotoxic T cells. The goal of immunotherapy for cancer is to overcome these barriers to an effective anticancer immune response. These biological therapies restore or increase the activities of specific immune-system components or counteract immunosuppressive signals produced by cancer cells.

What Are Monoclonal Antibodies (mAbs), and How Are They Used in Cancer Treatment?

Monoclonal antibodies, or mAbs, are laboratory-produced antibodies that bind to specific antigens expressed by cells, such as a protein that is present on the surface of cancer cells but is absent from (or expressed at lower levels by) normal cells.

To create mAbs, researchers inject mice with an antigen from human cells. They then harvest the antibody-producing cells from the mice and individually fuse them with a myeloma cell (cancerous B cell) to produce a fusion cell known as a hybridoma. Each hybridoma then divides to produce identical daughter cells or clones—hence the term "monoclonal"—and antibodies secreted by different clones are tested to identify the antibodies that bind most strongly to the antigen. Large quantities of antibodies can be produced by these immortal hybridoma cells. Because mouse antibodies can themselves elicit an immune response in humans, which would reduce their effectiveness, mouse antibodies are often "humanized" by replacing as much of the mouse portion of the antibody as possible with human portions. This is done through genetic engineering.

Some mAbs stimulate an immune response that destroys cancer cells. Similar to the antibodies produced naturally by B cells, these mAbs "coat" the cancer cell surface, triggering its destruction by the immune system. FDA-approved mAbs of this type include rituximab, which targets the CD20 antigen found on non-Hodgkin lymphoma (NHL) cells, and alemtuzumab, which targets the CD52 antigen found on B-cell chronic lymphocytic leukemia (CLL) cells. Rituximab may also trigger cell death (apoptosis) directly.

Another group of mAbs stimulates an anticancer immune response by binding to receptors on the surface of immune cells and inhibiting signals that prevent immune cells from attacking the body's own tissues, including cancer cells. One such MAb, ipilimumab, has been approved by the FDA for treatment of metastatic melanoma, and others are being investigated in clinical studies.

Other mAbs interfere with the action of proteins that are necessary for tumor growth. For example, bevacizumab targets vascular endothelial growth factor (VEGF), a protein secreted by tumor cells and other cells in the tumor's microenvironment that promotes the development of tumor blood vessels. When bound to bevacizumab, VEGF cannot interact with its cellular receptor, preventing the signaling that leads to the growth of new blood vessels.

Similarly, cetuximab and panitumumab target the epidermal growth factor receptor (EGFR), and trastuzumab targets the human epidermal growth factor receptor 2 (HER-2). mAbs that bind to cell surface growth factor receptors prevent the targeted receptors from sending their normal growth-promoting signals. They may also trigger apoptosis and activate the immune system to destroy tumor cells.

471

Another group of cancer therapeutic mAbs are the immunoconjugates. These mAbs, which are sometimes called immunotoxins or antibody-drug conjugates, consist of an antibody attached to a cell-killing substance, such as a plant or bacterial toxin, a chemotherapy drug, or a radioactive molecule. The antibody latches onto its specific antigen on the surface of a cancer cell, and the cell-killing substance is taken up by the cell. FDA-approved conjugated mAbs that work this way include 90Y-ibritumomab tiuxetan, which targets the CD20 antigen to deliver radioactive yttrium-90 to B-cell non-Hodgkin lymphoma cells, and ado-trastuzumab emtansine, which targets the HER-2 molecule to deliver the drug DM1, which inhibits cell proliferation, to HER-2 expressing metastatic breast cancer cells.

What Are Cytokines, and How Are They Used in Cancer Treatment?

Cytokines are signaling proteins that are produced by white blood cells. They help mediate and regulate immune responses, inflammation, and hematopoiesis (new blood cell formation). Two types of cytokines are used to treat patients with cancer: interferons (INFs) and interleukins (ILs). A third type, called hematopoietic growth factors, is used to counteract some of the side effects of certain chemotherapy regimens.

Researchers have found that one type of INF, INF-alfa, can enhance a patient's immune response to cancer cells by activating certain white blood cells, such as natural killer cells and dendritic cells. INF-alfa may also inhibit the growth of cancer cells or promote their death. INF-alfa has been approved for the treatment of melanoma, Kaposi sarcoma, and several hematologic cancers.

Like INFs, ILs play important roles in the body's normal immune response and in the immune system's ability to respond to cancer. Researchers have identified more than a dozen distinct ILs, including IL-2, which is also called T-cell growth factor. IL-2 is naturally produced by activated T cells. It increases the proliferation of white blood cells, including cytotoxic T cells and natural killer cells, leading to an enhanced anticancer immune response. IL-2 also facilitates the production of antibodies by B cells to further target cancer cells. Aldesleukin, IL-2 that is made in a laboratory, has been approved for the treatment of metastatic kidney cancer and metastatic melanoma. Researchers are currently investigating whether combining aldesleukin treatment with other types of biological therapies may enhance its anticancer effects.

Hematopoietic growth factors are a special class of naturally occurring cytokines. All blood cells arise from hematopoietic stem cells in the bone marrow. Because chemotherapy drugs target proliferating cells, including normal blood stem cells, chemotherapy depletes these stem cells and the blood cells that they produce. Loss of red blood cells, which transport oxygen and nutrients throughout the body, can cause anemia. A decrease in platelets, which are responsible for blood clotting, often leads to abnormal bleeding. Finally, lower white blood cell counts leave chemotherapy patients vulnerable to infections.

Several growth factors that promote the growth of these various blood cell populations have been approved for clinical use. Erythropoietin stimulates red blood cell formation, and IL-11 increases platelet production. Granulocyte-macrophage colony-stimulating factor (GM-CSF) and granulocyte colony-stimulating factor (G-CSF) both increase the number of white blood cells, reducing the risk of infections. Treatment with these factors allows patients to continue chemotherapy regimens that might otherwise be stopped temporarily or modified to reduce the drug doses because of low blood cell numbers.

G-CSF and GM-CSF can also enhance the immune system's specific anticancer responses by increasing the number of cancer-fighting T cells. Thus, GM-CSF and G-CSF are used in combination with other biological therapies to strengthen anticancer immune responses.

What Are Cancer Treatment Vaccines?

Cancer treatment vaccines are designed to treat cancers that have already developed rather than to prevent them in the first place. Cancer treatment vaccines contain cancer-associated antigens to enhance the immune system's response to a patient's tumor cells. The cancer-associated antigens can be proteins or another type of molecule found on the surface of or inside cancer cells that can stimulate B cells or killer T cells to attack them.

Some vaccines that are under development target antigens that are found on or in many types of cancer cells. These types of cancer vaccines are being tested in clinical trials in patients with a variety of cancers, including colorectal, lung, breast, and thyroid cancers. Other cancer vaccines target antigens that are unique to a specific cancer type. Still, other vaccines are designed against an antigen specific to one patient's tumor and need to be customized for each patient. The one cancer treatment vaccine that has received FDA approval, sipuleucel-T, is this type of vaccine. Because of the limited toxicity seen with cancer vaccines, they are also being tested in clinical trials in combination with other forms of therapy, such as hormonal therapy, chemotherapy, radiation therapy, and targeted therapies.

What Is Bacillus Calmette-GuéRin (BCG) Therapy?

Bacillus Calmette-Guérin (BCG) was the first biological therapy to be approved by the FDA. It is a weakened form of a live tuberculosis bacterium that does not cause disease in humans. It was first used medically as a vaccine against tuberculosis. When inserted directly into the bladder with a catheter, BCG stimulates a general immune response that is directed not only against the foreign bacterium itself but also against bladder cancer cells. How and why BCG exerts this anticancer effect is not well understood, but the efficacy of the treatment is well documented. Approximately 70 percent of patients with early-stage bladder cancer experience a remission after BCG therapy. BCG is also being studied in the treatment of other types of cancer.

What Is Oncolytic Virus Therapy?

Oncolytic virus therapy is an experimental form of biological therapy that involves the direct destruction of cancer cells. Oncolytic viruses (OVs) infect both cancer and normal cells, but they have little effect on normal cells. In contrast, they readily replicate, or reproduce, inside cancer cells and ultimately cause the cancer cells to die. Some viruses, such as reovirus, Newcastle disease virus, and mumps virus, are naturally oncolytic, whereas others, including measles virus, adenovirus, and vaccinia virus, can be adapted or modified to replicate efficiently only in cancer cells. In addition, OVs can be genetically engineered to preferentially infect and replicate in cancer cells that produce a specific cancer-associated antigen, such as EGFR or HER-2.

One of the challenges in using OVs is that they may themselves be destroyed by the patient's immune system before they have a chance to attack the cancer. Researchers have developed several strategies to overcome this challenge, such as administering a combination of immune-suppressing chemotherapy drugs like cyclophosphamide along with the virus or "cloaking" the virus within a protective envelope. But an immune reaction in the patient may actually have benefits: although it may hamper oncolytic virus therapy at the time of viral delivery, it may enhance cancer cell destruction after the virus has infected the tumor cells.

No oncolytic virus has been approved for use in the United States, although H101, a modified form of adenovirus, was approved in China in 2006 for the treatment of patients with head and neck cancer. Several OVs are currently being tested in clinical trials. Researchers are also investigating whether OVs can be combined with other types of cancer therapies or can be used to sensitize patients' tumors to additional therapy.

What Is Gene Therapy?

Still an experimental form of treatment, gene therapy attempts to introduce genetic material (DNA or RNA) into living cells. Gene therapy is being studied in clinical trials for many types of cancer.

In general, genetic material cannot be inserted directly into a person's cells. Instead, it is delivered to the cells using a carrier, or "vector." The vectors most commonly used in gene therapy are viruses, because they have the unique ability to recognize certain cells and insert genetic material into them. Scientists alter these viruses to make them more safe for humans (e.g., by inactivating genes that enable them to reproduce or cause disease) and/or to improve their ability to recognize and enter the target cell. A variety of liposomes (fatty particles) and nanoparticles are also being used as gene therapy vectors, and scientists are investigating methods of targeting these vectors to specific cell types.

Researchers are studying several methods for treating cancer with gene therapy. Some approaches target cancer cells, to destroy them or prevent their growth. Others target healthy cells to enhance their ability to fight cancer. In some cases, researchers remove cells from the patient, treat the cells with the vector in the laboratory, and return the cells to the patient. In others, the vector is given directly to the patient. Some gene therapy approaches being studied are described below.

- Replacing an altered tumor suppressor gene that produces a nonfunctional protein (or no protein) with a normal version of the gene. Because tumor suppressor genes (e.g., *TP53*) play a role in preventing cancer, restoring the normal function of these genes may inhibit cancer growth or promote cancer regression.

- Introducing genetic material to block the expression of an oncogene whose product promotes tumor growth. Short RNA or DNA molecules with sequences complementary to the gene's messenger RNA (mRNA) can be packaged into vectors or given to cells directly. These short molecules, called oligonucleotides, can bind to the target mRNA, preventing its translation into protein or even causing its degradation.

- Improving a patient's immune response to cancer. In one approach, gene therapy is used to introduce cytokine-producing genes into cancer cells to stimulate the immune response to the tumor.

- Inserting genes into cancer cells to make them more sensitive to chemotherapy, radiation therapy, or other treatments.

- Inserting genes into healthy blood-forming stem cells to make them more resistant to the side effects of cancer treatments, such as high doses of anticancer drugs.

- Introducing "suicide genes" into a patient's cancer cells. A suicide gene is a gene whose product is able to activate a "pro-drug" (an inactive form of a toxic drug), causing the toxic drug to be produced only in cancer cells in patients given the pro-drug. Normal cells, which do not express the suicide genes, are not affected by the pro-drug.

- Inserting genes to prevent cancer cells from developing new blood vessels (angiogenesis).

Proposed gene therapy clinical trials, or protocols, must be approved by at least two review boards at the researchers' institution before they can be conducted. Gene therapy protocols must also be approved by the FDA, which regulates all gene therapy products. In addition, gene therapy trials that are funded by the National Institutes of Health (NIH) must be registered with the NIH Recombinant DNA Advisory Committee (RAC).

What Is Adoptive T-Cell Transfer Therapy?

Adoptive cell transfer is an experimental anticancer therapy that attempts to enhance the natural cancer-fighting ability of a patient's T cells. In one form of this therapy, researchers first harvest cytotoxic T cells that have invaded a patient's tumor. They then identify the cells with the greatest antitumor activity and grow large populations of those cells in a laboratory. The patients are then treated to deplete their immune cells, and the laboratory-grown T cells are infused into the patients.

In another, more recently developed form of this therapy, which is also a kind of gene therapy, researchers isolate T cells from a small sample of the patient's blood. They genetically modify the cells by inserting the gene for a receptor that recognizes an antigen specific to the patient's cancer cells and grow large numbers of these modified cells in culture. The genetically modified cells are then infused into patients whose immune cells have been depleted. The receptor expressed by the modified T cells allows these cells to attach to antigens on the surface of the tumor cells, which activates the T cells to attack and kill the tumor cells.

Adoptive T-cell transfer was first studied for the treatment of metastatic melanoma because melanomas often cause a substantial immune response, with many tumor-invading cytotoxic T cells. Adoptive cell transfer with genetically modified T cells is also being investigated as a treatment for other solid tumors, as well as for hematologic cancers.

What Are the Side Effects of Biological Therapies?

The side effects associated with various biological therapies can differ by treatment type. However, pain, swelling, soreness, redness, itchiness, and rash at the site of infusion or injection are fairly common with these treatments.

Less common but more serious side effects tend to be more specific to one or a few types of biological therapy. For example, therapies intended to prompt an immune response against cancer can cause an array of flu-like symptoms, including fever, chills, weakness, dizziness, nausea or vomiting, muscle or joint aches, fatigue, headache, occasional breathing difficulties, and lowered or heightened blood pressure. Biological therapies that provoke an immune system response also pose a risk of severe or even fatal hypersensitivity (allergic) reactions.

Potential serious side effects of specific biological therapies are as follows:

Monoclonal Antibodies (mAbs)

- Flu-like symptoms

- Severe allergic reaction

- Lowered blood counts

- Changes in blood chemistry

- Organ damage (usually to heart, lungs, kidneys, liver, or brain)

Cytokines (Interferons, Interleukins, Hematopoietic Growth Factors)

- Flu-like symptoms
- Severe allergic reaction
- Lowered blood counts
- Changes in blood chemistry
- Organ damage (usually to heart, lungs, kidneys, liver, or brain)

Treatment Vaccines

- Flu-like symptoms
- Severe allergic reaction

Bacillus Calmette-GuéRin (BCG)

- Flu-like symptoms
- Severe allergic reaction
- Urinary side effects
- Pain or burning sensation during urination
- Increased urgency or frequency of urination
- Blood in the urine

Oncolytic Viruses

- Flu-like symptoms
- Tumor lysis syndrome: Severe, sometimes life-threatening alterations in blood chemistry following the release of materials formerly contained within cancer cells into the bloodstream

Gene Therapy

- Flu-like symptoms
- Secondary cancer: Techniques that insert DNA into a host cell chromosome can cause cancer to develop if the insertion inhibits expression of a tumor suppressor gene or activates an oncogene; researchers are working to minimize this possibility

- Mistaken introduction of a gene into healthy cells, including reproductive cells

- Overexpression of the introduced gene may harm healthy tissues

- Virus vector transmission to other individuals or into the environment

Chapter 39

Laser Treatment and Photodynamic Therapy

What Is Laser Light?

The term "laser" stands for light amplification by stimulated emission of radiation. Ordinary light, such as that from a light bulb, has many wavelengths and spreads in all directions. Laser light, on the other hand, has a specific wavelength. It is focused in a narrow beam and creates a very high-intensity light. This powerful beam of light may be used to cut through steel or to shape diamonds. Because lasers can focus very accurately on tiny areas, they can also be used for very precise surgical work or for cutting through tissue (in place of a scalpel).

What Is Laser Therapy, and How Is It Used in Cancer Treatment?

Laser therapy uses high-intensity light to treat cancer and other illnesses. Lasers can be used to shrink or destroy tumors or precancerous

This chapter contains text excerpted from the following sources: Text beginning with the heading "What Is Laser Light?" is excerpted from "Lasers in Cancer Treatment," National Cancer Institute (NCI), September 13, 2011. Reviewed May 2018; Text beginning with the heading "What Is Photodynamic Therapy?" is excerpted from "Photodynamic Therapy for Cancer," National Cancer Institute (NCI), September 6, 2011. Reviewed May 2018.

growths. Lasers are most commonly used to treat superficial cancers (cancers on the surface of the body or the lining of internal organs) such as basal cell skin cancer and the very early stages of some cancers, such as cervical, penile, vaginal, vulvar, and nonsmall cell lung cancer.

Lasers also may be used to relieve certain symptoms of cancer, such as bleeding or obstruction. For example, lasers can be used to shrink or destroy a tumor that is blocking a patient's trachea (windpipe) or esophagus. Lasers also can be used to remove colon polyps or tumors that are blocking the colon or stomach.

Laser therapy can be used alone, but most often it is combined with other treatments, such as surgery, chemotherapy, or radiation therapy. In addition, lasers can seal nerve endings to reduce pain after surgery and seal lymph vessels to reduce swelling and limit the spread of tumor cells.

How Is Laser Therapy Given to the Patient?

Laser therapy is often given through a flexible endoscope (a thin, lighted tube used to look at tissues inside the body). The endoscope is fitted with optical fibers (thin fibers that transmit light). It is inserted through an opening in the body, such as the mouth, nose, anus, or vagina. Laser light is then precisely aimed to cut or destroy a tumor.

Laser-induced interstitial thermotherapy (LITT), or interstitial laser photocoagulation (ILP), also uses lasers to treat some cancers. LITT is similar to a cancer treatment called hyperthermia, which uses heat to shrink tumors by damaging or killing cancer cells. During LITT, an optical fiber is inserted into a tumor. Laser light at the tip of the fiber raises the temperature of the tumor cells and damages or destroys them. LITT is sometimes used to shrink tumors in the liver.

Photodynamic therapy (PDT) is another type of cancer treatment that uses lasers. In PDT, a certain drug, called a photosensitizer or photosensitizing agent, is injected into a patient and absorbed by cells all over the patient's body. After a couple of days, the agent is found mostly in cancer cells. Laser light is then used to activate the agent and destroy cancer cells. Because the photosensitizer makes the skin and eyes sensitive to light afterward, patients are advised to avoid direct sunlight and bright indoor light during that time.

What Types of Lasers Are Used in Cancer Treatment?

Three types of lasers are used to treat cancer: carbon dioxide (CO_2) lasers, argon lasers, and neodymium:yttrium-aluminum-garnet (Nd:YAG) lasers. Each of these can shrink or destroy tumors and can be used with endoscopes. CO_2 and argon lasers can cut the skin's surface without going into deeper layers. Thus, they can be used to remove superficial cancers, such as skin cancer. In contrast, the Nd:YAG laser is more commonly applied through an endoscope to treat internal organs, such as the uterus, esophagus, and colon. Nd:YAG laser light can also travel through optical fibers into specific areas of the body during LITT. Argon lasers are often used to activate the drugs used in PDT.

What Are the Advantages of Laser Therapy?

Lasers are more precise than standard surgical tools (scalpels), so they do less damage to normal tissues. As a result, patients usually have less pain, bleeding, swelling, and scarring. With laser therapy, operations are usually shorter. In fact, laser therapy can often be done on an outpatient basis. It takes less time for patients to heal after laser surgery, and they are less likely to get infections. Patients should consult with their healthcare provider about whether laser therapy is appropriate for them.

What Are the Disadvantages of Laser Therapy?

Laser therapy also has several limitations. Surgeons must have specialized training before they can do laser therapy, and strict safety precautions must be followed. Laser therapy is expensive and requires bulky equipment. In addition, the effects of laser therapy may not last long, so doctors may have to repeat the treatment for a patient to get the full benefit.

What Is Photodynamic Therapy (PDT)?

Photodynamic therapy (PDT) is a treatment that uses a drug, called a photosensitizer or photosensitizing agent, and a particular type of light. When photosensitizers are exposed to a specific wavelength of light, they produce a form of oxygen that kills nearby cells. Each photosensitizer is activated by light of a specific wavelength. This wavelength determines how far the light can travel into the body. Thus, doctors use specific photosensitizers and wavelengths of light to treat different areas of the body with PDT.

How Is PDT Used to Treat Cancer?

In the first step of PDT for cancer treatment, a photosensitizing agent is injected into the bloodstream. The agent is absorbed by cells all over the body but stays in cancer cells longer than it does in normal cells. Approximately 24–72 hours after injection, when most of the agent has left normal cells but remains in cancer cells, the tumor is exposed to light. The photosensitizer in the tumor absorbs the light and produces an active form of oxygen that destroys nearby cancer cells.

In addition to directly killing cancer cells, PDT appears to shrink or destroy tumors in two other ways. The photosensitizer can damage blood vessels in the tumor, thereby preventing the cancer from receiving necessary nutrients. PDT also may activate the immune system to attack the tumor cells.

The light used for PDT can come from a laser or other sources. Laser light can be directed through fiber optic cables (thin fibers that transmit light) to deliver light to areas inside the body. For example, a fiber optic cable can be inserted through an endoscope (a thin, lighted tube used to look at tissues inside the body) into the lungs or esophagus to treat cancer in these organs. Other light sources include light-emitting diodes (LEDs), which may be used for surface tumors, such as skin cancer.

PDT is usually performed as an outpatient procedure. PDT may also be repeated and may be used with other therapies, such as surgery, radiation therapy, or chemotherapy.

Extracorporeal photopheresis (ECP) is a type of PDT in which a machine is used to collect the patient's blood cells, treat them outside the body with a photosensitizing agent, expose them to light, and then return them to the patient. The U.S. Food and Drug Administration (FDA) has approved ECP to help lessen the severity of skin symptoms of cutaneous T-cell lymphoma that has not responded to other therapies. Studies are underway to determine if ECP may have some application for other blood cancers, and also to help reduce rejection after transplants.

What Types of Cancer Are Currently Treated with PDT?

To date, the FDA has approved the photosensitizing agent called porfimer sodium, or Photofrin®, for use in PDT to treat or relieve the symptoms of esophageal cancer and nonsmall cell lung cancer. Porfimer sodium is approved to relieve symptoms of esophageal cancer when the cancer obstructs the esophagus or when the cancer cannot be satisfactorily treated with laser therapy alone. Porfimer sodium is used to treat nonsmall cell lung cancer in patients for whom the usual treatments are not appropriate, and to relieve symptoms in patients with nonsmall cell lung cancer that obstructs the airways. In 2003, the FDA approved porfimer sodium for the treatment of precancerous lesions in patients with Barrett esophagus, a condition that can lead to esophageal cancer.

What Are the Limitations of PDT?

The light needed to activate most photosensitizers cannot pass through more than about one-third of an inch of tissue (1 centimeter). For this reason, PDT is usually used to treat tumors on or just under the skin or on the lining of internal organs or cavities. PDT is also less effective in treating large tumors, because the light cannot pass far into these tumors. PDT is a local treatment and generally cannot be used to treat cancer that has spread (metastasized).

Does PDT Have Any Complications or Side Effects?

Porfimer sodium makes the skin and eyes sensitive to light for approximately 6 weeks after treatment. Thus, patients are advised to avoid direct sunlight and bright indoor light for at least 6 weeks. Photosensitizers tend to build up in tumors and the activating light is focused on the tumor. As a result, damage to healthy tissue is minimal. However, PDT can cause burns, swelling, pain, and scarring in nearby healthy tissue. Other side effects of PDT are related to the area that is treated. They can include coughing, trouble swallowing, stomach pain, painful breathing, or shortness of breath; these side effects are usually temporary.

Chapter 40

If You Are Considering Complementary and Alternative Medicine Treatments for Cancer

Complementary and alternative medicine (CAM) is the term for medical products and practices that are not part of standard medical care.

- **Standard medical care** is medicine that is practiced by health professionals who hold an M.D. (medical doctor) or D.O. (doctor of osteopathy) degree. It is also practiced by other health professionals, such as physical therapists, physician assistants, psychologists, and registered nurses. Standard medicine may also be called biomedicine or allopathic, Western, mainstream, orthodox, or regular medicine. Some standard medical care practitioners are also practitioners of CAM.

This chapter contains text excerpted from the following sources: Text in this chapter begins with excerpts from "Cancer Treatment—Complementary and Alternative Medicine," National Cancer Institute (NCI), April 10, 2015; Text beginning with the heading "Use of Complementary Health Approaches for Cancer" is excerpted from "Cancer: In Depth," National Center for Complementary and Integrative Health (NCCIH), July 2014. Reviewed May 2018; Text beginning with the heading "Using Trusted Resources" is excerpted from "Managing Cancer Care—Using Trusted Resources," National Cancer Institute (NCI), May 3, 2017.

- **Complementary medicine** is treatments that are used along with standard medical treatments but are not considered to be standard treatments. One example is using acupuncture to help lessen some side effects of cancer treatment.

- **Alternative medicine** is treatments that are used instead of standard medical treatments. One example is using a special diet to treat cancer instead of anticancer drugs that are prescribed by an oncologist.

- **Integrative medicine** is a total approach to medical care that combines standard medicine with the CAM practices that have been shown to be safe and effective. They treat the patient's mind, body, and spirit.

Are CAM Approaches Safe?

Some CAM therapies have undergone careful evaluation and have been found to be safe and effective. However, there are others that have been found to be ineffective or possibly harmful. Less is known about many CAM therapies, and research has been slower for a number of reasons:

- Time and funding issues

- Problems finding institutions and cancer researchers to work with on the studies

- Regulatory issues

CAM therapies need to be evaluated with the same long and careful research process used to evaluate standard treatments. Standard cancer treatments have generally been studied for safety and effectiveness through an intense scientific process that includes clinical trials with large numbers of patients.

Natural Does Not Mean Safe

CAM therapies include a wide variety of botanicals and nutritional products, such as dietary supplements, herbal supplements, and vitamins. Many of these "natural" products are considered to be safe because they are present in, or produced by, nature. However, that is not true in all cases. In addition, some may affect how well other medicines work in your body. For example, the herb St. John's wort, which some people use for depression, may cause certain anticancer drugs not to work as well as they should.

Herbal supplements may be harmful when taken by themselves, with other substances, or in large doses. For example, some studies have shown that kava-kava, an herb that has been used to help with stress and anxiety, may cause liver damage.

Vitamins can also have unwanted effects in your body. For example, some studies show that high doses of vitamins, even vitamin C, may affect how chemotherapy and radiation work. Too much of any vitamin is not safe, even in a healthy person.

Tell your doctor if you're taking any dietary supplements, no matter how safe you think they are. This is very important. Even though there may be ads or claims that something has been used for years, they do not prove that it's safe or effective.

Supplements do not have to be approved by the federal government before being sold to the public. Also, a prescription is not needed to buy them. Therefore, it's up to consumers to decide what is best for them.

National Cancer Institute (NCI) and the National Center for Complementary and Integrative Health (NCCIH) are currently sponsoring or cosponsoring various clinical trials that test CAM treatments and therapies in people. Some study the effects of complementary approaches used in addition to conventional treatments, and some compare alternative therapies with conventional treatments.

What Should Patients Do When Using or Considering CAM Therapies?

Cancer patients who are using or considering using complementary or alternative therapy should talk with their doctor or nurse. Some therapies may interfere with standard treatment or even be harmful. It is also a good idea to learn whether the therapy has been proven to do what it claims to do.

To find a CAM practitioner, ask your doctor or nurse to suggest someone. Or ask if someone at your cancer center, such as a social worker or physical therapist can help you. Choosing a CAM practitioner should be done with as much care as choosing a primary care provider. Patients, their families, and their healthcare providers can learn about new CAM therapies and practitioners from government agencies.

Use of Complementary Health Approaches for Cancer

Many people who've been diagnosed with cancer use complementary health approaches.

- According to the National Health Interview Survey (NHIS), which included a comprehensive survey on the use of complementary health approaches by Americans, 65 percent of respondents who had ever been diagnosed with cancer had used complementary approaches, as compared to 53 percent of other respondents. Those who had been diagnosed with cancer were more likely than others to have used complementary approaches for general wellness, immune enhancement, and pain management.

- Other surveys have also found that use of complementary health approaches is common among people who've been diagnosed with cancer, although estimates of use vary widely. Some data indicate that the likelihood of using complementary approaches varies with the type of cancer and with factors such as sex, age, and ethnicity. The results of surveys from 18 countries show that use of complementary approaches by people who had been diagnosed with cancer was more common in North America than in Australia/New Zealand or Europe and that use had increased since the 1970s and especially since 2000.

- Surveys have also shown that many people with cancer don't tell their healthcare providers about their use of complementary health approaches. In the NHIS, survey respondents who had been diagnosed with cancer told their healthcare providers about 15 percent of their herb use and 23 percent of their total use of complementary approaches. In other studies, between 32 and 69 percent of cancer patients and survivors who used dietary supplements or other complementary approaches reported that they discussed these approaches with their physicians. The differences in the reported percentages may reflect differences in the definitions of complementary approaches used in the studies, as well as differences in the communication practices of different groups of patients.

What the Science Says about the Safety and Side Effects of Complementary Health Approaches for Cancer

Delaying conventional cancer treatment can decrease the chances of remission or cure. Don't use unproven products or practices to postpone or replace conventional medical treatment for cancer.

Some complementary health approaches may interfere with cancer treatments or be unsafe for cancer patients. For example, the herb St. John's wort, which is sometimes used for depression, can make some cancer drugs less effective.

Other complementary approaches may be harmful if used inappropriately. For example, to make massage therapy safe for people with cancer, it may be necessary to avoid massaging places on the body that are directly affected by the disease or its treatment (for example, areas where the skin is sensitive following radiation therapy).

People who've been diagnosed with cancer should consult the healthcare providers who are treating them for cancer before using any complementary health approach for any purpose—whether or not it's cancer-related.

What the Science Says about the Effectiveness of Complementary Health Approaches for Cancer

No complementary health product or practice has been proven to cure cancer. Some complementary approaches may help people manage cancer symptoms or treatment side effects and improve their quality of life.

Incorporating Complementary Health Approaches Into Cancer Care

In 2009, the Society for Integrative Oncology (SIO) issued evidence-based clinical practice guidelines for healthcare providers to consider when incorporating complementary health approaches in the care of cancer patients. The guidelines point out that, when used in addition to conventional therapies, some of these approaches help to control symptoms and enhance patients' well-being. The guidelines warn, however, that unproven methods shouldn't be used in place of conventional treatment because delayed treatment of cancer reduces the likelihood of a remission or cure.

A comprehensive summary of research on complementary health approaches for cancer is beyond the scope of this chapter. The following sections provide an overview of the research status of some commonly used complementary approaches, highlighting results from a few reviews and studies focusing on preventing and treating the disease, as well as managing cancer symptoms and treatment side effects.

491

Complementary Health Approaches for Cancer Symptoms and Treatment Side Effects

Some complementary health approaches, such as acupuncture, massage therapy, mindfulness-based stress reduction, and yoga, may help people manage cancer symptoms or the side effects of treatment. However, some approaches may interfere with conventional cancer treatment or have other risks. People who have been diagnosed with cancer should consult their healthcare providers before using any complementary health approach.

- There is substantial evidence that acupuncture can help to manage treatment-related nausea and vomiting in cancer patients. There isn't enough evidence to judge whether acupuncture relieves cancer pain or other symptoms such as treatment-related hot flashes. Complications from acupuncture are rare, as long as the acupuncturist uses sterile needles and proper procedures. Chemotherapy and radiation therapy weaken the body's immune system, so it's especially important for acupuncturists to follow strict clean-needle procedures when treating cancer patients.

- Recent studies suggest that the herb ginger may help to control nausea related to cancer chemotherapy when used in addition to conventional anti-nausea medication.

- Studies suggest that massage therapy may help to relieve symptoms experienced by people with cancer, such as pain, nausea, anxiety, and depression. However, investigators haven't reached any conclusions about the effects of massage therapy because of the limited amount of rigorous research in this field. People with cancer should consult their healthcare providers before having massage therapy to find out if any special precautions are needed. The massage therapist shouldn't use deep or intense pressure without the healthcare providers' approval and may need to avoid certain sites, such as areas directly over a tumor or those where the skin is sensitive following radiation therapy.

- There is evidence that mindfulness-based stress reduction, a type of meditation training, can help cancer patients relieve anxiety, stress, fatigue, and general mood and sleep disturbances, thus improving their quality of life. Most participants in mindfulness studies have been patients with early-stage cancer, primarily breast cancer, so the evidence favoring mindfulness training is strongest for this group of patients.

- Preliminary evidence indicates that yoga may help to improve anxiety, depression, distress, and stress in people with cancer. It also may help to lessen fatigue in breast cancer patients and survivors. However, only a small number of yoga studies in cancer patients have been completed, and some of the research hasn't been of the highest quality. Because yoga involves physical activities, it's important for people with cancer to talk with their healthcare providers in advance to find out whether any aspects of yoga might be unsafe for them.

- Various studies suggest possible benefits of hypnosis, relaxation therapies, and biofeedback to help patients manage cancer symptoms and treatment side effects.

- A review of the research literature on herbal supplements and cancer concluded that although several herbs have shown promise for managing side effects and symptoms such as nausea and vomiting, pain, fatigue, and insomnia, the scientific evidence is limited, and many clinical trials haven't been well designed. Use of herbs for managing symptoms also raises concerns about potential negative interactions with conventional cancer treatments.

Complementary Health Approaches for Cancer Treatment

No complementary approach has cured cancer or caused it to go into remission. Some products or practices that have been advocated for cancer treatment may interfere with conventional cancer treatments or have other risks. People who've been diagnosed with cancer should consult their healthcare providers before using any complementary health approach.

- Studies on whether herbal supplements or substances derived from them might be of value in cancer treatment are in their early stages, and scientific evidence is limited. Herbal supplements may have side effects, and some may interact in harmful ways with drugs, including drugs used in cancer treatment.

- The effects of taking vitamin and mineral supplements, including antioxidant supplements, during cancer treatment are uncertain. NCI advises cancer patients to talk to their healthcare providers before taking any supplements.

- An NCCIH-supported trial of a standardized shark cartilage extract, taken in addition to chemotherapy and radiation therapy, showed no benefit in patients with advanced lung cancer. An earlier, smaller study in patients with advanced breast or colorectal cancers also showed no benefit from the addition of shark cartilage to conventional treatment.

- A systematic review of research on laetrile found no evidence that it's effective as a cancer treatment. Laetrile can be toxic, especially if taken orally, because it contains cyanide.

Using Trusted Resources

Health information, whether in print or online, should come from a trusted, credible source. Government agencies, hospitals, universities, and medical journals and books that provide evidence-based information are sources you can trust. Too often, other sources can provide misleading or incorrect information. If a source makes claims that are too good to be true, remember—they usually are.

There are many websites, books, and magazines that provide health information to the public, but not all of them are trustworthy. Use the resources provided below to safeguard yourself when reviewing sources of health information.

Websites

Online sources of health information should make it easy for people to learn who is responsible for posting the information. They should make clear the original source of the information, along with the medical credentials of the people who prepare or review the posted material.

Use the following questions to determine the credibility of health information published online.

- **Who manages this information?**

  The person or group that has published health information online should be easy to find somewhere on the page.

- **What are the letters at the end of the web address?**

  Government websites end in ".gov" and those ending with ".edu" are run by a university or other educational institution. These are sources that you can usually trust. If you see ".org" or ".com" at the end of a web address, it may also be a trusted site. However, check it closely to make sure.

- **Who is paying for the project, and what is their purpose?**

  You should be able to find this information in the "About Us" section.

- **What is the original source of the information that they have posted?**

  If the information was originally published in a research journal or a book, they should say which one(s) so that you can find it.

- **How is information reviewed before it gets posted?**

  Most health information publications have someone with medical or research credentials (e.g., someone who has earned an M.D., D.O., or Ph.D.) review the information before it gets posted, to make sure it is correct.

- **How current is the information?**

  Online health information sources should show you when the information was posted or last reviewed.

- **If they are asking for personal information, how will they use that information and how will they protect your privacy?**

  This is very important. Do not share personal information until you understand the policies under which it will be used and you are comfortable with any risk involved in sharing your information online.

Social Media

Social media sites (such as Facebook, Twitter) are good ways to stay connected. However, when you're seeking medical information, only follow social media from reputable sources. Many trusted organizations have social media accounts that link to their websites. For example, the National Cancer Institute has an official Facebook page and many Twitter accounts from its offices and departments.

When it comes to personal social media accounts, it's common for users to post their experiences with illness. This may include:

- How they're feeling physically
- Treatments they're going through
- Complementary therapies they're using, such as a type of diet or supplements
- What feelings they're having

But remember that everyone is different. Even someone with the exact same kind of cancer has a different body and health history from you. And never take recommendations for treatment or medicines from someone other than your doctor. You don't know where or how the user got their information. You also don't know if the information is current, or what the user's knowledge of cancer is.

Books

A number of books have been written about cancer, cancer treatment, and complementary and alternative medicine (CAM). Some books contain trustworthy content, while others do not.

It's important to know that information is always changing and that new research results are reported every day. Be aware that if a book is written by only one person, you may only be getting that one person's view.

If you go to the library, ask the staff for suggestions. Or if you live near a college or university, there may be a medical library available. Local bookstores may also have people on staff who can help you. If you find a book online, look very carefully at the author's credentials, background, and expertise. Questions you may want to ask yourself are:

- Is the author an expert on this subject?
- Do you know anyone else who has read the book?
- Has the book been reviewed by other experts?
- Was it published in the past 5 years?
- Does the book offer different points of view, or does it seem to hold one opinion?
- Has the author researched the topic in full?
- Are the references listed in the back?

Magazines

If you want to look for articles you can trust, search online medical journal databases or ask your librarian to help you look for medical journals, books, and other research that has been done by experts.

Articles in popular magazines are usually not written by experts. Rather, the authors speak with experts, gather information, and then write the article. If claims are made in a magazine, remember:

- The authors may not have expert knowledge in this area.

- They may not say where they found their information.

- The articles have not been reviewed by experts.

The publisher may have ties to advertisers or other organizations. Therefore, the article may be one-sided in the information or view(s) it presents.

When you read these articles, you can use the same process that the magazine writer uses:

- Speak with experts

- Ask lots of questions

- Then decide if the therapy is right for you

Where to Get More Help

Cancer Treatment Scams

A webpage (www.consumer.ftc.gov/articles/0104-cancer-treatment-scams) from the Federal Trade Commission (FTC) that advises people to ask their healthcare provider about products that claim to cure or treat cancer and offers tips for spotting treatment scams.

Protecting Yourself

A webpage (www.fda.gov/ForConsumers/ProtectYourself/default. htm) from the U.S. Food and Drug Administration (FDA) that includes links to several resources that have tips about buying medicines and other products online.

Evaluating Cancer Information on the Internet

Developed by the American Society of Clinical Oncology (ASCO), Cancer.Net (www.cancer.net/research-and-advocacy/

497

introduction-cancer-research/evaluating-cancer-information-internet) provides information, including common misconceptions about cancer and tips to evaluate the credibility of online cancer information.

Chapter 41

Cancer Clinical Trials

Clinical trials are research studies that involve people. Through clinical trials, doctors find new ways to improve treatments and the quality of life for people with disease.

Researchers design cancer clinical trials to test new ways to:

- Treat cancer

- Find and diagnose cancer

- Prevent cancer

- Manage symptoms of cancer and side effects from its treatment

Clinical trials are the final step in a long process that begins with research in a lab. Before any new treatment is used with people in clinical trials, researchers work for many years to understand its effects on cancer cells in the lab and in animals. They also try to figure out the side effects it may cause.

Any time you or a loved one needs treatment for cancer, clinical trials are an option to think about. Trials are available for all stages of cancer. It is a myth that they are only for people who have advanced cancer that is not responding to treatment.

This chapter contains text excerpted from the following sources: Text in this chapter begins with excerpts from "What Are Cancer Clinical Trials?" National Cancer Institute (NCI), June 27, 2016; Text beginning with the heading "Steps to Find a Clinical Trial" is excerpted from "Steps to Find a Clinical Trial," National Cancer Institute (NCI), June 23, 2016.

Every trial has a person in charge, usually a doctor, who is called the principal investigator. The principal investigator prepares a plan for the trial, called a protocol. The protocol explains what will be done during the trial. It also contains information that helps the doctor decide if this treatment is right for you. The protocol includes information about:

- The reason for doing the trial

- Who can join the trial (called "eligibility criteria")

- How many people are needed for the trial

- Any drugs or other treatments that will be given, how they will be given, the dose, and how often

- What medical tests will be done and how often

- What types of information will be collected about the people taking part

Why Are Clinical Trials Important?

People are living longer lives from successful cancer treatments that are the results of past clinical trials. Through clinical trials, doctors determine whether new treatments are safe and effective and work better than current treatments. Clinical trials also help National Cancer Institute (NCI) find new ways to prevent and detect cancer. And they help NCI improve the quality of life for people during and after treatment. When you take part in a clinical trial, you add to NCI's knowledge about cancer and help improve cancer care for future patients. Clinical trials are the key to making progress against cancer.

Where Trials Take Place

Cancer clinical trials take place in cities and towns across the United States and throughout the world. They take place in doctors' offices, cancer centers, medical centers, community hospitals and clinics, and veterans' and military hospitals. A single trial may take place in one or two places, or at hundreds of different sites.

You can search for clinical trials by using the Cancer.gov clinical trials search form. This form helps you find National Cancer Institute (NCI)-supported clinical trials that are taking place across the United States, Canada, and internationally. The list includes:

- All NCI network trials, including trials supported through the:
  - National Clinical Trials Network (NCTN)
  - NCI Community Oncology Research Program (NCORP)
  - Experimental Therapeutics Clinical Trials Network (ETCTN)
- Trials that are funded in full or in part by NCI, including trials taking place at NCI-designated cancer centers
- Trials at the National Institutes of Health (NIH) Clinical Center (CC) in Bethesda, Maryland

When you talk with your doctor about treatment options, ask about clinical trials. There may be one that is right for you taking place at your doctor's office or nearby cancer center.

Types of Clinical Trials

There are several types of cancer clinical trials, including treatment trials, prevention trials, screening trials, and supportive and palliative care trials. Each type of trial is designed to answer different research questions and will help researchers learn things that will help people in the future.

Treatment Trials

Most cancer clinical trials are treatment studies that involve people who have cancer. These trials test new treatments or new ways of using existing treatments, such as new:

- Drugs
- Vaccines
- Approaches to surgery or radiation therapy
- Combinations of treatments, including some that work to boost your immune system to help fight the cancer

Many newer treatment trials require people to have their tumors tested for genetic changes first to see if treatments targeting specific changes might work better for them than standard treatments.

Treatment trials are designed to answers questions such as:

- What is a safe dose of the new treatment?

501

- How should the new treatment be given?

- Does the new treatment help people with cancer live longer?

- Can the new treatment shrink tumors or prevent them from growing and spreading to new places in the body?

- What are the new treatment's side effects?

- Does the new treatment allow a better quality of life with fewer side effects?

- Does the new treatment help prevent the cancer from coming back once treatment is finished?

Prevention Trials

Cancer prevention trials are studies involving healthy people. In most prevention trials, the participants either do not have cancer but are at high risk for developing the disease or have had cancer and are at high risk for developing a new cancer. These studies look at cancer risk and ways to reduce that risk.

There are two kinds of prevention trials, action studies and agent studies.

- **Action studies** ("doing something")

  Focus on finding out whether actions people take—such as exercising more or eating more fruits and vegetables—can prevent cancer

- **Agent studies** ("taking something")

  Focus on finding out whether taking certain medicines, vitamins, minerals, or dietary supplements (or a combination of them) may lower the risk of a certain type of cancer. Agent studies are also called chemoprevention studies

Researchers who conduct these studies want to know:

- How safe it is for a person to take this agent or do this activity?

- Does the new approach prevent cancer?

Screening Trials

The goal of cancer screening trials is to test new ways to find disease early, when it may be more easily treated. An effective screening test will reduce the number of deaths from the cancer being screened.

Researchers who conduct cancer screening studies want to know:

- Does finding disease earlier, before people have any symptoms, save lives?

- Is one screening test better than another?

- Do a large number of people who receive the screening test undergo unnecessary follow-up tests and procedures?

Quality-of-Life / Supportive Care / Palliative Care Trials

These trials look at ways to improve the quality of life of cancer patients, especially those who have side effects from cancer and its treatment. They find new ways to help people cope with pain, nutrition problems, infection, nausea and vomiting, sleep disorders, depression, and other health problems.

Trials might test drugs, such as those that help with depression or nausea. Or, they might test activities, such as attending support groups, exercising, or talking with a counselor. Some trials test ways to help families and caregivers cope with their own needs, as well as those of the person with cancer.

Researchers who conduct these studies want to know:

- How does cancer and its treatment affect patients and their loved ones?

- What can improve the comfort and quality of life of people who have cancer?

Phases of Clinical Trials

Clinical trials to test new cancer treatments involve a series of steps, called phases. If a new treatment is successful in one phase, it will proceed to further testing in the next phase. During the early phases (phases 1 and 2), researchers figure out whether a new treatment is safe, what its side effects are, and the best dose of the new treatment. They also make sure that the treatment has some benefit, such as slowing tumor growth. In the later phase (phase 3), researchers study whether the treatment works better than the current standard therapy. They also compare the safety of the new treatment with that of current treatments. Phase 3 trials include large numbers of people to make sure that the result is valid.

There are also very early (phase 0) and later (phase 4) phase clinical trials. These trials are less common. Phase 0 trials are very small trials that help researchers decide if a new agent should be tested in a phase 1 trial. Phase 4 trials look at long-term safety and effectiveness. They take place after a new treatment has been approved and is on the market.

The following shows the number of patients that take part and the purpose of the most common phases. Although the trial phases are explained in the context of drug treatment trials, the same concepts apply to most types of clinical trials.

Phase One

Purpose

- To find a safe dose

- To decide how the new treatment should be given (by mouth, in a vein, etc.)

- To see how the new treatment affects the human body and fights cancer

Number of people taking part: 15–30

Phase Two

Purpose

- To determine if the new treatment has an effect on a certain cancer

- To see how the new treatment affects the body and fights cancer

Number of people taking part: Less than 100

Phase Three

Purpose

- To compare the new treatment (or new use of a treatment) with the current standard treatment

Number of people taking part: From 100 to several thousand

Some researchers design trials that combine two phases (phase 1/2 or phase 2/3 trials) in a single protocol. In this combined design, there is a seamless transition between trial phases, which may allow research questions to be answered more quickly or with fewer patients.

Finding a Clinical Trial

If you are thinking about joining a clinical trial as a treatment option, the best place to start is to talk with your doctor or another member of your healthcare team. Often, your doctor may know about a clinical trial that could be a good option for you. He or she may also be able to search for a trial for you, provide information, and answer questions to help you decide about joining a clinical trial.

Some doctors may not be aware of or recommend clinical trials that could be appropriate for you. If so, you may want to get a second opinion about your treatment options, including taking part in a clinical trial.

If you decide to look for trials on your own, the following steps can guide you in your search. This information should not be used in place of advice from your doctor or other members of your healthcare team. The following are the steps involved in finding a clinical trial.

Step One: Gather Details about Your Cancer

If you decide to look for a clinical trial, you must know certain details about your cancer diagnosis. You will need to compare these details with the eligibility criteria of any trial that interests you. Eligibility criteria are the guidelines for who can and cannot take part in a certain clinical trial. To help you gather details about your cancer, complete as much of the cancer details checklist as possible. Refer to the form during your search for a clinical trial. If you need help filling out the form, talk with your doctor, a nurse, or social worker at your doctor's office. The more information you can gather, the easier it will be to find a clinical trial to fit your situation.

Step Two: Find Clinical Trials

There are many lists of cancer clinical trials taking place in the United States. Some trials are funded by nonprofit organizations, including the U.S. government. Others are funded by for-profit groups, such as drug companies. Hospitals and academic medical centers also sponsor trials conducted by their own researchers. Because of the many types of sponsors, no single list contains every clinical trial.

Whichever website you use to search for clinical trials, be sure to bookmark or print a copy of the protocol summary for every trial that interests you.

A protocol summary should explain the goal of the trial and describe which treatments will be tested. It should also list the locations where the trial is taking place.

Keep in mind that protocol summaries are written for healthcare providers and use medical language to describe the trial that may be difficult to understand. For help understanding the protocol summary, call, email, or chat with a trained information specialist at the NCI Contact Center.

NCI-Supported Clinical Trials

NCI's website helps you find NCI-supported clinical trials that are taking place across the United States, Canada, and internationally. The list includes:

- All NCI network trials, including trials supported through the:
  - National Clinical Trials Network (NCTN)
  - NCI Community Oncology Research Program (NCORP)
  - Experimental Therapeutics Clinical Trials Network (ETCTN)
- Trials that are funded in full or in part by NCI, including trials taking place at NCI-Designated Cancer Centers
- Trials at the NIH Clinical Center in Bethesda, Maryland

If you need help with your search, you can call, email, or chat with a trained information specialist at the NCI Contact Center. They will need to know details about your cancer, so have your Cancer Details Checklist ready.

Other Lists of Trials

In addition to NCI's list of cancer clinical trials, you may want to check a few other trial lists. Other places to look for lists of cancer clinical trials include:

ClinicalTrials.gov

ClinicalTrials.gov, which is part of the U.S. National Library of Medicine (NLM), lists clinical trials for cancer and many other diseases and conditions. It contains trials that are in NCI's list of cancer trials as well as trials sponsored by pharmaceutical or biotech companies that may not be on NCI's list.

Cancer Centers and Clinics That Conduct Cancer Clinical Trials

Many cancer centers across the United States, including NCI-Designated Cancer Centers, sponsor or take part in cancer clinical trials.

The websites of these centers usually have a list of the clinical trials taking place at their institutions. Some of the trials included in these lists may not be on NCI's list.

Keep in mind that the amount of information about clinical trials on these websites can vary. You may have to contact a cancer center clinical trials office to get more information about the trials that interest you.

Drug and Biotechnology Companies

Many companies provide lists of the clinical trials that they sponsor on their websites. Sometimes, a company's website may refer you to the website of another organization that helps the company find patients for its trials. The other organization may be paid fees for this service.

The website of the Pharmaceutical Research and Manufacturers of America (PhRMA) includes a list of its member companies, many of which sponsor cancer clinical trials. PhRMA is a trade organization that represents drug and biotechnology companies in the United States.

Clinical Trial Listing Services

Some organizations provide lists of clinical trials as a part of their business. These organizations generally do not sponsor or take part in clinical trials. Some of them may receive fees from drug or biotechnology companies for listing their trials or helping find patients for their trials.

Keep the following points in mind about clinical trial listing services:

- The lists of trials provided by these organizations often draw from the trial lists that are available from the U.S. government (NCI and ClinicalTrials.gov).

- The websites of these organizations may not be updated regularly.

- The websites of these organizations may require you to register to search for clinical trials or to obtain trial contact information for trials that interest you.

Cancer Advocacy Groups

Cancer advocacy groups provide education, support, financial assistance, and advocacy to help patients and families who are dealing with cancer, its treatment, and survivorship. These organizations recognize that clinical trials are important to improving cancer care. They work to educate and empower people to find information and obtain access to appropriate treatment.

Advocacy groups work hard to know about the latest advances in cancer research. Some will have information about clinical trials that are enrolling patients.

To find trials, search the websites of advocacy groups for specific types of cancer. Many of these websites have lists of clinical trials or refer you to the websites of organizations that match patients to trials. Or, you can contact an advocacy group directly for help finding clinical trials.

Step Three: Take a Closer Look at the Trials That Interest You

Once you have completed the Cancer Details Checklist and found some trials that interest you, you should now:

- Take a closer look at the protocol summary for each trial

- Use the questions below to narrow your list to include only those trials for which you would like to get more information

Helpful Tip: Don't worry if you can't answer all of the questions below just yet. The idea is to narrow your list of potential trials, if possible. However, don't give up on trials you're not sure about. You may want to talk with your doctor or another healthcare team member during this process, especially if you find the protocol summaries hard to understand.

Questions to Ask about Each Trial

The below are some of the key questions to ask about each trial.

Trial Objective

What is the main purpose of the trial? Is it to cure your cancer? To slow its growth or spread? To lessen the severity of cancer symptoms or the side effects of treatment? To determine whether a new treatment is safe and well-tolerated? Read this information carefully to learn whether the trial's main objective matches your goals for treatment.

Eligibility Criteria

Do the details of your cancer diagnosis and your current overall state of health match the trial's eligibility criteria? Some treatment trials will not accept people who have already been treated for their cancer. Other treatment trials are looking for people who have already been treated for their cancer.

Helpful Hint: If you have just found out that you have cancer, the time to think about joining a trial is before you have any treatment. Talk with your doctor about how quickly you need to make a treatment decision.

Trial Location

Is the location of the trial manageable for you? Some trials take place at more than one location. Look carefully at how often you will need to receive treatment during the course of the trial. Decide how far and how often you are willing to travel. You will also need to ask whether the sponsoring organization will pay for some or all of your travel costs.

Study Length

How long will the trial run? Not all protocol summaries provide this information. If they do, consider the time involved and whether it will work for you and your family.

After thinking about these questions, if you are still interested in a clinical trial, then you are ready to contact the team running the trial.

Step Four: Contact the Team Running the Trial

There are a few ways to reach the clinical trial team.

- **Contact the trial team directly.** The protocol summary should include the phone number of a person or an office that you can contact for more information. You do not need to talk to the lead researcher (called the "protocol chair" or "principal investigator") at this time, even if his or her name is given along with the telephone number. Instead, call the number and ask to speak with the "trial coordinator." This person can answer questions from patients and their doctors. It is also the trial coordinator's job to decide whether you are likely to be eligible to join the trial. However, a final decision will probably not be made until you have met with a doctor who is part of the trial team.

- **Ask your doctor or another healthcare team member to contact the trial team for you.** The clinical trial coordinator will ask questions about your cancer diagnosis and your current general health that you may not be sure how to answer. So, you may want to ask your doctor or someone else on your healthcare team to contact the trial coordinator for you.

- **The trial team may contact you.** If you have registered to use the website of a clinical trial listing service and found a trial that interests you, the clinical trial team may contact you directly by using the phone number and email address you provide when you register.

Step Five: Ask Questions

Whether you or someone from your healthcare team speaks with the clinical trial team, this is the time to get answers to questions that will help you decide whether or not to take part in this particular clinical trial. Questions to Ask Your Doctor about Treatment Clinical Trials can help you think about questions you want to ask.

Talk with Your Doctor

To make a final decision, you will want to know the potential risks and benefits of all treatment options available to you. If you have any remaining questions or concerns, you should discuss them with your doctor. Ask your doctor some of the same questions that you asked the trial coordinator. You should also ask your doctor about the risks and benefits of standard treatment for your cancer. Then, you and your doctor can compare the risks and benefits of standard treatment with those of treatment in a clinical trial. You may decide that joining a trial is your best option, or you may decide not to join a trial. It's your choice.

Step Six: Make an Appointment

If you decide to join a clinical trial for which you are eligible, schedule a visit with the team running the trial.

Part Six

Coping with the Side Effects of Cancer and Cancer Treatments

Chapter 42

Side Effects of Cancer Treatment

Cancer treatments can cause side effects—problems that occur when treatment affects healthy tissues or organs. Ask your healthcare team what side effects you are likely to have. Learn about steps you can take, and supportive care you will receive, to feel better. Information about ways to prevent or manage specific cancer-related side effects is included in the list below:

Anemia

Anemia is a condition that can make you feel very tired, short of breath, and lightheaded. Other signs of anemia may include feeling dizzy or faint, headaches, a fast heartbeat, and/or pale skin.

Cancer treatments, such as chemotherapy and radiation therapy, as well as cancers that affect the bone marrow, can cause anemia. When you are anemic, your body does not have enough red blood cells (RBCs). Red blood cells are the cells that that carry oxygen from the lungs throughout your body to help it work properly. You will have blood tests to check for anemia. Treatment for anemia is also based on your symptoms and on what is causing the anemia.

This chapter includes text excerpted from "Side Effects of Cancer Treatment," National Cancer Institute (NCI), September 22, 2017.

Appetite Loss

Cancer treatments may lower your appetite or change the way food tastes or smells. Side effects such as mouth and throat problems, or nausea and vomiting can also make eating difficult. Cancer-related fatigue can also lower your appetite. Don't wait until you feel weak, have lost too much weight, or are dehydrated, to talk with your doctor or nurse. It's important to eat well, especially during treatment for cancer.

Bleeding and Bruising (Thrombocytopenia)

Some cancer treatments, such as chemotherapy and targeted therapy, can increase your risk of bleeding and bruising. These treatments can lower the number of platelets in the blood. Platelets are the cells that help your blood to clot and stop bleeding. When your platelet count is low, you may bruise or bleed a lot or very easily and have tiny purple or red spots on your skin. This condition is called thrombocytopenia. It is important to tell your doctor or nurse if you notice any of these changes.

Call your doctor or nurse if you have more serious problems, such as:

- Bleeding that doesn't stop after a few minutes; bleeding from your mouth, nose, or when you vomit; bleeding from your vagina when you are not having your period (menstruation); urine that is red or pink; stools that are black or bloody; or bleeding during your period that is heavier or lasts longer than normal.

- Head or vision changes such as bad headaches or changes in how well you see, or if you feel confused or very sleepy.

Constipation

Constipation is when you have infrequent bowel movements and stool that may be hard, dry, and difficult to pass. You may also have stomach cramps, bloating, and nausea when you are constipated.

Cancer treatments such as chemotherapy can cause constipation. Certain medicines (such as pain medicines), changes in diet, not drinking enough fluids, and being less active may also cause constipation.

Delirium

Delirium is a confused mental state that includes changes in awareness, thinking, judgment, sleeping patterns, as well as behavior.

Although delirium can happen at the end of life, many episodes of delirium are caused by medicine or dehydration and are reversible.

The symptoms of delirium usually occur suddenly (within hours or days) over a short period of time and may come and go. Although delirium may be mistaken for depression or dementia, these conditions are different and have different treatments.

Diarrhea

Diarrhea means having bowel movements that are soft, loose, or watery more often than normal. If diarrhea is severe or lasts a long time, the body does not absorb enough water and nutrients. This can cause you to become dehydrated or malnourished. Cancer treatments, or the cancer itself, may cause diarrhea or make it worse. Some medicines, infections, and stress can also cause diarrhea. Tell your healthcare team if you have diarrhea.

Diarrhea that leads to dehydration (the loss of too much fluid from the body) and low levels of salt and potassium (important minerals needed by the body) can be life-threatening. Call your healthcare team if you feel dizzy or lightheaded, have dark yellow urine or are not urinating, or have a fever of 100.5°F (38°C) or higher.

Edema (Swelling)

Edema, a condition in which fluid builds up in your body's tissues, may be caused by some types of chemotherapy, certain cancers, and conditions not related to cancer.

Signs of edema may include:

- Swelling in your feet, ankles, and legs

- Swelling in your hands and arms

- Swelling in your face or abdomen

- Skin that is puffy, shiny, or looks slightly dented after being pressed

- Shortness of breath, a cough, or irregular heartbeat

Some problems related to edema are serious. Call your doctor or nurse if you feel short of breath, have a heartbeat that seems different or is not regular, have sudden swelling or swelling that is getting worse or is moving up your arms or legs, you gain weight quickly, or you don't urinate at all or urinate only a little.

Fatigue

Fatigue is a common side effect of many cancer treatments, including chemotherapy, immunotherapy, radiation therapy, bone marrow transplant, and surgery. Conditions such as anemia, as well as pain, medications, and emotions, can also cause or worsen fatigue.

People often describe cancer-related fatigue as feeling extremely tired, weak, heavy, run down, and having no energy. Resting does not always help with cancer-related fatigue. Cancer-related fatigue is one of the most difficult side effects for many people to cope with.

Tell your healthcare team if you feel extremely tired and are not able to do your normal activities or are very tired even after resting or sleeping. There are many causes of fatigue. Keeping track of your levels of energy throughout the day will help your doctor to assess your fatigue. Write down how fatigue affects your daily activities and what makes the fatigue better or worse.

Fertility Issues in Girls and Women

Many cancer treatments can affect a girl's or woman's fertility. Most likely, your doctor will talk with you about whether or not cancer treatment may increase the risk of, or cause, infertility. However, not all doctors bring up this topic. Sometimes you, a family member, or parents of a child being treated for cancer may need to initiate this conversation.

Whether or not fertility is affected depends on factors such as:

- Your baseline fertility
- Your age at the time of treatment
- The type of cancer and treatment(s)
- The amount (dose) of treatment
- The length (duration) of treatment
- The amount of time that has passed since cancer treatment
- Other personal health factors

Hair Loss (Alopecia)

Some types of chemotherapy cause the hair on your head and other parts of your body to fall out. Radiation therapy can also cause hair loss on the part of the body that is being treated. Hair loss is called alopecia. Talk with your healthcare team to learn if the cancer treatment you will be receiving causes hair loss.

Infection and Neutropenia

An infection is the invasion and growth of germs in the body, such as bacteria, viruses, yeast, or other fungi. An infection can begin anywhere in the body, may spread throughout the body, and can cause one or more of these signs:

- Fever of 100.5°F (38°C) or higher or chills

- Cough or sore throat

- Diarrhea

- Ear pain, headache or sinus pain, or a stiff or sore neck

- Skin rash

- Sores or white coating in your mouth or on your tongue

- Swelling or redness, especially where a catheter enters your body

- Urine that is bloody or cloudy, or pain when you urinate

Infections during cancer treatment can be life-threatening and require urgent medical attention. Be sure to talk with your doctor or nurse before taking medicine—even aspirin, acetaminophen (such as Tylenol®), or ibuprofen (such as Advil®) for a fever. These medicines can lower a fever but may also mask or hide signs of a more serious problem.

Memory or Concentration Problems

Whether you have memory or concentration problems (sometimes described as a mental fog or chemo brain) depends on the type of treatment you receive, your age, and other health-related factors. Cancer treatments such as chemotherapy may cause difficulty with thinking, concentrating, or remembering things. So can some types of radiation therapy to the brain and immunotherapy.

These cognitive problems may start during or after cancer treatment. Some people notice very small changes, such as a bit more difficulty remembering things, whereas others have much greater memory or concentration problems.

Your doctor will assess your symptoms and advise you about ways to manage or treat these problems. Treating conditions such as poor nutrition, anxiety, depression, fatigue, and insomnia may also help.

Mouth and Throat Problems

Cancer treatments may cause dental, mouth, and throat problems. Radiation therapy to the head and neck may harm the salivary glands and tissues in your mouth and/or make it hard to chew and swallow safely. Some types of chemotherapy and immunotherapy can also harm cells in your mouth, throat, and lips. Drugs used to treat cancer and certain bone problems may also cause oral complications.

Mouth and throat problems may include:

- Changes in taste (dysgeusia) or smell

- Dry mouth (xerostomia)

- Infections and mouth sores

- Pain or swelling in your mouth (oral mucositis)

- Sensitivity to hot or cold foods

- Swallowing problems (dysphagia)

- Tooth decay (cavities)

Mouth problems are more serious if they interfere with eating and drinking because they can lead to dehydration and/or malnutrition. It's important to call your doctor or nurse if you have pain in your mouth, lips, or throat that makes it difficult to eat, drink, or sleep or if you have a fever of 100.5°F (38°C) or higher.

Nausea and Vomiting

Nausea is when you feel sick to your stomach, as if you are going to throw up. Vomiting is when you throw up. There are different types of nausea and vomiting caused by cancer treatment, including anticipatory, acute, and delayed nausea and vomiting. Controlling nausea and vomiting will help you to feel better and prevent more serious problems such as malnutrition and dehydration.

Your doctor or nurse will determine what is causing your symptoms and advise you on ways to prevent them. Medicines called antinausea drugs or antiemetics are effective in preventing or reducing many types of nausea and vomiting. The medicine is taken at specific times to prevent and/or control symptoms of nausea and vomiting. There are also practical steps you may be advised to take to feel better.

Nerve Problems (Peripheral Neuropathy)

Some cancer treatments cause peripheral neuropathy, a result of damage to the peripheral nerves. These nerves carry information from the brain to other parts of the body. Side effects depend on which peripheral nerves (sensory, motor, or autonomic) are affected.

Damage to sensory nerves (nerves that help you feel pain, heat, cold, and pressure) can cause:

- Tingling, numbness, or a pins-and-needles feeling in your feet and hands that may spread to your legs and arms

- Inability to feel a hot or cold sensation, such as a hot stove

- Inability to feel pain, such as from a cut or sore on your foot

Damage to motor nerves (nerves that help your muscles to move) can cause:

- Weak or achy muscles. You may lose your balance or trip easily. It may also be difficult to button shirts or open jars.

- Muscles that twitch and cramp or muscle wasting (if you don't use your muscles regularly)

- Swallowing or breathing difficulties (if your chest or throat muscles are affected)

Damage to autonomic nerves (nerves that control functions such as blood pressure, digestion, heart rate, temperature, and urination) can cause:

- Digestive changes such as constipation or diarrhea

- Dizzy or faint feeling, due to low blood pressure

- Sexual problems; men may be unable to get an erection and women may not reach orgasm

- Sweating problems (either too much or too little sweating)

- Urination problems, such as leaking urine or difficulty emptying your bladder

If you start to notice any of the problems listed above, talk with your doctor or nurse. Getting these problems diagnosed and treated early is the best way to control them, prevent further damage, and to reduce pain and other complications.

Pain

Cancer itself and the side effects of cancer treatment can sometimes cause pain. Pain is not something that you have to "put up with." Controlling pain is an important part of your cancer treatment plan. Pain can suppress the immune system, increase the time it takes your body to heal, interfere with sleep, and affect your mood.

Talk with your healthcare team about pain, especially if:

- The pain isn't getting better or going away with pain medicine

- The pain comes on quickly

- The pain makes it hard to eat, sleep, or perform your normal activities

- You feel new pain

- You have side effects from the pain medicine such as sleepiness, nausea, or constipation

Your doctor will work with you to develop a pain control plan that is based on your description of the pain. Taking pain medicine is an important part of the plan. Your doctor will talk with you about using drugs to control pain and prescribe medicine (including opioids and nonopioid medicines) to treat the pain.

Sexual Health Issues in Women

Women being treated for cancer may experience changes that affect their sexual life during, and sometimes after, treatment. While you may not have the energy or interest in sexual activity that you did before treatment, feeling close to and being intimate with your spouse or partner is probably still important.

Your doctor or nurse may talk with you about how cancer treatment might affect your sexual life, or you may need to be proactive and ask questions such as:

- What sexual changes or problems are common among women receiving this type of treatment?

- What methods of birth control or protection are recommended during treatment?

Whether or not your sexual health will be affected by treatment depends on factors such as:

- The type of cancer

- The type of treatment(s)

- The amount (dose) of treatment

- The length (duration) of treatment

- Your age at the time of treatment

- The amount of time that has passed since treatment

- Other personal health factors

Skin and Nail Changes

Cancer treatments may cause a range of skin and nail changes. Talk with your healthcare team to learn whether or not you will have these changes, based on the treatment you are receiving.

- Radiation therapy can cause the skin on the part of your body receiving radiation therapy to become dry and peel, itch (called pruritus), and turn red or darker. It may look sunburned or tan and be swollen or puffy.

- Chemotherapy may damage fast growing skin and nail cells. This can cause problems such as skin that is dry, itchy, red, and/or that peels. Some people may develop a rash or sun sensitivity, causing you to sunburn easily. Nail changes may include dark, yellow, or cracked nails and/or cuticles that are red and hurt. Chemotherapy in people who have received radiation therapy in the past can cause skin to become red, blister, peel, or hurt on the part of the body that received radiation therapy; this is called radiation recall.

- Biological therapy may cause itching (pruritus).

- Targeted therapy may cause a dry skin, a rash, and nail problems.

These skin problems are more serious and need urgent medical attention:

- Sudden or severe itching, a rash, or hives during chemotherapy. These may be signs of an allergic reaction.

- Sores on the part of your body where you are receiving treatment that become painful, wet, and/or infected. This is called a moist reaction and may happen in areas where the skin folds, such as around your ears, breast, or bottom.

Your doctor or nurse will talk with about possible skin and nail changes and advise you on ways to treat or prevent them.

Sleep Problems

Sleeping well is important for your physical and mental health. A good night's sleep not only helps you to think clearly, it also lowers your blood pressure, helps your appetite, and strengthens your immune system.

Sleep problems such as being unable to fall asleep and/or stay asleep, also called insomnia, are common among people being treated for cancer. Studies show that as many as half of all patients have sleep-related problems. These problems may be caused by the side effects of treatment, medicine, long hospital stays, or stress.

Talk with your healthcare team if you have difficulty sleeping, so you can get help you need. Sleep problems that go on for a long time may increase the risk of anxiety or depression. Your doctor will do an assessment, which may include a polysomnogram (recordings taken during sleep that show brain waves, breathing rate, and others activities such as heart rate) to correctly diagnose and treat sleep problems. Assessments may be repeated from time to time, since sleeping problems may change over time.

Urinary and Bladder Problems

Some cancer treatments, such as those listed below, may cause urinary and bladder problems:

- Radiation therapy to the pelvis (including reproductive organs, the bladder, colon, and rectum) can irritate the bladder and urinary tract. These problems often start several weeks after radiation therapy begins and go away several weeks after treatment has been completed.

- Some types of chemotherapy and immunotherapy can also affect or damage cells in the bladder and kidneys.

- Surgery to remove a woman's uterus, the tissue on the sides of the uterus, the cervix, and the top part of the vagina (radical hysterectomy) and bladder cancer surgery can also cause urinary problems. These types of surgery may also increase the risk of a urinary tract infection.

Chapter 43

Nausea and Vomiting

Nausea and vomiting are side effects of cancer therapy and affect most patients who have chemotherapy. Radiation therapy to the brain, gastrointestinal (GI) tract, or liver also causes nausea and vomiting. Nausea is an unpleasant feeling in the back of the throat and/or stomach that may come and go in waves. It may occur before vomiting.

Vomiting is throwing up the contents of the stomach through the mouth. Retching is the movement of the stomach and esophagus without vomiting and is also called dry heaves. Although treatments for nausea and vomiting have improved, nausea and vomiting are still serious side effects of cancer therapy because they cause the patient distress and may cause other health problems. Patients may have nausea more than vomiting.

Nausea is controlled by a part of the autonomic nervous system which controls involuntary body functions (such as breathing or digestion). Vomiting is a reflex controlled in part by a vomiting center in the brain. Vomiting can be triggered by smell, taste, anxiety, pain, motion, or changes in the body caused by inflammation, poor blood flow, or irritation of the stomach.

It is very important to prevent and control nausea and vomiting in patients with cancer so that they can continue treatment and perform

This chapter includes text excerpted from "Nausea and Vomiting Related to Cancer Treatment (PDQ®)—Patient Version," National Cancer Institute (NCI), June 6, 2017.

523

activities of daily life. Nausea and vomiting that are not controlled can cause the following:

- Chemical changes in the body
- Mental changes
- Loss of appetite
- Malnutrition
- Dehydration
- A torn esophagus
- Broken bones
- Reopening of surgical wounds

Different types of nausea and vomiting are caused by chemotherapy, radiation therapy, and other conditions. Nausea and vomiting can occur before, during, or after treatment. The types of nausea and vomiting include:

- **Acute:** Nausea and vomiting that happens within 24 hours after treatment starts.

- **Delayed:** Nausea and vomiting that happens more than 24 hours after chemotherapy. This is also called late nausea and vomiting.

- **Anticipatory:** Nausea and vomiting that happens before a chemotherapy treatment begins. If a patient has had nausea and vomiting after an earlier chemotherapy session, she may have anticipatory nausea and vomiting before the next treatment. This usually begins after the third or fourth treatment. The smells, sights, and sounds of the treatment room may remind the patient of previous times and may trigger nausea and vomiting before the chemotherapy session has even begun.

- **Breakthrough:** Nausea and vomiting that happen within five days after getting antinausea treatment. Different drugs or doses are needed to prevent more nausea and vomiting.

- **Refractory:** Nausea and vomiting that does not respond to drugs.

- **Chronic:** Nausea and vomiting that lasts for a period of time after treatment ends.

Causes

Many factors increase the risk of nausea and vomiting with chemotherapy. Nausea and vomiting with chemotherapy are more likely if the patient:

- Is treated with certain chemotherapy drugs
- Had severe or frequent periods of nausea and vomiting after past chemotherapy treatments
- Is female
- Is younger than 50 years
- Had motion sickness or vomiting with a past pregnancy
- Has a fluid and/or electrolyte imbalance (dehydration, too much calcium in the blood, or too much fluid in the body's tissues)
- Has a tumor in the gastrointestinal tract, liver, or brain
- Has constipation
- Is receiving certain drugs, such as opioids (pain medicine)
- Has an infection, including an infection in the blood
- Has kidney disease

Patients who drank large amounts of alcohol over time have a lower risk of nausea and vomiting after being treated with chemotherapy. Radiation therapy may also cause nausea and vomiting. The following treatment factors may affect the risk of nausea and vomiting:

- The part of the body where the radiation therapy is given. Radiation therapy to the gastrointestinal tract, liver, or brain, or whole body is likely to cause nausea and vomiting.
- The size of the area being treated
- The dose of radiation
- Receiving chemotherapy and radiation therapy at the same time

The following patient factors may cause nausea and vomiting with radiation therapy if the patient:

- Is younger than 55 years
- Is female

- Has anxiety

- Had severe or frequent periods of nausea and vomiting after past chemotherapy or radiation therapy treatments

Other conditions may also increase the risk of nausea and vomiting in patients with advanced cancer. Nausea and vomiting may also be caused by other conditions. In patients with advanced cancer, chronic nausea and vomiting may be caused by the following:

- Brain tumors or pressure on the brain

- Tumors of the gastrointestinal tract

- High or low levels of certain substances in the blood

- Medicines such as opioids

Anticipatory Nausea and Vomiting

Anticipatory nausea and vomiting may occur after several chemotherapy treatments. In some patients, after they have had several courses of treatment, nausea and vomiting may occur before a treatment session. This is called anticipatory nausea and vomiting. It is caused by triggers, such as odors in the therapy room. For example, a person who begins chemotherapy and smells an alcohol swab at the same time may later have nausea and vomiting at the smell of an alcohol swab. The more chemotherapy sessions a patient has, the more likely it is that anticipatory nausea and vomiting will occur.

Having three or more of the following may make anticipatory nausea and vomiting more likely:

- Having nausea and vomiting, or feeling warm or hot after the last chemotherapy session

- Being younger than 50 years

- Being female

- A history of motion sickness

- Having a high level of anxiety in certain situations

Other factors that may make anticipatory nausea and vomiting more likely include:

- Expecting to have nausea and vomiting before a chemotherapy treatment begins

- Doses and types of chemotherapy (some are more likely to cause nausea and vomiting)

- Feeling dizzy or lightheaded after chemotherapy

- How often chemotherapy is followed by nausea

- Having delayed nausea and vomiting after chemotherapy

- A history of morning sickness during pregnancy

The earlier that anticipatory nausea and vomiting is identified, the more effective treatment may be. When symptoms of anticipatory nausea and vomiting are diagnosed early, treatment is more likely to work. Psychologists and other mental health professionals with special training can often help patients with anticipatory nausea and vomiting. The following types of treatment may be used:

- Muscle relaxation with guided imagery

- Hypnosis

- Behavior changing methods

- Biofeedback

- Distraction (such as playing video games)

Antinausea drugs given for anticipatory nausea and vomiting do not seem to help.

Acute or Delayed Nausea and Vomiting

Acute and delayed nausea and vomiting are common in patients being treated with chemotherapy. Chemotherapy is the most common cause of nausea and vomiting that is related to cancer treatment. How often nausea and vomiting occur and how severe they are may be affected by the following:

- The specific drug being given

- The dose of the drug or if it is given with other drugs

- How often the drug is given

- The way the drug is given

- The individual patient

The following may make acute or delayed nausea and vomiting with chemotherapy more likely if the patient:

- Had chemotherapy in the past
- Had nausea and vomiting after a previous chemotherapy session
- Is dehydrated
- Is malnourished
- Had recent surgery
- Received radiation therapy
- Is female
- Is younger than 50 years
- Has a history of motion sickness
- Has a history of morning sickness

Patients who have acute nausea and vomiting with chemotherapy are more likely to have delayed nausea and vomiting as well. Acute and delayed nausea and vomiting with chemotherapy or radiation therapy are usually treated with drugs. Drugs may be given before each treatment, to prevent nausea and vomiting. After chemotherapy, drugs may be given to prevent delayed vomiting. Patients who are given chemotherapy several days in a row may need treatment for both acute and delayed nausea and vomiting. Some drugs last only a short time in the body and need to be given more often. Others last a long time and are given less often.

The following table shows drugs that are commonly used to prevent nausea and vomiting caused by chemotherapy and the type of drug.

Table 43.1. Drugs Used to Prevent Nausea and Vomiting Caused by Chemotherapy

Drug Name	Type of Drug
Chlorpromazine, prochlorperazine, promethazine	Phenothiazines
Droperidol, haloperidol	Butyrophenones
Metoclopramide, trimethobenzamide	Substituted benzamides
Dolasetron, granisetron, ondansetron, palonosetron	Serotonin receptor antagonists

Table 43.1. Continued

Drug Name	Type of Drug
Aprepitant, fosaprepitant, netupitant, rolapitant	Substance P/NK-1 antagonists
Dexamethasone, methylprednisolone	Corticosteroids
Alprazolam, lorazepam	Benzodiazepines
Olanzapine	Antipsychotic/monoamine antagonists
Cannabis, dronabinol, ginger, nabilone	Other

The following table shows drugs that are commonly used to prevent nausea and vomiting caused by radiation therapy and the type of drug:

Table 43.2. Drugs Used to Prevent Nausea and Vomiting Caused by Radiation Therapy

Drug Name	Type of Drug
Dolasetron, granisetron, ondansetron, palonosetron	Serotonin receptor antagonists
Dexamethasone	Corticosteroids
Metoclopramide, prochlorperazine	Dopamine receptor antagonists

It is not known whether it is best to give antinausea medicine for the first 5 days of radiation treatment or for the full treatment course. Talk with your doctor about the treatment plan that is best for you.

Treating Nausea and Vomiting without Drugs

Treatment without drugs is sometimes used to control nausea and vomiting. Nondrug treatments may help relieve nausea and vomiting, and may help antinausea drugs work better. These treatments include:

- Diet changes
- Acupuncture and acupressure
- Relaxation methods such as guided imagery and hypnosis
- Behavior therapy

Treatment-Related Nausea and Vomiting in Children

Nausea and vomiting in children treated with chemotherapy is a serious problem. Like adults, nausea in children receiving chemotherapy is more of a problem than vomiting. Children may have anticipatory, acute, and/or delayed nausea and vomiting.

Anticipatory nausea and vomiting may occur in children. Children who have nausea and vomiting after a chemotherapy treatment may have the same symptoms before their next treatment when the child sees, smells, or hears sounds from the treatment room. This is called anticipatory nausea and vomiting.

When the child's nausea and vomiting are well controlled during and after a chemotherapy treatment, the child may have less anxiety before the next treatment and less chance of having anticipatory symptoms.

Health professionals caring for children who have anticipatory nausea and vomiting have found that children may benefit from:

- Hypnosis

- Drugs used to treat anxiety in doses adjusted for the age and needs of the child

In children, acute nausea and vomiting are usually treated with drugs and other methods.

Drugs may be given before each treatment to prevent nausea and vomiting. After chemotherapy, drugs may be given to prevent delayed vomiting. Patients who are given chemotherapy several days in a row may need treatment for both acute and delayed nausea and vomiting. Some drugs last only a short time in the body and need to be given more often. Others last a long time and are given less often. The following table shows drugs that are commonly used to prevent nausea and vomiting caused by chemotherapy and the type of drug. Different types of drugs may be given together to treat acute and delayed nausea and vomiting.

Table 43.3. Drugs Used to Prevent Nausea and Vomiting Caused by Chemotherapy

Drug Name	Type of Drug
Chlorpromazine, prochlorperazine, promethazine	Phenothiazines
Metoclopramide	Substituted benzamides
Granisetron, ondansetron, palonosetron	Serotonin receptor antagonists
Aprepitant, fosaprepitant	Substance P/NK-1 antagonists
Dexamethasone, methylprednisolone	Corticosteroids

Table 43.3. Continued

Drug Name	Type of Drug
Lorazepam	Benzodiazepines
Olanzapine	Atypical antipsychotic
Dronabinol, nabilone	Other drugs

Nondrug treatments may help relieve nausea and vomiting, and may help antinausea drugs work better in children. These treatments include:

- Acupuncture

- Acupressure

- Guided imagery

- Music therapy

- Muscle relaxation training

- Child and family support groups

- Virtual reality games

Dietary support may include:

- Eating smaller meals more often

- Avoiding food smells and other strong odors

- Avoiding foods that are spicy, fatty, or highly salted

- Eating "comfort foods" that have helped prevent nausea in the past

- Taking antinausea drugs before meals

Delayed nausea may be hard to detect in children. Unlike in adults, delayed nausea and vomiting in children may be harder for parents and caregivers to see. A change in the child's eating pattern may be the only sign of a problem. In addition, most chemotherapy treatments for children are scheduled over several days. This makes the timing and risk of delayed nausea unclear.

Studies on the prevention of delayed nausea and vomiting in children are limited. Children are usually treated the same way as adults, with doses of drugs that prevent nausea adjusted for age.

Chapter 44

Fighting Cancer Fatigue

Fatigue is the most common side effect of cancer treatment. Cancer treatments such as chemotherapy, radiation therapy, and biologic therapy can cause fatigue in cancer patients. Fatigue is also a common symptom of some types of cancer. Patients describe fatigue as feeling tired, weak, worn-out, heavy, slow, or that they have no energy or get-up-and-go. Fatigue in cancer patients may be called cancer fatigue, cancer-related fatigue, and cancer treatment-related fatigue.

Fatigue related to cancer is different from fatigue that healthy people feel. When a healthy person is tired by day-to-day activities, their fatigue can be relieved by sleep and rest. Cancer-related fatigue is different. Cancer patients get tired after less activity than people who do not have cancer. Also, cancer-related fatigue is not completely relieved by sleep and rest and may last for a long time. Fatigue usually decreases after cancer treatment ends, but patients may still feel some fatigue for months or years.

Fatigue can decrease a patient's quality of life. It can affect all areas of life by making the patient too tired to take part in daily activities, relationships, social events, and community activities. Patients may miss work or school, spend less time with friends and family, or spend more time sleeping. In some cases, physical fatigue leads to mental fatigue and mood changes. This can make it hard for the patient to pay attention, remember things, and think clearly. Money may become a

This chapter includes text excerpted from "Fatigue (PDQ®)—Patient Version," National Cancer Institute (NCI), June 30, 2017.

problem if the patient needs to take leave from a job or stop working completely. Job loss can lead to the loss of health insurance. All these things can lessen the patient's quality of life and self-esteem. Getting help with fatigue may prevent some of these problems and improve quality of life.

Causes of Fatigue in Cancer Patients

Fatigue in cancer patients may have more than one cause. Doctors do not know all the reasons cancer patients have fatigue. Many conditions may cause fatigue at the same time. Fatigue in cancer patients may be caused by the following:

- Cancer treatment with chemotherapy, radiation therapy, and some biologic therapies

- Anemia (a lower than normal number of red blood cells (RBCs))

- Hormone levels that are too low or too high

- Trouble breathing or getting enough oxygen

- Heart trouble

- Infection

- Pain

- Stress

- Loss of appetite or not getting enough calories and nutrients

- Dehydration (loss of too much water from the body, such as from severe diarrhea or vomiting)

- Changes in how well the body uses food for energy

- Loss of weight, muscle, and/or strength

- Medicines that cause drowsiness

- Problems getting enough sleep

- Being less active

- Other medical conditions

Fatigue is common in people with advanced cancer who are not receiving cancer treatment. How cancer treatments cause fatigue is not known. Doctors are trying to better understand how cancer treatments such as surgery, chemotherapy, and radiation therapy cause fatigue. Some studies show that fatigue is caused by:

- The need for extra energy to repair and heal body tissue damaged by treatment

- The buildup of toxic substances that are left in the body after cells are killed by cancer treatment

- The effect of biologic therapy on the immune system

- Changes in the body's sleep-wake cycle

When they begin cancer treatment, many patients are already tired from medical tests, surgery, and the emotional stress of coping with the cancer diagnosis. After treatment begins, fatigue may get worse. Patients who are older, have advanced cancer, or receive more than one type of treatment (for example, both chemotherapy and radiation therapy) are more likely to have long-term fatigue. Different cancer treatments have different effects on a patient's energy level. The type and schedule of treatments can affect the amount of fatigue caused by cancer therapy.

Fatigue Caused by Chemotherapy

Patients treated with chemotherapy usually feel the most fatigue in the days right after each treatment. Then the fatigue decreases until the next treatment. Fatigue usually increases with each cycle. Some studies have shown that patients have the most severe fatigue about mid-way through all the cycles of chemotherapy. Fatigue decreases after chemotherapy is finished, but patients may not feel back to normal until a month or more after the last treatment. Many patients feel fatigued for months or years after treatment ends. Fatigue during chemotherapy may be increased by the following:

- Pain

- Depression

- Anxiety

- Anemia. Some types of chemotherapy stop the bone marrow from making enough new red blood cells, causing anemia (too few red blood cells to carry oxygen to the body).

- Lack of sleep caused by some anticancer drugs

535

Fatigue Caused by Radiation Therapy

Many patients receiving radiation therapy have fatigue that keeps them from being as active as they want to be. After radiation therapy begins, fatigue usually increases until mid-way through the course of treatments and then stays about the same until treatment ends. For many patients, fatigue improves after radiation therapy stops. However, in some patients, fatigue will last months or years after treatment ends. Some patients never have the same amount of energy they had before treatment. Cancer-related fatigue has been studied in patients with breast cancer. The amount of fatigue they felt and the time of day the fatigue was worst was different in different patients.

In women with breast cancer, fatigue was increased by the following:

- Working while receiving radiation therapy
- Having children at home
- Depression
- Anxiety
- Trouble sleeping
- Younger age
- Being underweight
- Having advanced cancer or other medical conditions

Fatigue Caused by Biologic Therapy

Biologic therapy often causes flu-like symptoms. These symptoms include being tired physically and mentally, fever, chills, muscle pain, headache, and not feeling well in general. Some patients may also have problems thinking clearly. Fatigue symptoms depend on the type of biologic therapy used.

Fatigue Caused by Surgery

Fatigue is often a side effect of surgery, but patients usually feel better with time. However, fatigue caused by surgery can be worse when the surgery is combined with other cancer treatments.

Anemia Is a Common Cause of Fatigue

Anemia affects the patient's energy level and quality of life. Anemia may be caused by the following:

- The cancer
- Cancer treatments
- A medical condition not related to the cancer

The effects of anemia on a patient depend on the following:

- How quickly the anemia occurs
- The patient's age
- The amount of plasma (fluid part of the blood) in the patient's blood
- Other medical conditions the patient has

Side Effects Related to Nutrition May Cause or Increase Fatigue

The body's energy comes from food. Fatigue may occur if the body does not take in enough food to give the body the energy it needs. For many patients, the effects of cancer and cancer treatments make it hard to eat well. In people with cancer, three major factors may affect nutrition:

- A change in the way the body is able to use food. A patient may eat the same amount as before having cancer, but the body may not be able to absorb and use all the nutrients from the food. This is caused by the cancer or its treatment.
- A decrease in the amount of food eaten because of low appetite, nausea, vomiting, diarrhea, or a blocked bowel
- An increase in the amount of energy needed by the body because of a growing tumor, infection, fever, or shortness of breath

Anxiety and Depression May Cause Fatigue in Cancer Patients

The emotional stress of cancer can cause physical problems, including fatigue. It's common for cancer patients to have changes in moods and attitudes. Patients may feel anxiety and fear before and after a cancer diagnosis. These feelings may cause fatigue. The effect of the disease on the patient's physical, mental, social, and financial well-being can increase emotional distress.

About 15–25 percent of patients who have cancer get depressed, which may increase fatigue caused by physical factors. The following are signs of depression:

- Feeling tired mentally and physically

- Loss of interest in life

- Problems thinking

- Loss of sleep

- Feeling a loss of hope

Some patients have more fatigue after cancer treatments than others do. Fatigue may be increased when it is hard for patients to learn and remember. During and after cancer treatment, patients may find they cannot pay attention for very long and have a hard time thinking, remembering, and understanding. This is called attention fatigue. Sleep helps to relieve attention fatigue, but sleep may not be enough when the fatigue is related to cancer. Taking part in restful activities and spending time outdoors may help relieve attention fatigue. Not sleeping well may cause fatigue. Some people with cancer are not able to get enough sleep. The following problems related to sleep may cause fatigue:

- Waking up during the night

- Not going to sleep at the same time every night

- Sleeping during the day and less at night

- Not being active during the day

Poor sleep affects people in different ways. For example, the time of day that fatigue is worse may be different. Some patients who have trouble sleeping may feel more fatigue in the morning. Others may have severe fatigue in both the morning and the evening. Even in patients who have poor sleep, fixing sleep problems does not always improve fatigue. A lack of sleep may not be the cause of the fatigue.

Patients may take medicines for cancer symptoms, such as pain, or conditions other than the cancer. These medicines may cause the patient to feel sleepy. Opioids, antidepressants, and antihistamines have this side effect. If many of these medicines are taken at the same time, fatigue may be worse. Taking opioids over time may lower the amount of sex hormones made in the testicles and ovaries. This can lead to fatigue as well as sexual problems and depression.

Assessment of Fatigue

An assessment is done to find out the level of fatigue and how it affects the patient's daily life. There is no test to diagnose fatigue, so it is important for the patient to tell family members and the healthcare team if fatigue is a problem. To assess fatigue, the patient is asked to describe how bad the fatigue is, how it affects daily activities, and what makes the fatigue better or worse. The doctor will look for causes of fatigue that can be treated.

A fatigue assessment is repeated to see if there is a pattern for when fatigue starts or becomes worse. Fatigue may be worse right after a chemotherapy treatment, for example. The same method of measuring fatigue is used at each assessment. This helps show changes in fatigue over time.

Treatments for Fatigue

Fatigue in cancer patients is often treated by relieving related conditions such as anemia and depression. Treatment of fatigue depends on the symptoms and whether the cause of fatigue is known. When the cause of fatigue is not known, treatment is usually given to relieve symptoms and teach the patient ways to cope with fatigue.

Treatment of Anemia

Treating anemia may help decrease fatigue. When known, the cause of the anemia is treated. When the cause is not known, treatment for anemia is supportive care and may include the following:

- **Change in diet:** Eating more foods rich in iron and vitamins may be combined with other treatments for anemia.

- **Transfusions of red blood cells:** Transfusions work well to treat anemia. Possible side effects of transfusions include an allergic reaction, infection, graft-versus-host disease (GvHD), immune system changes, and too much iron in the blood.

- **Medicine:** Drugs that cause the bone marrow to make more red blood cells may be used to treat anemia-related fatigue in patients receiving chemotherapy. Epoetin alfa and darbepoetin alfa are two of these drugs. This type of drug may shorten survival time, increase the risk of serious heart problems, and cause some tumors to grow faster or recur. The U.S. Food and Drug Administration (FDA) has not approved these drugs for the treatment of fatigue. Discuss the risks and benefits of these drugs with your doctor.

Treatment of Pain

If pain is making fatigue worse, the patient's pain medicine may be changed or the dose may be increased. If too much pain medicine is making fatigue worse, the patient's pain medicine may be changed or the dose may be decreased.

Treatment of Depression

Fatigue in patients who have depression may be treated with antidepressant drugs. Psychostimulant drugs may help some patients have more energy and a better mood, and help them think and concentrate. The use of psychostimulants for treating fatigue is still being studied. The FDA has not approved psychostimulants for the treatment of fatigue.

Psychostimulants have side effects, especially with long-term use. Different psychostimulants have different side effects. Patients who have heart problems or who take anticancer drugs that affect the heart may have serious side effects from psychostimulants. These drugs have warnings on the label about their risks. Talk to your doctor about the effects these drugs may have and use them only under a doctor's care. Some of the possible side effects include the following:

- Trouble sleeping
- Euphoria (feelings of extreme happiness)
- Headache
- Nausea
- Anxiety
- Mood changes
- Loss of appetite

- Nightmares

- Paranoia (feelings of fear and distrust of other people)

- Serious heart problems

The doctor may prescribe low doses of a psychostimulant to be used for a short time in patients with advanced cancer who have severe fatigue. Talk to your doctor about the risks and benefits of these drugs. The following drugs are being studied for fatigue related to cancer:

- Bupropion is an antidepressant that is being studied to treat fatigue in patients with or without depression.

- Dexamethasone is an anti-inflammatory drug being studied in patients with advanced cancer. In one clinical trial, patients who received dexamethasone reported less fatigue than the group that received a placebo. More trials are needed to study the link between inflammation and fatigue.

The following dietary supplements are being studied for fatigue related to cancer:

- L-carnitine is a supplement that helps the body make energy and lowers inflammation that may be linked to fatigue.

- Ginseng is an herb used to treat fatigue which may be taken in capsules of ground ginseng root. In a clinical trial, cancer patients who were either in treatment or had finished treatment, received either ginseng or placebo. The group receiving ginseng had less fatigue than the placebo group.

Ways to Increase Energy and Cope with Fatigue

Treatment of fatigue may include teaching the patient ways to increase energy and cope with fatigue in daily life.

Exercise

Exercise (including walking) may help people with cancer feel better and have more energy. The effect of exercise on fatigue in cancer patients is being studied. One study reported that breast cancer survivors who took part in enjoyable physical activity had less fatigue and pain and were better able to take part in daily activities. In clinical trials, some patients reported the following benefits from exercise:

- More physical energy
- Better appetite
- More able to do the normal activities of daily living
- Better quality of life
- More satisfaction with life
- A greater sense of well-being
- More able to meet the demands of cancer and cancer treatment

Moderate activity for 3–5 hours a week may help cancer-related fatigue. You are more likely to follow an exercise plan if you choose a type of exercise that you enjoy. The healthcare team can help you plan the best time and place for exercise and how often to exercise. Patients may need to start with light activity for short periods of time and build up to more exercise little by little. Studies have shown that exercise can be safely done during and after cancer treatment.

Mind and body exercises such as qigong, tai chi, and yoga may help relieve fatigue. These exercises combine activities like movement, stretching, balance, and controlled breathing with spiritual activity such as meditation.

A Schedule of Activity and Rest

Changes in daily routine make the body use more energy. A regular routine can improve sleep and help the patient have more energy to be active during the day. A program of regular times for activity and rest help to make the most of a patient's energy. A healthcare professional can help patients plan an exercise program and decide which activities are the most important to them.

The following sleep habits may help decrease fatigue:

- Lie in bed for sleep only
- Take naps for no longer than one hour
- Avoid noise (like television and radio) during sleep

Cancer patients should not try to do too much. Health professionals have information about support services to help with daily activities and responsibilities.

Talk Therapy

Therapists use talk therapy (counseling) to treat certain emotional or behavioral disorders. This kind of therapy helps patients change how they think and feel about certain things. Talk therapy may help decrease a cancer patient's fatigue by working on problems related to cancer that make fatigue worse, such as:

- Stress from coping with cancer
- Fear that the cancer may come back
- Feeling hopeless about fatigue
- Not enough social support
- A pattern of sleep and activity that changes from day to day

Self-Care for Fatigue

Learning about the risk of cancer-related fatigue and how to reduce fatigue may help you cope with it better and improve quality of life. For example, some patients in treatment worry that having fatigue means the treatment is not working. Anxiety over this can make fatigue even worse. Some patients may feel that reporting fatigue is complaining. Knowing that fatigue is a normal side effect that should be reported and treated may make it easier to manage.

Working with the healthcare team to learn about the following may help patients cope with fatigue:

- How to cope with fatigue as a normal side effect of treatment
- The possible medical causes of fatigue such as not enough fluids, electrolyte imbalance, breathing problems, or anemia
- How patterns of rest and activity affect fatigue
- How to schedule important daily activities during times of less fatigue, and give up less important activities
- The kinds of activities that may help you feel more alert (walking, gardening, bird-watching)
- The difference between fatigue and depression
- How to avoid or change situations that cause stress
- How to avoid or change activities that cause fatigue
- How to change your surroundings to help decrease fatigue

- Exercise programs that are right for you and decrease fatigue
- The importance of eating enough food and drinking enough fluids
- Physical therapy for patients who have nerve problems or muscle weakness
- Respiratory therapy for patients who have trouble breathing
- How to tell if treatments for fatigue are working

Fatigue after Cancer Treatment Ends

Fatigue continues to be a problem for many cancer survivors long after treatment ends and the cancer is gone. Studies show that some patients continue to have moderate-to-severe fatigue years after treatment. Long-term therapies such as tamoxifen can also cause fatigue. In children who were treated for brain tumors and cured, fatigue may continue after treatment. The causes of fatigue after treatment ends are different than the causes of fatigue during treatment. Treating fatigue after treatment ends also may be different from treating it during cancer therapy. Since fatigue may greatly affect the quality of life for cancer survivors, long-term follow-up care is important.

Chapter 45

Controlling Cancer-Related Pain

Cancer, treatment for cancer, or diagnostic tests may cause you to feel pain. Pain is one of the most common symptoms in cancer patients. Pain can be caused by cancer, treatment for cancer, or a combination of factors. Tumors, surgery, intravenous chemotherapy, radiation therapy, targeted therapy, supportive care therapies such as bisphosphonates, and diagnostic procedures may cause you pain.

Younger patients are more likely to have cancer pain and pain flares than older patients. Patients with advanced cancer have more severe pain, and many cancer survivors have pain that continues after cancer treatment ends. Pain control can improve your quality of life. It can be controlled in most patients who have cancer. Although cancer pain cannot always be relieved completely, there are ways to lessen pain in most patients. It can improve your quality of life all through your cancer treatment and after it ends.

Pain can be managed before, during, and after diagnostic and treatment procedures. Many diagnostic and treatment procedures are painful. It helps to start pain control before the procedure begins. Some drugs may be used to help you feel calm or fall asleep. Treatments such as imagery or relaxation can also help control pain and anxiety related

This chapter includes text excerpted from "Cancer Pain (PDQ®)—Patient Version," National Cancer Institute (NCI), August 31, 2017.

to treatment. Knowing what will happen during the procedure and having a relative or friend stay with you may also help lower anxiety.

Specific Types of Pain from Cancer Treatment

Different cancer treatments may cause specific types of pain. Patients may have different types of pain depending on the treatments they receive, including:

- Spasms, stinging, and itching caused by intravenous chemotherapy

- Mucositis (sores or inflammation in the mouth or other parts of the digestive system) caused by chemotherapy or targeted therapy

- Skin pain, rash, or hand-foot syndrome (redness, tingling, or burning in the palms of the hands and/or the soles of feet) caused by chemotherapy or targeted therapy

- Pain in joints and muscles throughout the body caused by paclitaxel or aromatase inhibitor therapy

- Osteonecrosis of the jaw caused by bisphosphonates given for cancer that has spread to the bone

- Pain syndromes caused by radiation, including:
    - Pain from brachytherapy
    - Pain from the position the patient stays in during radiation therapy
    - Mucositis
    - Inflammation of the mucous membranes in areas that were treated with radiation
    - Dermatitis (inflammation of the skin in areas that were treated with radiation)
    - Pain flares (a temporary worsening of pain in the treated area)

Cancer pain may affect quality of life and ability to function even after treatment ends. Pain that is severe or continues after cancer treatment ends increases the risk of anxiety and depression. Patients may be disabled by their pain, unable to work, or feel that they are losing support once their care moves from their oncology team back to their primary care team. Feelings of anxiety and depression can worsen cancer pain and make it harder to control.

Each patient needs a personal plan to control cancer pain. Each person's diagnosis, cancer stage, response to pain, and personal likes and dislikes are different. For this reason, each patient needs a personal plan to control cancer pain. You, your family, and your healthcare team can work together to manage your pain. As part of your pain control plan, your healthcare provider can give you and your family members written instructions to control your pain at home. Find out who you should call if you have questions.

Assessment of Cancer Pain

You and your healthcare team work together to assess cancer pain. It's important that the cause of the pain is found early and treated quickly. Your healthcare team will help you measure pain levels often, including at the following times:

- After starting cancer treatment

- When there is new pain

- After starting any type of pain treatment

To learn about your pain, the healthcare team will ask you to describe the pain with the following questions:

- When did the pain start?

- How long does the pain last?

- Where is the pain? You will be asked to show exactly where the pain is on your body or on a drawing of a body.

- How strong is the pain?

- Have there been changes in where or when the pain occurs?

- What makes the pain better or worse?

- Is the pain worse during certain times of the day or night?

- Is there breakthrough pain (intense pain that flares up quickly even when pain control medicine is being used)?

- Do you have symptoms, such as trouble sleeping, fatigue, depression, or anxiety?

- Does pain get in the way of activities of daily life, such as eating, bathing, or moving around?

Your healthcare team will also take into account:

- Past and current pain treatments

- Prognosis (chance of recovery)

- Other conditions you may have, such as kidney, liver, or heart disease

- Past and current use of nicotine, alcohol, or sleeping pills

- Personal or family history of substance abuse

- Personal history of childhood sexual abuse

- Your own choices

This information will be used to decide how to help relieve your pain. This may include drugs or other treatments. In some cases, patients are referred to pain specialists or palliative care specialists. Your healthcare team will work with you to decide whether the benefits of treatment outweigh any risks and how much improvement you should expect. After pain control is started, the doctor will continue to assess how well it is working for you and make changes if needed.

A family member or caregiver may be asked to give answers for a patient who has a problem with speech, language, or understanding.

Physical and neurological exams will be done to help plan pain control.

The following exams will be done:

- **Physical exam and history:** An exam of the body to check general signs of health, including checking for signs of disease, such as lumps or anything else that seems unusual. A history of your health habits and past illnesses and treatments will also be taken.

- **Neurological exam:** A series of questions and tests to check the brain, spinal cord, and nerve function. The exam checks your mental status, coordination, and ability to walk normally, and how well the muscles, senses, and reflexes work. This may also be called a neuro exam or a neurologic exam.

Your healthcare team will also assess your psychological, social, and spiritual needs.

Using Drugs to Control Cancer Pain

The doctor will prescribe drugs based on whether the pain is mild, moderate, or severe. Your doctor will prescribe drugs to help relieve your pain. These drugs need to be taken at scheduled times to keep a constant level of the drug in the body to help keep the pain from coming back. Drugs may be taken by mouth or given in other ways, such as by infusion or injection.

Your doctor may prescribe extra doses of a drug that can be taken as needed for pain that occurs between scheduled doses of the drug. The doctor will adjust the drug dose for your needs.

A scale from 0–10 is used to measure how severe the pain is and decide which pain medicine to use. On this scale:

- 0 means no pain

- 1–3 means mild pain

- 4–6 means moderate pain

- 7–10 means severe pain

Acetaminophen and nonsteroidal anti-inflammatory drugs (NSAIDs) may be used to relieve mild pain.

Acetaminophen and NSAIDs help relieve mild pain. They may be given with opioids for moderate to severe pain.

Pain relievers of this type include:

- Acetaminophen

- Celecoxib

- Diclofenac

- Ibuprofen

- Ketoprofen

- Ketorolac

Patients, especially older patients, who are taking acetaminophen or NSAIDs need to be closely watched for side effects.

Opioids are used to relieve moderate to severe pain. It works very well to relieve moderate to severe pain. Some patients with cancer pain stop getting pain relief from opioids if they take them for a long time. This is called tolerance. Larger doses or a different opioid may be needed if your body stops responding to the same dose. Tolerance of an opioid is a physical dependence on it. This is not the same as addiction (psychological dependence).

Since 1999, there have been four times the number of prescriptions written for opioids and four times the number of deaths caused by drug overdose in the United States. Although most patients who are prescribed opioids for cancer pain use them safely, a small percentage of patients may become addicted to opioids. Your doctor will carefully prescribe and monitor your opioid doses so that you are treated for pain safely.

There are several types of opioids:

- Buprenorphine

- Codeine

- Diamorphine

- Fentanyl

- Hydrocodone

- Hydromorphone

- Methadone

- Morphine (the most commonly used opioid for cancer pain)

- Oxycodone

- Oxymorphone

- Tapentadol

- Tramadol

The doctor will prescribe drugs and the times they should be taken in order to best control your pain. Also, it is important that patients and family caregivers know how to safely use, store, and dispose of opioids.

Most patients with cancer pain will need to receive opioids on a regular schedule. Receiving opioids on a regular schedule helps relieve the pain and keeps it from getting worse. The amount of time between doses depends on which opioid you are using. The correct dose is the amount of opioid that controls your pain with the fewest side effects. The dose will be slowly adjusted until there is a good balance between pain relief and side effects. If opioid tolerance does occur, the dose may be increased or a different opioid may be needed.

Opioids may be given by the following ways:

- **Mouth:** If your stomach and intestines work normally, medicine is usually given by mouth. Opioids given orally are easy to use and usually low cost. Oral opioids are sometimes placed under the tongue (sublingual route) or on the inside of the cheek (buccal route) to be absorbed.

- **Rectum:** If you cannot take opioids by mouth, they may be given as rectal suppositories.

- **Skin patches:** Opioid patches are placed on the skin (transdermal route).

- **Nose spray:** Opioids may be given in the form of a nasal spray.

- **Intravenous (IV) line:** Opioids are given into a vein only when simpler and less costly methods cannot be used, don't work, or are not wanted by the patient. Patient-controlled analgesia (PCA) pumps are one way to control pain through your IV line. A PCA pump allows you to control the amount of drug that is used. With a PCA pump, you can receive a preset opioid dose by pressing a button on a computerized pump that is connected to a small tube. Once the pain is controlled, the doctor may prescribe regular opioid doses based on the amount you used with the PCA pump.

- **Subcutaneous injection:** Opioids are given by injection into the fatty layer of tissue just under the skin.

- **Intraspinal injection:** Intraspinal opioids are injected into the fluid around the spinal cord. These may be combined with a local anesthetic to help some patients who have pain that is very hard to control.

There are common side effects caused by opioids. Your doctor will discuss the side effects with you before opioid treatment begins and will watch you for side effects. The following are the most common side effects:

- Constipation

- Nausea

- Drowsiness

- Dry mouth

Nausea and drowsiness most often occur when opioid treatment is first started and usually get better within a few days.

Opioids slow down the muscle contractions and movement in the stomach and intestines, which can cause hard stools. To keep the stool soft and prevent constipation, it's important to drink plenty of fluids. Unless there are problems such as a blocked bowel or diarrhea, you will be given a treatment plan to follow to prevent constipation and information on how to avoid problems with your intestines while taking opioids.

Other side effects of opioid treatment include the following:

- Vomiting

- Low blood pressure

- Dizziness

- Trouble sleeping

- Trouble thinking clearly

- Delirium or hallucinations

- Trouble urinating

- Problems with breathing

- Severe itching

- Problems with sexual function

- Hot flashes

- Depression

- Hypoglycemia

Talk with your doctor about side effects that bother you or become severe. Your doctor may decrease the dose of the opioid, change to a different opioid, or change the way the opioid is given to help decrease the side effects.

Other drugs may be given while you are taking opioids for pain relief. These are drugs that help the opioids work better, treat symptoms, and relieve certain types of pain. The following types of drugs may be used:

- Antidepressants

- Anticonvulsants

- Local anesthetics

- Corticosteroids

- Stimulants

- Bisphosphonates and denosumab

There are big differences in how patients respond to these drugs. Side effects are common and should be reported to your doctor.

Bisphosphonates (pamidronate, zoledronic acid, and ibandronate) are drugs that are sometimes used when cancer has spread to the bones. They are given as an intravenous infusion and combined with other treatments to decrease pain and reduce risk of broken bones. However, bisphosphonates sometimes cause severe side effects. Talk to your doctor if you have severe muscle or bone pain. Bisphosphonate therapy may need to be stopped.

The use of bisphosphonates is also linked to the risk of bisphosphonate-associated osteonecrosis (BON). Denosumab is another drug that may be used when cancer has spread to the bones. It is given as a subcutaneous injection and may help prevent and relieve pain.

Other Treatments for Cancer Pain

Most cancer pain can be controlled with drug treatments, but some patients have too many side effects from drugs or have pain in a certain part of the body that needs to be treated in a different way. You can talk to your doctor to help decide which methods work best to relieve your pain. These other treatments include:

Nerve Blocks

A nerve block is the injection of either a local anesthetic or a drug into or around a nerve to block pain. Nerve blocks help control pain that can't be controlled in other ways. Nerve blocks may also be used to find where the pain is coming from, to predict how the pain will respond to long-term treatments, and to prevent pain after certain procedures.

Neurological Treatments

Surgery can be done to insert a device that delivers drugs or stimulates the nerves with mild electric current. In rare cases, surgery may be done to destroy a nerve or nerves that are part of the pain pathway.

Cordotomy

Cordotomy is a less common surgical procedure that is used to relieve pain by cutting certain nerves in the spinal cord. This blocks pain and also hot/cold feelings. This procedure may be chosen for patients who are near the end of life and have severe pain that cannot be relieved in other ways.

Palliative Care

Certain patients are helped by palliative care services. Palliative care providers may also be called supportive care providers. They work in teams that include doctors, nurses, mental health specialists, social workers, chaplains, pharmacists, and dietitians. Some of the goals of palliative care are to:

- Improve quality of life for patients and their families

- Manage pain and nonpain symptoms

- Support patients who need higher doses of opioids, have a history of substance abuse, or are coping with emotional and social problems

Radiation Therapy

Radiation therapy is used to relieve pain in patients with skin lesions, tumors, or cancer that has spread to the bone. This is called palliative radiation therapy. It may be given as local therapy directly to the tumor or to larger areas of the body. Radiation therapy helps drugs and other treatments work better by shrinking tumors that are causing pain. Radiation therapy may help patients with bone pain move more freely and with less pain.

The following types of radiation therapy may be used:

External Radiation Therapy

External radiation therapy uses a machine outside the body to send high-energy X-rays or other types of radiation toward the cancer. External radiation therapy relieves pain from cancer that has spread to the bone. Radiation therapy may be given in a single dose or divided into several smaller doses given over a period of time. The decision whether to have a single or divided dose may depend on how easy it is to get the treatments and how much they cost. Patients may have a pain flare (a temporary worsening of pain in the treated area) after receiving palliative radiation therapy for cancer that has spread to the bone, but this side effect is only temporary.

Radiopharmaceuticals

Radiopharmaceuticals are drugs that have a radioactive substance that may be used to diagnose or treat disease, including cancer. Radiopharmaceuticals may also be used to relieve pain from cancer that has spread to the bone. A single dose of a radioactive agent injected into a vein may relieve pain when cancer has spread to several areas of bone and/or when there are too many areas to treat with external radiation therapy.

Physical Medicine and Rehabilitation

Patients with cancer and pain may lose their strength, freedom of movement, and ability to manage their daily activities. Physical therapy or occupational therapy may help these patients.

Physical medicine uses physical methods, such as exercise and machines to prevent and treat disease or injury. Physical methods to treat weakness, muscle wasting, and muscle and bone pain include the following:

- Exercise to strengthen and stretch weak muscles, loosen stiff joints, help coordination and balance, and strengthen the heart

- Changing position (for patients who are not able to move on their own)

- Limiting the movement of painful areas or broken bones

Some patients may be referred to a physiatrist (a doctor who specializes in physical medicine) who can develop a personal plan for them. Some physiatrists are also trained in procedures to treat and manage pain.

Complementary Therapies

Complementary and alternative therapies combined with standard treatment may be used to treat pain. They may also be called integrative therapies. Acupuncture, support groups, and hypnosis are a few integrative therapies that have been used to relieve pain.

Acupuncture

Acupuncture is an integrative therapy that applies needles, heat, pressure, and other treatments to one or more places on the skin called acupuncture points. Acupuncture may be used to control pain, including pain related to cancer.

Hypnosis

Hypnosis may help you relax and may be combined with other thinking and behavior methods. Hypnosis to relieve pain works best in people who are able to concentrate and use imagery and who are willing to practice the technique.

Support Groups

Support groups help many patients. Religious counseling may also help by offering spiritual care and social support.

Chapter 46

Gastrointestinal Effects of Cancer Treatment

The gastrointestinal (GI) tract is part of the digestive system, which processes nutrients (vitamins, minerals, carbohydrates, fats, proteins, and water) in foods that are eaten and helps pass waste material out of the body. The GI tract includes the stomach and intestines (bowels). The stomach is a J-shaped organ in the upper abdomen. Food moves from the throat to the stomach through a hollow, muscular tube called the esophagus. After leaving the stomach, partly-digested food passes into the small intestine and then into the large intestine. The colon (large bowel) is the first part of the large intestine and is about 5 feet long. Together, the rectum and anal canal make up the last part of the large intestine and are 6–8 inches long. The anal canal ends at the anus (the opening of the large intestine to the outside of the body).

GI complications are common in cancer patients. Complications are medical problems that occur during a disease, or after a procedure or treatment. They may be caused by the disease, procedure, or treatment, or may have other causes.

- Constipation

- Fecal impaction

- Bowel obstruction

This chapter includes text excerpted from "Gastrointestinal Complications (PDQ®)—Patient Version," National Cancer Institute (NCI), March 2, 2018.

- Diarrhea

- Radiation enteritis

Constipation

With constipation, bowel movements are difficult or don't happen as often as usual. Constipation is the slow movement of stool through the large intestine. The longer it takes for the stool to move through the large intestine, the more it loses fluid and the drier and harder it becomes. The patient may be unable to have a bowel movement, have to push harder to have a bowel movement, or have fewer than their usual number of bowel movements.

Causes

Certain medicines, changes in diet, not drinking enough fluids, and being less active are common causes of constipation. Constipation is a common problem for cancer patients. Cancer patients may become constipated by any of the usual factors that cause constipation in healthy people. These include older age, changes in diet and fluid intake, and not getting enough exercise. In addition to these common causes of constipation, there are other causes in cancer patients.

Other causes of constipation include:

Medicines

- Opioids and other pain medicines. This is one of the main causes of constipation in cancer patients.

- Chemotherapy

- Medicines for anxiety and depression

- Antacids

- Diuretics (drugs that increase the amount of urine made by the body)

- Supplements such as iron and calcium

- Sleep medicines

- Drugs used for anesthesia (to cause loss of feeling for surgery or other procedures)

Diet

- Not drinking enough water or other fluids. This is a common problem for cancer patients.
- Not eating enough food, especially high-fiber food

Bowel Movement Habits

- Not going to the bathroom when the need for a bowel movement is felt
- Using laxatives and/or enemas too often

Conditions That Prevent Activity and Exercise

- Spinal cord injury or pressure on the spinal cord from a tumor or other cause
- Broken bones
- Fatigue
- Weakness
- Long periods of bed rest or not being active
- Heart problems
- Breathing problems
- Anxiety
- Depression

Intestinal Disorders

- Irritable colon
- Diverticulitis (inflammation of small pouches in the colon called diverticula)
- Tumor in the intestine

Muscle and Nerve Disorders

- Brain tumors
- Spinal cord injury or pressure on the spinal cord from a tumor or other cause

- Paralysis (loss of ability to move) of both legs
- Stroke or other disorders that cause paralysis of part of the body
- Peripheral neuropathy (pain, numbness, tingling) of feet
- Weakness of the diaphragm (the breathing muscle below the lungs) or abdominal muscles. This makes it hard to push to have a bowel movement

Changes in Body Metabolism

- Having a low level of thyroid hormone, potassium, or sodium in the blood
- Having too much nitrogen or calcium in the blood

Environment

- Having to go farther to get to a bathroom
- Needing help to go to the bathroom
- Being in unfamiliar places
- Having little or no privacy
- Feeling rushed
- Living in extreme heat that causes dehydration
- Needing to use a bedpan or bedside commode

Narrow Colon

- Scars from radiation therapy or surgery
- Pressure from a growing tumor

Treatment

Treating constipation is important to make the patient comfortable and to prevent more serious problems. It's easier to prevent constipation than to relieve it. The healthcare team will work with the patient to prevent constipation. Patients who take opioids may need to start taking laxatives right away to prevent constipation.

Constipation can be very uncomfortable and cause distress. If left untreated, constipation may lead to fecal impaction. This is a serious condition in which stool will not pass out of the colon or rectum. It's important to treat constipation to prevent fecal impaction.

Prevention and treatment are not the same for every patient. Do the following to prevent and treat constipation:

- Keep a record of all bowel movements.

- Drink eight 8-ounce glasses of fluid each day. Patients who have certain conditions, such as kidney or heart disease, may need to drink less.

- Get regular exercise. Patients who cannot walk may do abdominal exercises in bed or move from the bed to a chair.

- Increase the amount of fiber in the diet by eating more of the following:

  - Fruits, such as raisins, prunes, peaches, and apples

  - Vegetables, such as squash, broccoli, carrots, and celery

  - Whole grain cereals, whole grain breads, and bran

It's important to drink more fluids when eating more high-fiber foods, to avoid making constipation worse. Patients who have had a small or large intestinal obstruction or have had intestinal surgery (for example, a colostomy) should not eat a high-fiber diet.

- Drink a warm or hot drink about one half-hour before the usual time for a bowel movement.

- Find privacy and quiet when it is time for a bowel movement.

- Use the toilet or a bedside commode instead of a bedpan.

- Take only medicines that are prescribed by the doctor. Medicines for constipation may include bulking agents, laxatives, stool softeners, and drugs that cause the intestine to empty.

- Use suppositories or enemas only if ordered by the doctor. In some cancer patients, these treatments may lead to bleeding, infection, or other harmful side effects.

When constipation is caused by opioids, treatment may be drugs that stop the effects of the opioids or other medicines, stool softeners, enemas, and/or manual removal of stool.

Fecal Impaction

Fecal impaction is a mass of dry, hard stool that will not pass out of the colon or rectum. Patients with fecal impaction may not have gastrointestinal (GI) symptoms. Instead, they may have problems with circulation, the heart, or breathing. If fecal impaction is not treated, it can get worse and cause death.

Causes

A common cause of fecal impaction is using laxatives too often. Repeated use of laxatives in higher and higher doses makes the colon less able to respond naturally to the need to have a bowel movement. This is a common reason for fecal impaction. Other causes include:

- Opioid pain medicines
- Little or no activity over a long period
- Diet changes
- Constipation that is not treated

Certain types of mental illness may lead to fecal impaction.

Symptoms

Symptoms of fecal impaction include being unable to have a bowel movement and pain in the abdomen or back.

The following may be symptoms of fecal impaction:

- Being unable to have a bowel movement
- Having to push harder to have a bowel movement of small amounts of hard, dry stool
- Having fewer than the usual number of bowel movements
- Having pain in the back or abdomen
- Urinating more or less often than usual, or being unable to urinate
- Breathing problems, rapid heartbeat, dizziness, low blood pressure, and swollen abdomen
- Having sudden, explosive diarrhea (as stool moves around the impaction)
- Leaking stool when coughing
- Nausea and vomiting
- Dehydration
- Being confused and losing a sense of time and place, with rapid heartbeat, sweating, fever, and high or low blood pressure

These symptoms should be reported to the healthcare provider. Assessment includes a physical exam and questions like those asked in the assessment of constipation.

The doctor will ask questions similar to those for the assessment of constipation:

- How often do you have a bowel movement? When and how much?

- When was your last bowel movement? What was it like (how much, hard or soft, color)?

- Was there any blood in your stool?

- Has your stomach hurt or have you had any cramps, nausea, vomiting, gas, or feeling of fullness near the rectum?

- Do you use laxatives or enemas regularly?

- What do you usually do to relieve constipation? Does this usually work?

- What kind of food do you eat?

- How much and what type of fluids do you drink each day?

- What medicines are you taking? How much and how often?

- Is this constipation a recent change in your normal habits?

- How many times a day do you pass gas?

The doctor will do a physical exam to find out if the patient has a fecal impaction. The following tests and procedures may be done:

- Physical exam

- X-rays

- Digital rectal exam (DRE)

- Sigmoidoscopy

- Blood tests

- Electrocardiogram (EKG)

Treatment

A fecal impaction is usually treated with an enema. The main treatment for impaction is to moisten and soften the stool so it can be removed or passed out of the body. This is usually done with an enema. Enemas are given only as prescribed by the doctor since too many enemas can damage the intestine. Stool softeners or glycerin suppositories may be given to make the stool softer and easier to pass. Some patients may need to have stool manually removed from the rectum after it is softened.

Laxatives that cause the stool to move are not used because they can also damage the intestine.

Bowel Obstruction

A bowel obstruction is a blockage of the small or large intestine by something other than fecal impaction. Bowel obstructions (blockages) keep the stool from moving through the small or large intestines. They may be caused by a physical change or by conditions that stop the intestinal muscles from moving normally. The intestine may be partly or completely blocked. Most obstructions occur in the small intestine.

Physical Changes

- The intestine may become twisted or form a loop, closing it off and trapping stool.

- Inflammation, scar tissue from surgery, and hernias can make the intestine too narrow.

- Tumors growing inside or outside the intestine can cause it to be partly or completely blocked.

If the intestine is blocked by physical causes, it may decrease blood flow to blocked parts. Blood flow needs to be corrected or the affected tissue may die.

Conditions That Affect the Intestinal Muscle

- Paralysis (loss of ability to move)

- Blocked blood vessels going to the intestine

- Too little potassium in the blood

The most common cancers that cause bowel obstructions are cancers of the colon, stomach, and ovary. Other cancers, such as lung and breast cancers and melanoma, can spread to the abdomen and cause bowel obstruction. Patients who have had surgery on the abdomen or radiation therapy to the abdomen have a higher risk of a bowel obstruction. Bowel obstructions are most common during the advanced stages of cancer.

Assessment includes a physical exam and imaging tests.

The following tests and procedures may be done to diagnose a bowel obstruction:

- Physical exam
- Complete blood count (CBC)
- Electrolyte panel
- Urinalysis
- Abdominal X-ray
- Barium enema

Treatment is different for acute and chronic bowel obstructions.

Acute Bowel Obstruction

Acute bowel obstructions occur suddenly, may have not occurred before, and are not long-lasting. Treatment may include the following:

- **Fluid replacement therapy:** A treatment to get the fluids in the body back to normal amounts. Intravenous (IV) fluids may be given and medicines may be prescribed.

- **Electrolyte correction:** A treatment to get the right amounts of chemicals in the blood, such as sodium, potassium, and chloride. Fluids with electrolytes may be given by infusion.

- **Blood transfusion:** A procedure in which a person is given an infusion of whole blood or parts of blood.

- **Nasogastric or colorectal tube:** A nasogastric tube is inserted through the nose and esophagus into the stomach. A colorectal tube is inserted through the rectum into the colon. This is done to decrease swelling, remove fluid and gas buildup, and relieve pressure.

- **Surgery:** Surgery to relieve the obstruction may be done if it causes serious symptoms that are not relieved by other treatments.

Patients with symptoms that keep getting worse will have follow-up exams to check for signs and symptoms of shock and to make sure the obstruction isn't getting worse.

Chronic, Malignant Bowel Obstruction (MBO)

Chronic bowel obstructions keep getting worse over time. Patients who have advanced cancer may have chronic bowel obstructions that cannot be removed with surgery. The intestine may be blocked or narrowed in more than one place or the tumor may be too large to remove completely. Treatments include the following:

- **Surgery:** The obstruction is removed to relieve pain and improve the patient's quality of life.

- **Stent:** A metal tube inserted into the intestine to open the area that is blocked.

- **Gastrostomy tube:** A tube inserted through the wall of the abdomen directly into the stomach. The gastrostomy tube can relieve fluid and air buildup in the stomach and allow medications and liquids to be given directly into the stomach by pouring them down the tube. A drainage bag with a valve may also be attached to the gastrostomy tube. When the valve is open, the patient may be able to eat or drink by mouth and the food drains directly into the bag. This gives the patient the experience of tasting the food and keeping the mouth moist. Solid food is avoided because it may block the tubing to the drainage bag.

- **Medicines:** Injections or infusions of medicines for pain, nausea, and vomiting, and/or to make the intestines empty. This may be prescribed for patients who cannot be helped with a stent or gastrostomy tube.

Diarrhea

Diarrhea is frequent, loose, and watery bowel movements. Acute diarrhea lasts more than 4 days but less than 2 weeks. Symptoms of acute diarrhea may be loose stools and passing more than 3 unformed stools in one day. Diarrhea is chronic (long term) when it goes on for longer than 2 months. Diarrhea can occur at any time during cancer treatment. It can be physically and emotionally stressful for patients who have cancer. In cancer patients, the most common cause of diarrhea is cancer treatment.

Causes of diarrhea in cancer patients include the following:

- Cancer treatments, such as chemotherapy, targeted therapy, radiation therapy, bone marrow transplant, and surgery.

- Some chemotherapy and targeted therapy drugs cause diarrhea by changing how nutrients are broken down and absorbed in the small intestine. More than half of patients who receive chemotherapy have diarrhea that needs to be treated.

- Radiation therapy to the abdomen and pelvis can cause inflammation of the bowel. Patients may have problems digesting food and have gas, bloating, cramps, and diarrhea. These symptoms may last up to 8–12 weeks after treatment or may not happen for months or years. Treatment may include diet changes, medicines, or surgery.

- Patients who are having radiation therapy and chemotherapy often have severe diarrhea. Hospital treatment may not be needed. Treatment may be given at an outpatient clinic or with home care. Intravenous (IV) fluids may be given or medicines may be prescribed.

- Patients who have a donor bone marrow transplant may develop graft-versus-host disease (GVHD). Stomach and intestinal symptoms of GVHD include nausea and vomiting, severe abdominal pain and cramps, and watery, green diarrhea. Symptoms may show up 1 week to 3 months after the transplant.

- Surgery on the stomach or intestines

- Cancer itself
- Stress and anxiety from being diagnosed with cancer and having cancer treatment
- Medical conditions and diseases other than cancer
- Infections
- Antibiotic therapy for certain infections. Antibiotic therapy can irritate the lining of the bowel and cause diarrhea that often does not get better with treatment.
- Laxatives
- Fecal impaction in which the stool leaks around the blockage
- Certain foods that are high in fiber or fat

Assessment includes a physical exam, lab tests, and questions about diet and bowel movements.

Because diarrhea can be life-threatening, it is important to find out the cause so treatment can begin as soon as possible. The doctor may ask the following questions to help plan treatment:

- How often have you had bowel movements in the past 24 hours?

- When was your last bowel movement? What was it like (how much, how hard or soft, what color)? Was there any blood?

- Was there any blood in your stool or any rectal bleeding?

- Have you been dizzy, very drowsy, or had any cramps, pain, nausea, vomiting, or fever?

- What have you eaten? What and how much have you had to drink in the past 24 hours?

- Have you lost weight recently? How much?

- How often have you urinated in the past 24 hours?

- What medicines are you taking? How much and how often?

- Have you traveled recently?

Tests and procedures may include the following:

- Physical exam and history

- Digital rectal exam (DRE)

- Fecal occult blood test

- Stool tests

- Complete blood count (CBC)

- Electrolyte panel

- Urinalysis

- Abdominal X-ray

Treatment of diarrhea depends on what is causing it. The doctor may make changes in medicines, diet, and/or fluids.

- A change in the use of laxatives may be needed

- Medicine to treat diarrhea may be prescribed to slow down the intestines, decrease fluid secreted by the intestines, and help nutrients be absorbed

- Diarrhea caused by cancer treatment may be treated by changes in diet. Eat small frequent meals and avoid the following foods:
  - Milk and dairy products
  - Spicy foods
  - Alcohol
  - Foods and drinks that have caffeine
  - Certain fruit juices
  - Foods and drinks that cause gas
  - Foods high in fiber or fat
- A diet of bananas, rice, apples, and toast (the BRAT diet) may help mild diarrhea.
- Drinking more clear liquids may help decrease diarrhea. It is best to drink up to 3 quarts of clear fluids a day. These include water, sports drinks, broth, weak decaffeinated tea, caffeine-free soft drinks, clear juices, and gelatin. For severe diarrhea, the patient may need intravenous (IV) fluids or other forms of IV nutrition.
- Diarrhea caused by graft-versus-host-disease (GVHD) is often treated with a special diet. Some patients may need long-term treatment and diet management.
- Probiotics may be recommended. Probiotics are live microorganisms used as a dietary supplement to help with digestion and normal bowel function. A bacterium found in yogurt called *Lactobacillus acidophilus* is the most common probiotic.
- Patients who have diarrhea with other symptoms may need fluids and medicine given by IV.

Radiation Enteritis

Radiation enteritis is inflammation of the intestine caused by radiation therapy. It is a condition in which the lining of the intestine becomes swollen and inflamed during or after radiation therapy to the abdomen, pelvis, or rectum. The small and large intestine are very sensitive to radiation. The larger the dose of radiation, the more damage may be done to normal tissue. Most tumors in the abdomen and pelvis need large doses of radiation. Almost all patients receiving radiation to the abdomen, pelvis, or rectum will have enteritis.

Radiation therapy to kill cancer cells in the abdomen and pelvis affects normal cells in the lining of the intestines. Radiation therapy stops the growth of cancer cells and other fast-growing cells. Since normal cells in the lining of the intestines grow quickly, radiation treatment to that area can stop those cells from growing. This makes it hard for tissue to repair itself. As cells die and are not replaced, gastrointestinal problems occur over the next few days and weeks.

Doctors are studying whether the order that radiation therapy, chemotherapy, and surgery are given affects how severe enteritis will be.

Symptoms may begin during radiation therapy or months to years later.

Radiation enteritis may be acute or chronic:

- Acute radiation enteritis occurs during radiation therapy and may last up to 8–12 weeks after treatment stops.

- Chronic radiation enteritis may appear months to years after radiation therapy ends, or it may begin as acute enteritis and keep coming back.

The total dose of radiation and other factors affect the risk of radiation enteritis. Only 5–15 percent of patients treated with radiation to the abdomen will have chronic problems. The amount of time enteritis lasts and how severe it depends on the following:

- The total dose of radiation received

- The amount of normal intestine treated

- The tumor size and how much it has spread

- If chemotherapy was given at the same time as the radiation therapy

- If radiation implants were used

- If the patient has high blood pressure, diabetes, pelvic inflammatory disease (PID), or poor nutrition

- If the patient has had surgery to the abdomen or pelvis

Acute and chronic enteritis have symptoms that are a lot alike. Patients with acute enteritis may have the following symptoms:

- Nausea

- Vomiting

- Abdominal cramps

- Frequent urges to have a bowel movement

- Rectal pain, bleeding, or mucus in the stool

- Watery diarrhea

- Feeling very tired

Symptoms of acute enteritis usually go away 2–3 weeks after treatment ends. Symptoms of chronic enteritis usually appear 6–18 months after radiation therapy ends. It can be hard to diagnose. The doctor will first check to see if the symptoms are being caused by a recurrent tumor in the small intestine. The doctor will also need to know the patient's full history of radiation treatments.

Patients with chronic enteritis may have the following signs and symptoms:

- Abdominal cramps

- Bloody diarrhea

- Frequent urges to have a bowel movement

- Greasy and fatty stools

- Weight loss

- Nausea

Assessment of radiation enteritis includes a physical exam and questions for the patient.

Patients will be given a physical exam and be asked questions about the following:

- The usual pattern of bowel movements

- The pattern of diarrhea:

  - When it started

  - How long it has lasted

  - How often it occurs

  - Amount and type of stools

  - Other symptoms of diarrhea (such as gas, cramping, bloating, urgency, bleeding, and rectal soreness)

- Nutrition health:
  - Height and weight
  - Usual eating habits
  - Changes in eating habits
  - Amount of fiber in the diet
  - Signs of dehydration (such as poor skin tone, increased weakness, or feeling very tired)
- Stress levels and ability to cope
- Changes in lifestyle caused by the enteritis

Treatment depends on whether the radiation enteritis is acute or chronic.

Acute Radiation Enteritis

Treatment of acute enteritis includes treating the symptoms. The symptoms usually get better with treatment, but if symptoms get worse, then cancer treatment may have to be stopped for a while.

Treatment of acute radiation enteritis may include the following:

- Medicines to stop diarrhea
- Opioids to relieve pain
- Steroid foams to relieve rectal inflammation
- Pancreatic enzyme replacement for patients who have pancreatic cancer. A decrease in pancreatic enzymes can cause diarrhea
- Diet changes. Intestines damaged by radiation therapy may not make enough of certain enzymes needed for digestion, especially lactase. Lactase is needed to digest lactose, which is found in milk and milk products. A lactose-free, low-fat, and low-fiber diet may help to control symptoms of acute enteritis
  - Foods to avoid:
    - Milk and milk products, except buttermilk, yogurt, and lactose-free milkshake supplements, such as Ensure
    - Whole-bran bread and cereal
    - Nuts, seeds, and coconut

- Fried, greasy, or fatty foods
- Fresh and dried fruit and some fruit juices (such as prune juice).
- Raw vegetables
- Rich pastries
- Popcorn, potato chips, and pretzels
- Strong spices and herbs
- Chocolate, coffee, tea, and soft drinks with caffeine
- Alcohol and tobacco

- Foods to choose:
  - Fish, poultry, and meat that are broiled or roasted
  - Bananas
  - Applesauce and peeled apples
  - Apple and grape juices
  - White bread and toast
  - Macaroni and noodles
  - Baked, boiled, or mashed potatoes
  - Cooked vegetables that are mild, such as asparagus tips, green and waxed beans, carrots, spinach, and squash
  - Mild processed cheese. Processed cheese may not cause problems because the lactose is removed when it is made
  - Buttermilk, yogurt, and lactose-free milkshake supplements, such as Ensure
  - Eggs
  - Smooth peanut butter

- Helpful hints:
  - Eat food at room temperature
  - Drink about 12 eight-ounce glasses of fluid a day
  - Let sodas lose their fizz before drinking them

- Add nutmeg to food. This helps slow down movement of digested food in the intestines.

- Start a low-fiber diet on the first day of radiation therapy

Chronic Radiation Enteritis

Treatment of chronic radiation enteritis may include the following:

- Same treatments as for acute radiation enteritis symptoms

- Surgery. Few patients need surgery to control their symptoms. Two types of surgery may be used:

  - **Intestinal bypass:** A procedure in which the doctor creates a new pathway for the flow of intestinal contents around the damaged tissue.

  - **Total intestinal resection:** Surgery to completely remove the intestines.

Doctors look at the patient's general health and the amount of damaged tissue before deciding if surgery will be needed. Healing after surgery is often slow and long-term tube feeding may be needed. Even after surgery, many patients still have symptoms.

Chapter 47

Lymphedema

Lymphedema is the buildup of fluid in soft body tissues when the lymph system is damaged or blocked. Fluid builds up in soft body tissues and causes swelling. It is a common problem that may be caused by cancer and cancer treatment. Lymphedema usually affects an arm or leg, but it can also affect other parts of the body. Lymphedema can cause long-term physical, psychological, and social problems for patients.

The Lymph System

The lymph system is a network of lymph vessels, tissues, and organs that carry lymph throughout the body. The parts of the lymph system that play a direct part in lymphedema include the following:

- **Lymph:** A clear fluid that contains lymphocytes (white blood cells (WBCs)) that fight infection and the growth of tumors. Lymph also contains plasma, the watery part of the blood that carries the blood cells.

- **Lymph vessels:** A network of thin tubes that helps lymph flow through the body and returns it to the bloodstream.

- **Lymph nodes:** Small, bean-shaped structures that filter lymph and store white blood cells that help fight infection and disease.

This chapter includes text excerpted from "Lymphedema (PDQ®)—Patient Version," National Cancer Institute (NCI), May 29, 2015.

Lymph nodes are located along the network of lymph vessels found throughout the body. Clusters of lymph nodes are found in the underarm, pelvis, neck, abdomen, and groin.

The spleen, thymus, tonsils, and bone marrow are also part of the lymph system but do not play a direct part in lymphedema.

Common Occurrence of Lymphedema

Lymphedema occurs when lymph is not able to flow through the body the way that it should. When the lymph system is working as it should, lymph flows through the body and is returned to the bloodstream.

- Fluid and plasma leak out of the capillaries (smallest blood vessels) and flow around body tissues so the cells can take up nutrients and oxygen.

- Some of this fluid goes back into the bloodstream. The rest of the fluid enters the lymph system through tiny lymph vessels. These lymph vessels pick up the lymph and move it toward the heart. The lymph is slowly moved through larger and larger lymph vessels and passes through lymph nodes where waste is filtered from the lymph.

- The lymph keeps moving through the lymph system and collects near the neck, then flows into one of two large ducts:

  - The right lymph duct collects lymph from the right arm and the right side of the head and chest

  - The left lymph duct collects lymph from both legs, the left arm, and the left side of the head and chest

- These large ducts empty into veins under the collar bones, which carry the lymph to the heart, where it is returned to the bloodstream.

When part of the lymph system is damaged or blocked, fluid cannot drain from nearby body tissues. Fluid builds up in the tissues and causes swelling.

Types of Lymphedema

Lymphedema may be either primary or secondary:

- Primary lymphedema is caused by the abnormal development of the lymph system. Symptoms may occur at birth or later in life.

- Secondary lymphedema is caused by damage to the lymph system. The lymph system may be damaged or blocked by infection, injury, cancer, removal of lymph nodes, radiation to the affected area, or scar tissue from radiation therapy or surgery.

Symptoms of Lymphedema

Other conditions may cause the same symptoms. A doctor should be consulted if any of the following problems occur:

- Swelling of an arm or leg, which may include fingers and toes

- A full or heavy feeling in an arm or leg

- A tight feeling in the skin

- Trouble moving a joint in the arm or leg

- Thickening of the skin, with or without skin changes such as blisters or warts

- A feeling of tightness when wearing clothing, shoes, bracelets, watches, or rings

- Itching of the legs or toes

- A burning feeling in the legs

- Trouble sleeping

- Loss of hair

Daily activities and the ability to work or enjoy hobbies may be affected by lymphedema. These symptoms may occur very slowly over time or more quickly if there is an infection or injury to the arm or leg.

Risk Factors for Lymphedema

Lymphedema can occur after any cancer or treatment that affects the flow of lymph through the lymph nodes, such as removal of lymph nodes. It may develop within days or many years after treatment. Most lymphedema develops within three years of surgery. Risk factors for lymphedema include the following:

- Removal and/or radiation of lymph nodes in the underarm, groin, pelvis, or neck. The risk of lymphedema increases with the number of lymph nodes affected. There is less risk with the removal of only the sentinel lymph node (the first lymph node to receive lymphatic drainage from a tumor).

- Being overweight or obese

- Slow healing of the skin after surgery

- A tumor that affects or blocks the left lymph duct or lymph nodes or vessels in the neck, chest, underarm, pelvis, or abdomen

- Scar tissue in the lymph ducts under the collarbones, caused by surgery or radiation therapy

Lymphedema often occurs in breast cancer patients who had all or part of their breast removed and axillary (underarm) lymph nodes removed. Lymphedema in the legs may occur after surgery for uterine cancer, lymphoma, or melanoma. It may also occur with vulvar cancer or ovarian cancer.

How Lymphedema Is Diagnosed

It is important to make sure there are no other causes of swelling, such as infection or blood clots. The following tests and procedures may be used to diagnose lymphedema:

- **Physical exam and history:** An exam of the body to check general signs of health, including checking for signs of disease, such as lumps or anything else that seems unusual. A history of the patient's health habits and past illnesses and treatments will also be taken.

- **Lymphoscintigraphy:** A method used to check the lymph system for disease. A very small amount of a radioactive substance that flows through the lymph ducts and can be taken up by lymph nodes is injected into the body. A scanner or probe is used to follow the movement of this substance. Lymphoscintigraphy is used to find the sentinel lymph node (the first node to receive lymph from a tumor) or to diagnose certain diseases or conditions, such as lymphedema.

- **Magnetic resonance imaging (MRI):** A procedure that uses a magnet, radio waves, and a computer to make a series of detailed pictures of areas inside the body—This procedure is also called nuclear magnetic resonance imaging (NMRI).

The swollen arm or leg is usually measured and compared to the other arm or leg. Measurements are taken over time to see how well treatment is working. A grading system is also used to diagnose and describe lymphedema. Grades 1, 2, 3, and 4 are based on size of the affected limb and how severe the signs and symptoms are.

Stages of Lymphedema

- **Stage I:** The limb (arm or leg) is swollen and feels heavy. Pressing on the swollen area leaves a pit (dent). This stage of lymphedema may go away without treatment.

- **Stage II:** The limb is swollen and feels spongy. A condition called tissue fibrosis may develop and cause the limb to feel hard. Pressing on the swollen area does not leave a pit.

- **Stage III:** This is the most advanced stage. The swollen limb may be very large. Stage III lymphedema rarely occurs in breast cancer patients. Stage III is also called lymphostatic elephantiasis.

Managing Lymphedema

Patients can take steps to prevent lymphedema or keep it from getting worse. Taking preventive steps may keep lymphedema from developing. Healthcare providers can teach patients how to prevent and take care of lymphedema at home. If lymphedema has developed, these steps may keep it from getting worse.

Preventive Steps

Tell your healthcare right away if you have any of the symptoms. The chance of improving the condition is better if treatment begins early. Untreated lymphedema can lead to problems that cannot be reversed.

Bacteria can enter the body through a cut, scratch, insect bite, or other skin injury. Fluid that is trapped in body tissues by lymphedema makes it easy for bacteria to grow and cause infection. Look for signs of infection, such as redness, pain, swelling, heat, fever, or red streaks below the surface of the skin. Call your doctor right away if any of these signs appear. Careful skin and nail care helps prevent infection:

- Use cream or lotion to keep the skin moist.

- Treat small cuts or breaks in the skin with an antibacterial ointment.

- Avoid needle sticks of any type into the limb (arm or leg) with lymphedema. This includes shots or blood tests.

- Use a thimble for sewing.

- Avoid testing bath or cooking water using the limb with lymphedema. There may be less feeling (touch, temperature, pain) in the affected arm or leg, and skin might burn in water that is too hot.

- Wear gloves when gardening and cooking.

- Wear sunscreen and shoes when outdoors.

- Cut toenails straight across. See a podiatrist (foot doctor) as needed to prevent ingrown nails and infections.

- Keep feet clean and dry and wear cotton socks.

Avoid blocking the flow of fluids through the body. It is important to keep body fluids moving, especially through an affected limb or in areas where lymphedema may develop.

- Do not cross legs while sitting.

- Change sitting position at least every 30 minutes.

- Wear only loose jewelry and clothes without tight bands or elastic.

- Do not carry handbags on the arm with lymphedema.

- Do not use a blood pressure cuff on the arm with lymphedema.

- Do not use elastic bandages or stockings with tight bands.

Keep blood from pooling in the affected limb.

- Keep the limb with lymphedema raised higher than the heart when possible.

- Do not swing the limb quickly in circles or let the limb hang down. This makes blood and fluid collect in the lower part of the arm or leg.

- Do not apply heat to the limb.

Studies have shown that carefully controlled exercise is safe for patients with lymphedema. Exercise does not increase the chance that lymphedema will develop in patients who are at risk for lymphedema. In the past, these patients were advised to avoid exercising the affected limb. Studies have now shown that slow, carefully controlled exercise is safe and may even help keep lymphedema from developing. Studies have also shown that, in breast-cancer survivors, upper-body exercise does not increase the risk that lymphedema will develop.

Treatment of Lymphedema

Damage to the lymph system cannot be repaired. Treatment is given to control the swelling caused by lymphedema and keep other problems from developing or getting worse. Physical (nondrug) therapies are the standard treatment. Treatment may be a combination of several of the physical methods. The goal of these treatments is to help patients continue with activities of daily living, to decrease pain, and to improve the ability to move and use the limb (arm or leg) with lymphedema. Drugs are not usually used for long-term treatment of lymphedema.

Treatment of lymphedema may include the following:

Pressure Garments

Pressure garments are made of fabric that puts a controlled amount of pressure on different parts of the arm or leg to help move fluid and keep it from building up. Some patients may need to have these garments custom-made for a correct fit. Wearing a pressure garment during exercise may help prevent more swelling in an affected limb. It is important to use pressure garments during air travel, because lymphedema can become worse at high altitudes. Pressure garments are also called compression sleeves and lymphedema sleeves or stockings.

Exercise

Both light exercise and aerobic exercise (physical activity that causes the heart and lungs to work harder) help the lymph vessels move lymph out of the affected limb and decrease swelling.

- **Talk with a certified lymphedema therapist before beginning exercise.** Patients who have lymphedema or who are at risk for lymphedema should talk with a certified lymphedema therapist before beginning an exercise routine.

- **Wear a pressure garment if lymphedema has developed.**
  Patients who have lymphedema should wear a well-fitting pressure
  garment during all exercise that uses the affected limb or body
  part. When it is not known for sure if a woman has lymphedema,
  upper-body exercise without a garment may be more helpful than
  no exercise at all. Patients who do not have lymphedema do not
  need to wear a pressure garment during exercise.

- **Breast cancer survivors should begin with light upper-
  body exercise and increase it slowly.** Some studies with
  breast cancer survivors show that upper-body exercise is
  safe in women who have lymphedema or who are at risk for
  lymphedema. Weight-lifting that is slowly increased may keep
  lymphedema from getting worse. Exercise should start at a very
  low level, increase slowly over time, and be overseen by the
  lymphedema therapist. If exercise is stopped for a week or longer,
  it should be started again at a low level and increased slowly.

If symptoms (such as swelling or heaviness in the limb) change or
increase for a week or longer, talk with the lymphedema therapist. It
is likely that exercising at a low level and slowly increasing it again
over time is better for the affected limb than stopping the exercise
completely.

More studies are needed to find out if weight-lifting is safe for cancer survivors with lymphedema in the legs.

Bandages

Once the lymph fluid is moved out of a swollen limb, bandaging
(wrapping) can help prevent the area from refilling with fluid. Bandages also increase the ability of the lymph vessels to move lymph
along. Lymphedema that has not improved with other treatments is
sometimes helped with bandaging.

Skin Care

The goal of skin care is to prevent infection and to keep skin from
drying and cracking.

Combined Therapy

Combined physical therapy is a program of massage, bandaging, exercises, and skin care managed by a trained therapist. At the

beginning of the program, the therapist gives many treatments over a short time to decrease most of the swelling in the limb with lymphedema. Then the patient continues the program at home to keep the swelling down. Combined therapy is also called complex decongestive therapy (CDT).

Compression Device

Compression devices are pumps connected to a sleeve that wraps around the arm or leg and applies pressure on and off. The sleeve is inflated and deflated on a timed cycle. This pumping action may help move fluid through lymph vessels and veins and keep fluid from building up in the arm or leg. Compression devices may be helpful when added to combined therapy. The use of these devices should be supervised by a trained professional because too much pressure can damage lymph vessels near the surface of the skin.

Weight Loss

In patients who are overweight, lymphedema related to breast cancer may improve with weight loss.

Laser Therapy

Laser therapy may help decrease lymphedema swelling and skin hardness after a mastectomy. A hand-held, battery-powered device is used to aim low-level laser beams at the area with lymphedema.

Drug Therapy

Lymphedema is not usually treated with drugs. Antibiotics may be used to treat and prevent infections. Other types of drugs, such as diuretics or anticoagulants (blood thinners), are usually not helpful and may make the lymphedema worse.

Surgery

Lymphedema caused by cancer is rarely treated with surgery.

Massage Therapy

Massage therapy (manual therapy) for lymphedema should begin with someone specially trained in treating lymphedema. In this type of massage, the soft tissues of the body are lightly rubbed, tapped, and stroked. It is a very light touch, almost like a brushing. Massage may help move lymph out of the swollen area into an area with working lymph vessels. Patients can be taught to do this type of massage therapy themselves.

When done correctly, massage therapy does not cause medical problems. Massage should not be done on any of the following:

- Open wounds, bruises, or areas of broken skin

- Tumors that can be seen on the skin surface

- Areas with deep vein thrombosis (blood clot in a vein)

- Sensitive soft tissue where the skin was treated with radiation therapy

Treatment of Severe Lymphedema

Sometimes severe lymphedema does not get better with treatment or it develops several years after surgery. If there is no known reason, doctors will try to find out if the problem is something other than the original cancer or cancer treatment, such as another tumor. Lymphangiosarcoma is a rare, fast-growing cancer of the lymph vessels. It is a problem that occurs in some breast cancer patients and appears an average of 10 years after a mastectomy. Lymphangiosarcoma begins as purple lesions on the skin, which may be flat or raised. A computed tomography (CT) scan or MRI is used to check for lymphangiosarcoma. Lymphangiosarcoma usually cannot be cured.

Chapter 48

The Effects of Cancer Treatments on Blood Cells

Chapter Contents

Section 48.1

Anemia

This section includes text excerpted from "Side
Effects: Anemia and Cancer Treatment," National
Cancer Institute (NCI), February 13, 2018.

Anemia is a condition that can make you feel very tired, short of
breath, and lightheaded. Other signs of anemia may include feeling
dizzy or faint, headaches, a fast heartbeat, and/or pale skin. Cancer
treatments, such as chemotherapy and radiation therapy, as well as
cancers that affect the bone marrow, can cause anemia. When you
are anemic, your body does not have enough red blood cells (RBCs).
Red blood cells are the cells that that carry oxygen from the lungs
throughout your body to help it work properly. You will have blood
tests to check for anemia. Treatment for anemia is also based on your
symptoms and on what is causing the anemia.

Ways to Manage Anemia

Here are some steps you can take if you have fatigue caused by
anemia:

- **Save your energy and ask for help.** Choose the most
  important things to do each day. When people offer to help, let
  them do so. They can take you to the doctor, make meals, or do
  other things you are too tired to do.

- **Balance rest with activity.** Take short naps during the day,
  but keep in mind that too much bed rest can make you feel
  weak. You may feel better if you take short walks or exercise a
  little every day.

- **Eat and drink well.** Talk with your doctor, nurse, or a
  registered dietitian to learn what foods and drinks are best
  for you. You may need to eat foods that are high in protein or
  iron.

Talking with Your Healthcare Team about Anemia

Prepare for your visit by making a list of questions to ask. Consider adding these questions to your list:

- What is causing the anemia?

- What problems should I call you about?

- What steps can I take to feel better?

- Would medicine, iron pills, a blood transfusion, or other treatments help me?

- Would you give me the name of a registered dietitian who could also give me advice?

Section 48.2

Neutropenia

This section includes text excerpted from "Side Effects: Infection and Neutropenia during Cancer Treatment," National Cancer Institute (NCI), April 29, 2015.

An infection is the invasion and growth of germs in the body, such as bacteria, viruses, yeast, or other fungi. An infection can begin anywhere in the body, may spread throughout the body, and can cause one or more of these signs:

- Fever of 100.5°F (38°C) or higher or chills

- Cough or sore throat

- Diarrhea

- Ear pain, headache or sinus pain, or a stiff or sore neck

- Skin rash

- Sores or white coating in your mouth or on your tongue

- Swelling or redness, especially where a catheter enters your body

- Urine that is bloody or cloudy, or pain when you urinate

Call your healthcare team if you have signs of an infection. Infections during cancer treatment can be life-threatening and require urgent medical attention. Be sure to talk with your doctor or nurse before taking medicine—even aspirin, acetaminophen (such as Tylenol®), or ibuprofen (such as Advil®) for a fever. These medicines can lower a fever but may also mask or hide signs of a more serious problem.

Some types of cancer and treatments such as chemotherapy may increase your risk of infection. This is because they lower the number of white blood cells (WBCs), the cells that help your body to fight infection. During chemotherapy, there will be times in your treatment cycle when the number of white blood cells (called neutrophils) is particularly low and you are at increased risk of infection. Stress, poor nutrition, and not enough sleep can also weaken the immune system, making infection more likely. You will have blood tests to check for neutropenia (a condition in which there is a low number of neutrophils). Medicine may sometimes be given to help prevent infection or to increase the number of white blood cells.

Ways to Prevent Infection

Your healthcare team will talk with you about these and other ways to prevent infection:

- **Wash your hands often and well.** Use soap and warm water to wash your hands well, especially before eating. Have people around you wash their hands well too.

- **Stay extra clean.** If you have a catheter, keep the area around it clean and dry. Clean your teeth well and check your mouth for sores or other signs of an infection each day. If you get a scrape or cut, clean it well. Let your doctor or nurse know if your bottom is sore or bleeds, as this could increase your risk of infection.

- **Avoid germs.** Stay away from people who are sick or have a cold. Avoid crowds and people who have just had a live vaccine, such as one for chicken pox, polio, or measles. Follow food safety guidelines; make sure the meat, fish, and eggs you eat are well cooked. Keep hot foods hot and cold foods cold. You may be advised to eat only fruits and vegetables that can be peeled, or to wash all raw fruits and vegetables very well.

Talking with Your Healthcare Team about Infection

Prepare for your visit by making a list of questions to ask. Consider adding these questions to your list:

- Am I at increased risk of infection during treatment? When am I at increased risk?

- What steps should I take to prevent infection?

- What signs of infection should I look for?

- Which signs signal that I need urgent medical care at the emergency room? Which should I call you about?

Section 48.3

Thrombocytopenia

This section includes text excerpted from "Side Effects: Bleeding and Bruising (Thrombocytopenia) and Cancer Treatment," National Cancer Institute (NCI), April 29, 2015.

Some cancer treatments, such as chemotherapy and targeted therapy, can increase your risk of bleeding and bruising. These treatments can lower the number of platelets in the blood. Platelets are the cells that help your blood to clot and stop bleeding. When your platelet count is low, you may bruise or bleed a lot or very easily and have tiny purple or red spots on your skin. This condition is called thrombocytopenia. It is important to tell your doctor or nurse if you notice any of these changes.

Call your doctor or nurse if you have more serious problems, such as:

- Bleeding that doesn't stop after a few minutes; bleeding from your mouth, nose, or when you vomit; bleeding from your vagina when you are not having your period (menstruation); urine that

589

is red or pink; stools that are black or bloody; or bleeding during your period that is heavier or lasts longer than normal.

- Head or vision changes such as bad headaches or changes in how well you see, or if you feel confused or very sleepy.

Ways to Manage Bleeding and Bruising

Steps to take if you are at increased risk of bleeding and bruising:

Avoid certain medicines. Many over-the-counter (OTC) medicines contain aspirin or ibuprofen, which can increase your risk of bleeding. When in doubt, be sure to check the label. Get a list of medicines and products from your healthcare team that you should avoid taking. You may also be advised to limit or avoid alcohol if your platelet count is low.

- **Take extra care to prevent bleeding.** Brush your teeth gently, with a very soft toothbrush. Wear shoes, even when you are inside. Be extra careful when using sharp objects. Use an electric shaver, not a razor. Use lotion and a lip balm to prevent dry, chapped skin and lips. Tell your doctor or nurse if you are constipated or notice bleeding from your rectum.

- **Care for bleeding or bruising.** If you start to bleed, press down firmly on the area with a clean cloth. Keep pressing until the bleeding stops. If you bruise, put ice on the area.

Talking with Your Healthcare Team about Bleeding and Bruising

Prepare for your visit by making a list of questions to ask. Consider adding these questions to your list:

- What steps can I take to prevent bleeding or bruising?

- How long should I wait for the bleeding to stop before I call you or go the emergency room?

- Do I need to limit or avoid things that could increase my risk of bleeding, such as alcohol or sexual activity?

- What medicines, vitamins, or herbs should I avoid? Could I get a list from you of medicines to avoid?

Chapter 49

Fever, Sweats, and Hot Flashes

Hot flashes and night sweats may be side effects of cancer or its treatment. Sweating is the body's way of lowering body temperature by causing heat loss through the skin. In patients with cancer, sweating may be caused by fever, a tumor, or cancer treatment. Hot flashes can also cause too much sweating. They may occur in natural menopause or in patients who have been treated for breast cancer. Hot flashes combined with sweats that happen while sleeping are often called night sweats or hot flushes. Hot flashes and night sweats affect quality of life in many patients with cancer. A treatment plan to help manage hot flashes and night sweats is based on the patient's condition and goals of care. For some patients, relieving symptoms and improving quality of life is the most important goal.

Causes of Hot Flashes and Night Sweats in Patients with Cancer

In patients with cancer, hot flashes and night sweats may be caused by the tumor, its treatment, or other conditions. Sweating happens

This chapter includes text excerpted from "Hot Flashes and Night Sweats (PDQ®)—Patient Version," National Cancer Institute (NCI), March 16, 2018.

with disease conditions such as fever and may occur without disease in warm climates, during exercise, and during hot flashes in menopause. Sweating helps balance body temperature by allowing heat to evaporate through the skin.

Hot flashes and night sweats are common in patients with cancer and in cancer survivors. They are more common in women but can also occur in men.

Many patients treated for breast cancer have hot flashes. Menopause in women can have natural, surgical, or chemical causes. Chemical menopause in women with cancer is caused by certain types of chemotherapy, radiation, or hormone therapy with androgen (a male hormone).

Treatment for breast cancer can cause menopause or menopause-like effects, including severe hot flashes.

Certain types of drugs can cause night sweats. Drugs that may cause night sweats include the following:

- Tamoxifen

- Aromatase inhibitors

- Opioids

- Tricyclic antidepressants (TCAs)

- Steroids

Drug Treatment for Hot Flashes and Night Sweats in Patients with Cancer

Sweats caused by fever are controlled by treating the cause of the fever. Sweats caused by a tumor are usually controlled by treatment of the tumor. Hot flashes during natural or treatment-related menopause can be controlled with estrogen replacement therapy (ERT). However, many women are not able to take estrogen replacement (for example, women who have or had breast cancer). Hormone replacement therapy (HRT) that combines estrogen with progestin may increase the risk of breast cancer or breast cancer recurrence.

Other drugs may be useful in some patients. Studies of nonestrogen drugs to treat hot flashes in women with a history of breast cancer have reported that many of them do not work as well as estrogen replacement or have side effects. Megestrol (a drug like progesterone), certain antidepressants, anticonvulsants, and clonidine (a drug used to treat high blood pressure) are nonestrogen drugs used to control hot flashes. Some antidepressants may change how other drugs, such as tamoxifen, work in the body. Side effects of drug therapy may include the following:

- Antidepressants used to treat hot flashes over a short period of time may cause nausea, drowsiness, dry mouth, and changes in appetite.

- Anticonvulsants used to treat hot flashes may cause drowsiness, dizziness, and trouble concentrating.

- Clonidine may cause dry mouth, drowsiness, constipation, and insomnia.

Patients may respond in different ways to drug therapy. It is important that the patient's healthcare providers know about all medicines, dietary supplements, and herbs the patient is taking. Drugs that may relieve night-time hot flashes or night sweats and improve sleep at the same time are being studied in clinical trials.

If one medicine does not improve symptoms, switching to another medicine may help.

Nondrug Treatment for Hot Flashes and Night Sweats in Patients with Cancer

Treatments that change how patients deal with stress, anxiety, and negative emotions may help manage hot flashes. These are called psychological interventions. Psychological interventions help patients gain a sense of control and develop coping skills to manage symptoms. Staying calm and managing stress may lower levels of a hormone called serotonin that can trigger hot flashes.

Psychological interventions may help hot flashes and related problems when used together with drug treatment.

Hypnosis may help relieve hot flashes. It is a trance-like state that allows a person to be more aware, focused, and open to suggestion. Under hypnosis, the person can concentrate more clearly on a specific thought, feeling, or sensation without becoming distracted.

Hypnosis is a newer treatment for hot flashes that has been shown to be helpful. In hypnosis, a therapist helps the patient to deeply relax and focus on cooling thoughts. This may lower stress levels, balance body temperature, and calm the heart rate and breathing rate.

Comfort measures may be used to treat night sweats related to cancer. Since body temperature goes up before a hot flash, doing the following may control body temperature and help control symptoms:

- Wear loose-fitting clothes made of cotton.

- Use fans and open windows to keep air moving.

- Practice relaxation training and slow, deep breathing.

Herbs and dietary supplements should be used with caution. Studies of vitamin E for the relief of hot flashes show that it is only slightly better than a placebo (pill that has no effect). Most studies of soy and black cohosh show they are no better than a placebo in reducing hot flashes. Soy contains estrogen-like substances; the effect of soy on the risk of breast cancer growth or recurrence is not clear. Studies of ground flaxseed to treat hot flashes have shown mixed results.

Claims are made about several other plant-based and natural products as remedies for hot flashes. These include dong quai, milk thistle, red clover, licorice root extract, and chaste tree berry. Since little is known about how these products work or whether they affect the risk of breast cancer, women should be cautious about using them.

Acupuncture has been studied in the treatment of hot flashes. Pilot studies of acupuncture and randomized clinical trials that compare true acupuncture and sham (inactive) treatment have been done in patients with hot flashes and results are mixed. A review of many studies combined showed that acupuncture had slight or no effects in breast cancer patients with hot flashes.

Chapter 50

Treatment-Related Neuropathy

Cancer Treatment and Neuropathy[1]

Some cancer treatments cause peripheral neuropathy, a result of damage to the peripheral nerves. These nerves carry information from the brain to other parts of the body. Side effects depend on which peripheral nerves (sensory, motor, or autonomic) are affected.

Damage to sensory nerves (nerves that help you feel pain, heat, cold, and pressure) can cause:

- Tingling, numbness, or a pins-and-needles feeling in your feet and hands that may spread to your legs and arms

- Inability to feel a hot or cold sensation, such as a hot stove

- Inability to feel pain, such as from a cut or sore on your foot

---

This chapter includes text excerpted from documents published by two public domain sources. Text under headings marked 1 are excerpted from "Cancer Treatment—Side Effects—Nerve Problems (Peripheral Neuropathy) and Cancer Treatment," National Cancer Institute (NCI), December 4, 2017; Text under heading marked 2 is excerpted from "Peripheral Neuropathy Fact Sheet," National Institute of Neurological Disorders and Stroke (NINDS), December 2014. Reviewed May 2018.

Damage to motor nerves (nerves that help your muscles to move) can cause:

- Weak or achy muscles. You may lose your balance or trip easily. It may also be difficult to button shirts or open jars

- Muscles that twitch and cramp or muscle wasting (if you don't use your muscles regularly)

- Swallowing or breathing difficulties (if your chest or throat muscles are affected)

Damage to autonomic nerves (nerves that control functions such as blood pressure, digestion, heart rate, temperature, and urination) can cause:

- Digestive changes such as constipation or diarrhea

- Dizzy or faint feeling, due to low blood pressure

- Sexual problems; men may be unable to get an erection and women may not reach orgasm

- Sweating problems (either too much or too little sweating)

- Urination problems, such as leaking urine or difficulty emptying your bladder

If you start to notice any of the problems listed above, talk with your doctor or nurse. Getting these problems diagnosed and treated early is the best way to control them, prevent further damage, and to reduce pain and other complications.

What Are the Symptoms of Peripheral Nerve Damage?[1]

Symptoms vary depending on whether motor, sensory, or autonomic nerves are damaged. Motor nerves control voluntary movement of muscles such as those used for walking, grasping things, or talking. Sensory nerves transmit information such as the feeling of a light touch or the pain from a cut. Autonomic nerves control organ activities that are regulated automatically such as breathing, digesting food, and heart and gland functions. Some neuropathies may affect all three types of nerves; others primarily affect one or two types. Doctors may use terms such as predominantly motor neuropathy, predominantly sensory neuropathy, sensory-motor neuropathy, or autonomic neuropathy to describe the types of nerves involved in an individual's condition.

Motor nerve damage is most commonly associated with muscle weakness. Other symptoms may include painful cramps and fasciculations (uncontrolled muscle twitching visible under the skin), muscle atrophy (severe shrinkage of muscle size), and decreased reflexes.

Sensory nerve damage causes a variety of symptoms because sensory nerves have a broad range of functions. Larger sensory fibers enclosed in myelin register vibration, light touch, and position sense. Damage to large sensory fibers impairs touch, resulting in a general decrease in sensation. Since this is felt most in the hands and feet, people may feel as if they are wearing gloves and stockings even when they are not. This damage to larger sensory fibers may contribute to the loss of reflexes. Loss of position sense often makes people unable to coordinate complex movements like walking or fastening buttons, or to maintain their balance when their eyes are shut.

Smaller sensory fibers without myelin sheaths transmit pain and temperature sensations. Damage to these fibers can interfere with the ability to feel pain or changes in temperature. People may fail to sense that they have been injured from a cut or that a wound is becoming infected. Others may not detect pain that warns of impending heart attack or other acute conditions. Loss of pain sensation is a particularly serious problem for people with diabetes, contributing to the high rate of lower limb amputations among this population.

Neuropathic pain is a common, often difficult to control symptom of sensory nerve damage and can seriously affect emotional well-being and overall quality of life. Often worse at night, neuropathic pain seriously disrupts sleep and adds to the emotional burden of sensory nerve damage. Neuropathic pain can often be associated with an over sensitization of pain receptors in the skin, so that people feel severe pain (allodynia) from stimuli that are normally painless. For example, some may experience pain from bed sheets draped lightly over the body. Over many years, sensory neuropathy may lead to changes in the skin, hair, as well as to joint and bone damage. Unrecognized injuries due to poor sensation contribute to these changes, so it is important for people with neuropathy to inspect numb areas for injury or damage.

Autonomic nerve damage symptoms are diverse since the parasympathetic and sympathetic nerves of the peripheral nervous system control nearly every organ in the body. Common symptoms of autonomic nerve damage include an inability to sweat normally, which may lead to heat intolerance; a loss of bladder control; and an inability to control muscles that expand or contract blood vessels to regulate blood pressure. A drop in blood pressure when a person moves suddenly from a seated to a standing position (a condition known as postural or orthostatic hypotension) may result in dizziness, lightheadedness, or fainting. Irregular heartbeats may also occur.

Gastrointestinal symptoms may accompany autonomic neuropathy. Malfunction of nerves controlling intestinal muscle contractions can lead to diarrhea, constipation, or incontinence. Many people also have problems eating or swallowing if autonomic nerves controlling these functions are affected.

What Treatments Are Available?[2]

Address Underlying Conditions

The first step in treating peripheral neuropathy is to address any contributing causes such as infection, toxin exposure, medication-related toxicity, vitamin deficiencies, hormonal deficiencies, autoimmune disorders, or compression that can lead to neuropathy. Peripheral nerves have the ability to regenerate axons, as long as the nerve cell itself has not died, which may lead to functional recovery over time. Correcting an underlying condition often can result in the neuropathy resolving on its own as the nerves recover or regenerate.

The adoption of healthy lifestyle habits such as maintaining optimal weight, avoiding exposure to toxins, exercising, eating a balanced diet, correcting vitamin deficiencies, and limiting or avoiding alcohol consumption can reduce the effects of peripheral neuropathy. Exercise can reduce cramps, improve muscle strength, and prevent muscle wasting. Various dietary strategies can improve gastrointestinal symptoms. Timely treatment of injuries can help prevent permanent damage. Smoking cessation is particularly important because smoking constricts the blood vessels that supply nutrients to the peripheral nerves and can worsen neuropathic symptoms. Self-care skills such as meticulous foot care and careful wound treatment in people with diabetes and others who have an impaired ability to feel pain can alleviate symptoms and improve quality of life. Such changes often create conditions that encourage nerve regeneration.

Systemic diseases frequently require more complex treatments. Strict control of blood glucose levels has been shown to reduce neuropathic symptoms and help people with diabetic neuropathy avoid further nerve damage.

Inflammatory and autoimmune conditions leading to neuropathy can be controlled in several ways. Immunosuppressive drugs such as prednisone, cyclosporine, or azathioprine may be beneficial. Plasmapheresis—a procedure in which blood is removed, cleansed of immune system cells and antibodies, and then returned to the body—can help reduce inflammation or suppress immune system activity. Large intravenously administered doses of immunoglobulins (antibodies that alter the immune system, and agents such as rituximab that target specific inflammatory cells) also can suppress abnormal immune system activity.

Symptom Management

Neuropathic pain, or pain caused by the injury to a nerve or nerves, is often difficult to control. Mild pain may sometimes be alleviated by over-the-counter (OTC) analgesics such as nonsteroidal anti-inflammatory drugs (NSAIDs). More chronic and discomforting pain may need to be addressed through the care of a physician. Medications that are used for chronic neuropathic pain fall under several classes of drugs: antidepressants, anticonvulsant medications, antiarrhythmic medications, and narcotic agents. The antidepressant and anticonvulsant medications modulate pain through their mechanism of action on the peripheral nerves, spinal cord, or brain and tend to be the most effective types of medications to control neuropathic pain. Antidepressant medications include tricyclic antidepressants such as amitriptyline or newer serotonin-norepinephrine reuptake inhibitors such as duloxetine hydrochloride or venlafaxine. Anticonvulsant medications that are frequently used include gabapentin, pregabalin, topiramate, and carbamazepine, although other medications used for treating epilepsy may also be useful. Mexiletine is an antiarrhythmic medication that may be used for treatment of chronic painful neuropathies.

For pain that does not respond to the previously described medications, the addition of narcotic agents may be considered. Because the use of prescription obtained pain relievers that contain opioids can lead to dependence and addiction, their use is recommended only after other means of controlling the pain have failed. One of the newest narcotic medications approved for the treatment of diabetic neuropathy is tapentadol, a drug with both opioid activity and norepinephrine-reuptake inhibition activity of an antidepressant.

Topically administered medications are another option for neuropathic pain. Two agents are topical lidocaine, an anesthetic agent, and capsaicin, a substance found in hot peppers that modifies peripheral pain receptors. Topical agents are generally most appropriate for localized chronic pain such as herpes zoster neuralgia (shingles) pain. Their usefulness for treating diffuse chronic diabetic neuropathy is more limited.

Transcutaneous electrical nerve stimulation (TENS) is a noninvasive intervention used for pain relief in a range of conditions, and a number of studies have described its use for neuropathic pain. The therapy involves attaching electrodes to the skin at the site of pain or near associated nerves and then administering a gentle electrical current. Although data from controlled clinical trials are not available to broadly establish its efficacy for peripheral neuropathies, TENS has been shown in some studies to improve peripheral neuropathy symptoms associated with diabetes.

Other complementary approaches may provide additional support and pain relief. For example, mechanical aids such as hand or foot braces can help reduce pain and physical disability by compensating for muscle weakness or alleviating nerve compression. Orthopedic shoes can improve gait disturbances and help prevent foot injuries in people with a loss of pain sensation. Acupuncture, massage, and herbal medications also are considered in the treatment of neuropathic pain.

Surgical intervention can be considered for some types of neuropathies. Injuries to a single nerve caused by focal compression such as at the carpal tunnel of the wrist, or other entrapment neuropathies, may respond well to surgery that releases the nerve from the tissues compressing it. Some surgical procedures reduce pain by destroying the nerve; this approach is appropriate only for pain caused by a single nerve and when other forms of treatment have failed to provide relief. Peripheral neuropathies that involve more diffuse nerve damage, such as diabetic neuropathy, are not amenable to surgical intervention.

Ways to Prevent or Manage Problems Related to Nerve Changes[1]

You may be advised to take these steps:

- **Prevent falls.** Have someone help you prevent falls around the house. Move rugs out of your path so you will not trip on them. Put rails on the walls and in the bathroom, so you can hold on to them and balance yourself. Put bath mats in the shower or tub. Wear sturdy shoes with soft soles. Get up slowly after sitting or lying down, especially if you feel dizzy.

- **Take extra care in the kitchen and shower.** Use potholders in the kitchen to protect your hands from burns. Be careful when handling knives or sharp objects. Ask someone to check the water temperature, to make sure it's not too hot.

- **Protect your hands and feet.** Wear shoes, both inside and outside. Check your arms, legs, and feet for cuts or scratches everyday. When it's cold, wear warm clothes to protect your hands and feet.

- **Ask for help and slow down.** Let people help you with difficult tasks. Slow down and give yourself more time to do things.

- **Ask about pain medicine and integrative medicine practices.** You may be prescribed pain medicine. Sometimes practices such as acupuncture, massage, physical therapy, yoga, and others may also be advised to lower pain. Talk with your healthcare team to learn what is advised for you.

Talking with Your Healthcare Team[1]

Prepare for your visit by making a list of questions to ask. Consider adding these questions to your list:

- What symptoms or problems might I have? Which ones should I call you about?

- When will these problems start? How long might they last?

- What medicine, treatments, and integrative medicine practices could help me to feel better?

- What steps can I take to feel better? What precautions should I take to stay safe?

- Could you refer me to a specialist

Chapter 51

Cancer Treatment and Physical Appearance

Chapter Contents

Section 51.1

Hair Loss (Alopecia)

This section includes text excerpted from "Side
Effects: Hair Loss (Alopecia) and Cancer Treatment,"
National Cancer Institute (NCI), December 4, 2017.

Some types of chemotherapy cause the hair on your head and other
parts of your body to fall out. Radiation therapy can also cause hair
loss on the part of the body that is being treated. Hair loss is called
alopecia. Talk with your healthcare team to learn if the cancer treatment you will be receiving causes hair loss. Your doctor or nurse will
share strategies that have help others, including those listed below.

Ways to Manage Hair Loss

Talk with your healthcare team about ways to manage before and
after hair loss:

- **Treat your hair gently.** You may want to use a hairbrush with
  soft bristles or a wide-tooth comb. Do not use hair dryers, irons,
  or products such as gels or clips that may hurt your scalp. Wash
  your hair with a mild shampoo. Wash it less often and be very
  gentle. Pat it dry with a soft towel.

- **You have choices.** Some people choose to cut their hair short
  to make it easier to deal with when it starts to fall out. Others
  choose to shave their head. If you choose to shave your head,
  use an electric shaver so you won't cut yourself. If you plan to
  buy a wig, get one while you still have hair so you can match it
  to the color of your hair. If you find wigs to be itchy and hot, try
  wearing a comfortable scarf or turban.

- **Protect and care for your scalp.** Use sunscreen or wear a
  hat when you are outside. Choose a comfortable scarf or hat that
  you enjoy and that keeps your head warm. If your scalp itches
  or feels tender, using lotions and conditioners can help it feel
  better.

- **Talk about your feelings.** Many people feel angry, depressed, or embarrassed about hair loss. It can help to share these feelings with someone who understands. Some people find it helpful to talk with other people who have lost their hair during cancer treatment. Talking openly and honestly with your children and close family members can also help you all. Tell them that you expect to lose your hair during treatment.

Ways to Care for Your Hair When It Grows Back

- **Be gentle.** When your hair starts to grow back, you will want to be gentle with it. Avoid too much brushing, curling, and blow-drying. You may not want to wash your hair as frequently.

- **After chemotherapy.** Hair often grows back in 2–3 months after treatment has ended. Your hair will be very fine when it starts to grow back. Sometimes your new hair can be curlier or straighter—or even a different color. In time, it may go back to how it was before treatment.

- **After radiation therapy.** Hair often grows back in 3–6 months after treatment has ended. If you received a very high dose of radiation your hair may grow back thinner or not at all on the part of your body that received radiation.

Talking with Your Healthcare Team about Hair Loss

Prepare for your visit by making a list of questions to ask. Consider adding these questions to your list:

- Is treatment likely to cause my hair to fall out?

- How should I protect and care for my head? Are there products that you recommend? Ones I should avoid?

- Where can I get a wig or hairpiece?

- What support groups could I meet with that might help?

- When will my hair grow back?

Section 51.2

Nail and Skin Care

This section includes text excerpted from "Side
Effects: Skin and Nail Changes during Cancer Treatment,"
National Cancer Institute (NCI), April 29, 2015.

Cancer treatments may cause a range of skin and nail changes. Talk with your healthcare team to learn whether or not you will have these changes, based on the treatment you are receiving.

- Radiation therapy can cause the skin on the part of your body receiving radiation therapy to become dry and peel, itch (called pruritus), and turn red or darker. It may look sunburned or tan and be swollen or puffy.

- Chemotherapy may damage fast-growing skin and nail cells. This can cause problems such as skin that is dry, itchy, red, and/ or that peels. Some people may develop a rash or sun sensitivity, causing you to sunburn easily. Nail changes may include dark, yellow, or cracked nails and/or cuticles that are red and hurt. Chemotherapy in people who have received radiation therapy in the past can cause skin to become red, blister, peel, or hurt on the part of the body that received radiation therapy; this is called radiation recall.

- Biological therapy may cause itching (pruritus).

- Targeted therapy may cause a dry skin, a rash, and nail problems.

These skin problems are more serious and need urgent medical attention:

- Sudden or severe itching, a rash, or hives during chemotherapy. These may be signs of an allergic reaction.

- Sores on the part of your body where you are receiving treatment that become painful, wet, and/or infected. This is called a moist reaction and may happen in areas where the skin folds, such as around your ears, breast, or bottom.

Your doctor or nurse will talk with about possible skin and nail changes and advise you on ways to treat or prevent them.

Ways to Manage Skin and Nail Changes

Depending on what treatment you are receiving, you may be advised to take these steps to protect your skin, prevent infection, and reduce itching:

- **Use only recommended skin products.** Use mild soaps that are gentle on your skin. Ask your nurse to recommend specific lotions and creams. Ask when and how often to use them. Ask what skin products to avoid. For example, you may be advised to not use powders or antiperspirants before radiation therapy.

- **Protect your skin.** Ask about lotions or antibiotics for dry, itchy, infected or swollen skin. Don't use heating pads, ice packs, or bandages on the area receiving radiation therapy. Shave less often and use an electric razor or stop shaving if your skin is sore. Wear sunscreen and lip balm or a loose-fitting long-sleeved shirt, pants, and a hat with a wide brim when outdoors.

- **Prevent or treat dry, itchy skin (pruritus).** Your doctor will work to assess the cause of pruritus. There are also steps you can take to feel better. Avoid products with alcohol or perfume, which can dry or irritate your skin. Take short showers or baths in lukewarm, not hot, water. Put on lotion after drying off from a shower, while your skin is still slightly damp. Keep your home cool and humid. Eat a healthy diet and drink plenty of fluids to help keep your skin moist and healthy. Applying a cool washcloth or ice to the affected area may also help. Acupuncture also helps some people.

- **Prevent or treat minor nail problems.** Keep your nails clean and cut short. Wear gloves when you wash the dishes, work in the garden, or clean the house. Check with your nurse about products that can help your nails.

If your skin hurts in the area where you get treatment, tell your doctor or nurse. Your skin might have a moist reaction. Most often this happens in areas where the skin folds, such as behind the ears or under the breasts. It can lead to an infection if not properly treated. Ask your doctor or nurse how to care for these areas.

Talking with Your Healthcare Team about Skin and Nail Changes

Prepare for your visit by making a list of questions to ask. Consider adding these questions to your list:

- What symptoms or problems should I call you about?
- What steps can I take to feel better?
- What brands of soap and lotion are best for me to use? What products can help my nails stay healthy?
- What skin and nail products should I avoid?
- When will these problems go away?

Chapter 52

Cognitive-Related Effects of Cancer Treatment

Cognition is the process of gaining knowledge and understanding through thought, experience, and the senses. The thinking process includes being able to do the following:

- Focus on the important information, thoughts, and actions.

- Pay attention to a task or activity for a long period of time.

- Predict what may happen, plan, and solve problems.

- Take in new information quickly.

- Have a sense of where objects are around you.

- Understand and communicate by speaking or writing.

- Learn and remember new information.

This chapter is about cognitive changes that occur in cancer patients and cancer survivors who do not or did not have cancer in the central nervous system (CNS) (brain or spinal cord). Memory and thinking problems may occur in cancer patients and cancer survivors. Changes in memory and thinking are common in cancer patients and cancer

This chapter includes text excerpted from "Cognitive Impairment in Adults with Non-Central Nervous System Cancers (PDQ®)—Patient Version," National Cancer Institute (NCI), March 20, 2018.

survivors and are to be expected. Your thinking process may change, making it harder for you to pay attention and remember information the same way as you did before your cancer treatment. Talk to your doctor about memory and thinking problems that may happen with your type of cancer or after treatment.

Signs of Cognitive Problems

Possible signs of cognitive problems include trouble learning or remembering. Other conditions may also cause cognitive problems. Talk to your doctor if you have any of the following problems:

- Trouble focusing on one thing
- Being unable to complete tasks
- Memory loss
- Trouble understanding what people are saying
- Trouble remembering names and common words
- Being unable to recognize familiar objects
- Trouble following instructions
- Being unable to manage your money well. For example, you may have trouble paying bills or balancing your checkbook.
- Disorganized behavior or thinking
- Loss of motivation
- Change in how you see the world around you

Causes of Cognitive Problems

Cancer treatments or other diseases may cause cognitive problems. Factors that may cause cognitive problems in cancer patients and cancer survivors include the following:

- Older age
- Being weak or frail
- Cancer treatments, such as chemotherapy or radiation therapy, or other medications, and their side effects
- Being postmenopausal
- Having emotional distress, such as anxiety or depression

- Having certain symptoms, such as pain, fatigue, or trouble sleeping

- Having other diseases or conditions

- Using alcohol or other substances that change your mental state

Your doctor will do an exam to check for signs of disease. Your doctor will also ask you about factors that cause cognitive problems, and your education, job, and daily activities.

Treatment for Cognitive Problems

Treatment of cognitive problems may include activities that help your attention, memory, and thinking.

Cognitive Rehabilitation

The goal of cognitive rehabilitation is to improve your memory, thinking, organization, and decision-making skills. Cognitive rehabilitation includes the following:

- Learning how the brain works

- Learning ways to take in new information and perform new tasks or behaviors

- Using tools to help stay organized, such as calendars or electronic diaries

- Doing activities over and over, usually on a computer, that become more challenging over time

Movement Therapy

Movement therapy or exercises, such as tai chi, qigong, or yoga, may help improve your thinking and ability to focus.

Attention Restoration

Attention restoring activities may help you to focus and concentrate. These include walking, gardening, bird watching, and caring for pets.

Meditation

Meditation may help improve your cognitive function. Meditation is a mind-body practice in which a person focuses his or her attention on something, such as an object, word, phrase, or breathing. This will help keep you from being distracted or having stressful thoughts or feelings. Mindfulness-based stress reduction is a type of meditation that focuses on bringing attention and awareness to each moment.

Several drugs have been studied to treat cognitive problems in cancer patients and survivors, such as psychostimulants and erythropoietin-stimulating agents, but results are mixed. More research is needed.

Part Seven

Women's Issues in Cancer Survivorship

Chapter 53

Life after Cancer Treatment

All cancer survivors should have follow-up care. Knowing what to expect after cancer treatment can help you and your family make plans, lifestyle changes, and important decisions.

Some common questions you may have are:

- Should I tell the doctor about symptoms that worry me?

- Which doctors should I see after treatment?

- How often should I see my doctor?

- What tests do I need?

- What can be done to relieve pain, fatigue, or other problems after treatment?

- How long will it take for me to recover and feel more like myself?

- Is there anything I can or should be doing to keep cancer from coming back?

- Will I have trouble with health insurance?

- Are there any support groups I can go to?

Coping with these issues can be a challenge. Yet many say that getting involved in decisions about their medical care and lifestyle

---

This chapter includes text excerpted from "Facing Forward—Life after Cancer Treatment," National Cancer Institute (NCI), May 2014. Reviewed May 2018.

was a good way for them to regain some of the control they felt they lost during cancer treatment. Research has shown that people who feel more in control feel and function better than those who do not. Being an active partner with your doctor and getting help from other members of your healthcare team is the first step.

What Is Follow-Up Care?

Once you have finished your cancer treatment, you should receive a follow-up cancer care plan. Follow-up care means seeing a doctor for regular medical checkups. Your follow-up care plan depends on the type of cancer and type of treatment you had, along with your overall health. It is usually different for each person who has been treated for cancer.

In general, survivors usually return to the doctor every 3–4 months during the first 2–3 years after treatment, and once or twice a year after that. At these visits, your doctor will look for side effects from treatment and check if your cancer has returned (recurred) or spread (metastasized) to another part of your body.

At these visits, your doctor will:

- Review your medical history
- Give you a physical exam

Your doctor may run follow-up tests such as:

- Blood tests
- Magnetic resonance imaging (MRI) or computed tomography (CT) scans. These scans take detailed pictures of areas inside the body at different angles.
- Endoscopy. This test uses a thin, lighted tube to examine the inside of the body.

At your first follow-up visit, talk with your doctor about your follow-up care plan.

Medical Records and Follow-Up Care

Be sure to ask your oncologist for a written summary of your treatment. In the summary, he or she can suggest what aspects of your health need to be followed. Then, share this summary with any new doctors you see, especially your primary care doctor, as you discuss your follow-up care plan.

Many people keep their medical records in a binder or folder and refer to them as they see new doctors. This keeps key facts about your cancer treatment in the same place. Other kinds of health information you should keep include:

- The date you were diagnosed

- The type of cancer you were treated for

- Pathology report(s) that describe the type and stage of cancer

- Places and dates of specific treatment, such as:

  - Details of all surgeries

  - Sites and total amounts of radiation therapy

  - Names and doses of chemotherapy and all other drugs

  - Key lab reports, X-ray reports, CT scans, and MRI reports

- List of signs to watch for and possible long-term effects of treatment

- Contact information for all health professionals involved in your treatment and follow-up care

- Any problems that occurred during or after treatment

- Information about supportive care you received (such as special medicines, emotional support, and nutritional supplements)

Which Doctor Should I See Now? How Often?

You will need to decide which doctor will provide your follow-up cancer care and which one(s) you will see for other medical care. For follow-up cancer care, this may be the same doctor who provided your cancer treatment. For regular medical care, you may decide to see your main provider, such as a family doctor. For specific concerns, you may want to see a specialist. This is a topic you can discuss with your doctors. They can help you decide how to make transitions in care.

Depending on where you live, it may make more sense to get follow-up cancer care from your family doctor, rather than your oncologist. It's important to note that some insurance plans pay for follow-up care only with certain doctors and for a set number of visits.

In coming up with your schedule, you may want to check your health insurance plan to see what follow-up care it allows. No matter what your health coverage situation is, try to find doctors you feel comfortable with. Always tell any new doctors you see about your history of cancer. The type of cancer you had and your treatment can affect decisions about your care in the future. They may not know about your cancer unless you tell them.

A Survivor's Wellness Plan

After cancer treatment, many survivors want to find ways to reduce the chances of their cancer coming back. Some worry that the way they eat, the stress in their lives, or their exposure to chemicals may put them at risk. Cancer survivors find that this is a time when they take a good look at how they take care of themselves. This is an important start to living a healthy life. When you meet with your doctor about follow-up care, you should also ask about developing a wellness plan that includes ways you can take care of your physical, emotional, social, and spiritual needs. If you find that it's hard to talk with your doctor about these issues, it may be helpful to know that the more you do it, the easier it becomes. And your doctor may suggest other members of the healthcare team for you to talk with, such as a social worker, clergy member, or nurse.

Changes You May Want to Think about Making

- **Quit smoking.** Research shows that smoking can increase the chances of getting cancer at the same site or another site.

- **Cut down on how much alcohol you drink.** Research shows that drinking alcohol increases your chances of getting certain types of cancers.

- **Eat well.** Healthy food choices and physical activity may help reduce the risk of cancer or recurrence. Talk with your doctor or a nutritionist to find out about any special dietary needs that you may have. The American Cancer Society (ACS) and the American Institute for Cancer Research (AICR) have developed similar diet and fitness guidelines that may help reduce the risk of cancer:

  - Eat a plant-based diet and have at least 5–9 servings of fruit and vegetables daily. Try to include beans in your diet, and eat whole grains (such as cereals, breads, and pasta) several times daily.

  - Choose foods low in fat and low in salt.

  - Get to and stay at a healthy weight.

- **Exercise and stay active.** Several recent reports suggest that staying active after cancer can help lower the risk of recurrence and can lead to longer survival. Moderate exercise (walking, biking, swimming) for about 30 minutes every—or almost every—day can:

  - Reduce anxiety and depression

  - Improve mood and boost self-esteem

  - Reduce fatigue, nausea, pain, and diarrhea

It is important to start an exercise program slowly and increase activity over time, working with your doctor or a specialist (such as a physical therapist) if needed. If you need to stay in bed during your recovery, even small activities like stretching or moving your arms or legs can help you stay flexible, relieve muscle tension, and help you feel better. Some people may need to take special care in exercising. Talk with your doctor before you begin any exercise program.

Talking with Your Doctor

During cancer treatment, you had a lot of practice in getting the most out of every doctor's visit. These same skills now apply to you as a survivor and are especially helpful if you are changing doctors or going back to a family or primary care doctor you may not have seen for a while.

It is important to be able to talk openly with your doctor. Both of you need information to manage your care. Be sure to tell your doctor if you are having trouble doing everyday activities, and talk about new symptoms to watch for and what to do about them. If you are concerned that the treatment you had puts you at a higher risk for having health problems, be sure to discuss this with your doctor as you develop your follow-up plan.

At each visit, mention any health issues you are having, such as:

- New symptoms

- Pain that troubles you

- Physical problems that get in the way of your daily life or that bother you, such as fatigue, trouble sleeping, sexual problems, or weight gain or loss

- Other health problems you have, such as heart disease, diabetes, or arthritis

619

- Medicines, vitamins, or herbs you are taking and other treatments you are using

- Emotional problems, such as anxiety or depression, that you may have now or that you've had in the past

- Changes in your family's medical history, such as relatives with cancer

- Things you want to know more about, such as new research or side effects

Just because you have certain symptoms, it doesn't always mean the cancer has come back. Symptoms can be due to other problems that need to be addressed.

Guidelines for Follow-Up Care

The following programs or organizations provide helpful follow-up care guidelines for some cancers. You can use them as you talk with your doctor—they aren't meant to contradict or take the place of your doctor's knowledge or judgment. Ask your oncologist for a treatment summary and a survivorship care plan. Both documents are recommended by the National Cancer Institute (NCI) and other cancer organizations.

- **Cancer.Net.** The American Society of Clinical Oncology (ASCO) has a series of follow-up care guides focused on breast and colorectal cancer. They can be viewed at www.cancer.net/ survivorship.

- **Children's Oncology Group Long-Term Follow-up Guidelines.** The Children's Oncology Group (COG) offers long-term follow-up guidelines for survivors of childhood, adolescent, and young adult cancers at www. survivorshipguidelines.org.

- **Journey Forward.** The Journey Forward is a program centered on its Survivorship Care Plan. By using an online Care Plan Builder, the oncologist creates a full medical summary and recommendations for follow-up care to be shared with patients and their primary care providers. It was created by the National Coalition for Cancer Survivorship (NCCS), University of California at Los Angeles (UCLA) Cancer Survivorship Center, Genentech, and WellPoint, Inc.

- **Life after Cancer Care.** M.D. Anderson's Cancer Center website lists follow-up guidelines for 15 different disease sites at www.mdanderson.org/patients-family/life-after-cancer.

- **Livestrong Care Plan.** Developed by Livestrong and the University of Pennsylvania, the Livestrong Care Plan gives individuals a specific survivor care plan, based on the information they enter into the online program.

- **National Comprehensive Cancer Network (NCCN).** The NCCN website includes information about follow-up care for cancer, along with guidance on making formal survivorship plans.

Services to Think About

Talk with your doctor to help you locate services such as these:

- **Couples counseling.** You and your partner work with trained specialists who can help you talk about problems, learn about each other's needs, and find ways to cope. Counseling may include issues related to sex and intimacy.

- **Faith or spiritual counseling.** Some members of the clergy are trained to help you cope with cancer concerns, such as feeling alone, fear of death, searching for meaning, and doubts about faith.

- **Family support programs.** Your whole family may be involved in the healing process. In these programs, you and your family members take part in therapy sessions with trained specialists who can help you talk about problems, learn about each other's needs, and find answers.

- **Genetic counseling.** Trained specialists can advise you on whether to have genetic testing for cancer and how to deal with the results. It can be helpful for you and for family members who have concerns about their own health.

- **Home care services.** State and local governments offer many services that you may find useful after cancer treatment. For example, a nurse or physical therapist may be able to come to your home. You may also be able to get help with housework or cooking. Check the phone book under the categories Social Services, Health Services, or Aging Services.

- **Individual counseling.** Trained mental health specialists can help you deal with your feelings, such as anger, sadness, and concern for your future.

- **Long-term follow-up clinics.** All doctors can offer follow-up care, but there are also clinics that specialize in long-term follow-up after cancer. These clinics most often see people who are no longer being treated by an oncologist and who are considered disease-free. Ask your doctor if there are any follow-up cancer clinics in your area.

- **Nutritionists/Dietitians.** They can help you with gaining or losing weight and with healthy eating.

- **Occupational therapists.** They can help you regain, develop, and build skills that are important for day-to-day living. They can help you relearn how to do daily activities, such as bathing, dressing, or feeding yourself, after cancer treatment.

- **Oncology social workers.** These professionals are trained to counsel you about ways to cope with treatment issues and family problems related to your cancer. They can tell you about resources and connect you with services in your area.

- **Ostomy information and support.** The United Ostomy Association of America (UOAA) provides education, information, and support for people with intestinal/urinary diversions. Call 800-826-0826, or visit online at www.ostomy.org.

- **Pain clinics (also called Pain and Palliative Care Services).** These are centers with professionals from many different fields who are specially trained in helping people get relief from pain.

- **Physical therapists.** Physical therapists are trained to understand how different parts of your body work together. They can teach you about proper exercises and body motions that can help you gain strength and move better after treatment. They can also advise you about proper postures that help prevent injuries.

- **Quitting smoking (Smoking Cessation Services).** Research shows that the more support you have in quitting smoking, the greater your chance for success. Ask your doctor, nurse, social worker, or hospital about available programs, or call NCI's Smoking Quitline at 877-44-U-QUIT (877-448-7848).

- **Speech therapists.** Speech therapists can evaluate and treat any speech, language, or swallowing problems you may have after treatment.

- **Stress management programs.** These programs teach ways to help you relax and take more control over stress. Hospitals, clinics, or local cancer organizations may offer these programs and classes.

- **Support groups for survivors.** In-person and online groups enable survivors to interact with others in similar situations.

- **Survivor wellness programs.** These types of programs are growing in number, and they are meant for people who have finished their cancer treatment and are interested in redefining their life beyond cancer.

- **Vocational rehabilitation specialists.** If you have disabilities or other special needs, these specialists can help you find suitable jobs. They offer services such as counseling, education and skills training, and help in obtaining and using assistive technology and tools.

Chapter 54

Nutrition in Cancer Care

Good nutrition is important for cancer patients. Nutrition is a process in which food is taken in and used by the body for growth, to keep the body healthy, and to replace tissue. Good nutrition is important for good health. Eating the right kinds of foods before, during, and after cancer treatment can help the patient feel better and stay stronger. A healthy diet includes eating and drinking enough of the foods and liquids that have important nutrients (vitamins, minerals, protein, carbohydrates, fat, and water) the body needs.

Healthy eating habits are important during and after cancer treatment. Nutrition therapy is used to help cancer patients keep a healthy body weight, maintain strength, keep body tissue healthy, and decrease side effects both during and after treatment.

A registered dietitian (or nutritionist) is a part of the team of health professionals that help with cancer treatment and recovery. A dietitian will work with patients, their families, and the rest of the medical team to manage the patient's diet during and after cancer treatment. Cancer and cancer treatments may cause side effects that affect nutrition. For many patients, the effects of cancer and cancer treatments make it hard to eat well. Cancer treatments that affect nutrition include:

- Chemotherapy

- Hormone therapy

This chapter includes text excerpted from "Nutrition in Cancer Care (PDQ®)—Patient Version," National Cancer Institute (NCI), March 16, 2018.

- Radiation therapy

- Surgery

- Immunotherapy

- Stem cell transplant

When the head, neck, esophagus, stomach, intestines, pancreas, or liver are affected by the cancer treatment, it is hard to take in enough nutrients to stay healthy.

Cancer and cancer treatments may affect taste, smell, appetite, and the ability to eat enough food or absorb the nutrients from food. This can cause malnutrition, which is a condition caused by a lack of key nutrients. Alcohol abuse and obesity may increase the risk of malnutrition.

Malnutrition can cause the patient to be weak, tired, and unable to fight infection or finish cancer treatment. Malnutrition may be made worse if the cancer grows or spreads. Eating the right amount of protein and calories is important for healing, fighting infection, and having enough energy.

Anorexia and cachexia are common causes of malnutrition in cancer patients. Anorexia is the loss of appetite or desire to eat. It is a common symptom in patients with cancer. Anorexia may occur early in the disease or later, if the cancer grows or spreads. Some patients already have anorexia when they are diagnosed with cancer. Most patients who have advanced cancer will have anorexia. Anorexia is the most common cause of malnutrition in cancer patients.

Cachexia is a condition marked by weakness, weight loss, and fat and muscle loss. It is common in patients with tumors that affect eating and digestion. It can occur in cancer patients who are eating well, but are not storing fat and muscle because of tumor growth.

Some tumors change the way the body uses certain nutrients. The body's use of protein, carbohydrates, and fat may be affected, especially by tumors of the stomach, intestines, or head and neck. A patient may seem to be eating enough, but the body may not be able to absorb all the nutrients from the food.

Cancer patients may have anorexia and cachexia at the same time.

Effects of Cancer Treatment on Nutrition

Chemotherapy and Hormone Therapy

Chemotherapy and hormone therapy affect nutrition in different ways. Chemotherapy affects cells all through the body. Chemotherapy uses drugs to stop the growth of cancer cells, either by killing the cells or by stopping them from dividing. Healthy cells that normally grow and divide quickly may also be killed. These include cells in the mouth and digestive tract.

Hormone therapy adds, blocks, or removes hormones. It may be used to slow or stop the growth of certain cancers. Some types of hormone therapy may cause weight gain.

Chemotherapy and hormone therapy cause different nutrition problems. Side effects from chemotherapy may cause problems with eating and digestion. When more than one chemotherapy drug is given, each drug may cause different side effects or when drugs cause the same side effect, the side effect may be more severe.

The following side effects are common:

- Loss of appetite
- Nausea
- Vomiting
- Dry mouth
- Sores in the mouth or throat
- Changes in the way food tastes
- Trouble swallowing
- Feeling full after eating a small amount of food
- Constipation
- Diarrhea

Patients receiving hormone therapy may need changes in their diet to prevent weight gain.

Radiation Therapy

Radiation therapy kills cancer cells and healthy cells in the treatment area. How severe the side effects are depends on the following:

- The part of the body that is treated
- The total dose of radiation and how it is given

Radiation therapy may affect nutrition. Radiation therapy to any part of the digestive system has side effects that cause nutrition problems. Most of the side effects begin 2–3 weeks after radiation therapy begins and go away a few weeks after it is finished. Some side effects can continue for months or years after treatment ends.

The following are some of the more common side effects:

- For radiation therapy to the brain or head and neck

  - Loss of appetite

  - Nausea

  - Vomiting

  - Dry mouth or thick saliva. Medication may be given to treat a dry mouth

  - Sore mouth and gums

  - Changes in the way food tastes

  - Trouble swallowing

  - Pain when swallowing

  - Being unable to fully open the mouth

- For radiation therapy to the chest

  - Loss of appetite

  - Nausea

  - Vomiting

  - Trouble swallowing

  - Pain when swallowing

  - Choking or breathing problems caused by changes in the upper esophagus

- For radiation therapy to the abdomen, pelvis, or rectum

  - Nausea

  - Vomiting

  - Bowel obstruction

  - Colitis

  - Diarrhea

Radiation therapy may also cause tiredness, which can lead to a decrease in appetite.

Surgery

Surgery increases the body's need for nutrients and energy. The body needs extra energy and nutrients to heal wounds, fight infection, and recover from surgery. If the patient is malnourished before surgery, it may cause problems during recovery, such as poor healing or infection. For these patients, nutrition care may begin before surgery.

Surgery to the head, neck, esophagus, stomach, or intestines may affect nutrition.

Most cancer patients are treated with surgery. Surgery that removes all or part of certain organs can affect a patient's ability to eat and digest food.

The following are nutrition problems caused by surgery:

- Loss of appetite

- Trouble chewing

- Trouble swallowing

- Feeling full after eating a small amount of food

Immunotherapy

Immunotherapy may affect nutrition. The side effects of immunotherapy are different for each patient and the type of immunotherapy drug given.

The following nutrition problems are common:

- Tiredness

- Fever

- Nausea

- Vomiting

- Diarrhea

Stem Cell Transplant

Patients who receive a stem cell transplant have special nutrition needs.

Chemotherapy, radiation therapy, and other medicines used before or during a stem cell transplant may cause side effects that keep a patient from eating and digesting food as usual.

Common side effects include the following:

- Mouth and throat sores

- Diarrhea

Patients who receive a stem cell transplant have a high risk of infection. Chemotherapy or radiation therapy given before the transplant decrease the number of white blood cells, which fight infection. It is important that these patients learn about safe food handling and avoid foods that may cause infection.

After a stem cell transplant, patients are at risk for acute or chronic graft-versus-host disease (GVHD). GVHD may affect the gastrointestinal tract or liver and change the patient's ability to eat or absorb nutrients from food.

Nutrition Assessment in Cancer Care

The healthcare team may ask questions about diet and weight history. Screening is used to look for health problems that affect the risk of poor nutrition. This can help find out if the patient is likely to become malnourished, and if nutrition therapy is needed.

The healthcare team may ask questions about the following:

- Weight changes over the past year

- Changes in the amount and type of food eaten

- Problems that have affected eating, such as loss of appetite, nausea, vomiting, diarrhea, constipation, mouth sores, dry mouth, changes in taste and smell, or pain

- Ability to walk and do other activities of daily living (dressing, getting into or out of a bed or chair, taking a bath or shower, and using the toilet)

A physical exam is done to check the body for general health and signs of disease. The patient is checked for signs of loss of weight, fat, and muscle, and for fluid buildup in the body.

Counseling and diet changes are made to improve the patient's nutrition. A registered dietitian can work with patients and their families to counsel them on ways to improve the patient's nutrition. The registered dietitian gives care based on the patient's nutrition and diet needs. Changes to the diet are made to help decrease symptoms from cancer or cancer treatment. These changes may be in the types and amount of food, how often a patient eats, and how food is eaten (for example, at a certain temperature or taken with a straw).

A registered dietitian works with other members of the healthcare team to check the patient's nutritional health during cancer treatment and recovery. In addition to the dietitian, the healthcare team may include the following:

- Physician

- Nurse

- Social worker

- Psychologist

The goal of nutrition therapy for patients who have advanced cancer depends on the overall plan of care. The goal of nutrition therapy in patients with advanced cancer is to give patients the best possible quality of life and control symptoms that cause distress. Patients with advanced cancer may be treated with anticancer therapy and palliative care, palliative care alone, or may be in hospice care. Nutrition goals will be different for each patient. Some types of treatment may be stopped if they are not helping the patient. As the focus of care goes from cancer treatment to hospice or end-of-life care, nutrition goals may become less aggressive, and a change to care meant to keep the patient as comfortable as possible.

Types of Nutrition Support

Nutrition support helps patients who cannot eat or digest food normally. It is best to take in food by mouth whenever possible. Some patients may not be able to take in enough food by mouth because of problems from cancer or cancer treatment. Nutrition support can be given in different ways. In addition to counseling by a dietitian, and changes to the diet, nutrition therapy includes nutritional supplement drinks, and enteral and parenteral nutrition support. Nutritional supplement drinks help cancer patients get the nutrients they need. They provide energy, protein, fat, carbohydrates, fiber, vitamins, and minerals. They are not meant to be the patient's only source of nutrition. A patient who is not able to take in the right amount of calories and nutrients by mouth may be fed using the following:

- **Enteral nutrition:** Nutrients are given through a tube inserted into the stomach or intestines

- **Parenteral nutrition:** Nutrients are infused into the bloodstream

The nutrients are given in liquid formulas that have water, protein, fats, carbohydrates, vitamins, and/or minerals. Nutrition support can improve a patient's quality of life during cancer treatment, but may cause problems that should be considered before making the decision to use it. The patient and healthcare team should discuss the harms and benefits of each type of nutrition support.

Enteral Nutrition

Enteral nutrition is also called tube feeding. It is giving the patient nutrients in liquid form (formula) through a tube that is placed into the stomach or small intestine. The following types of feeding tubes may be used:

- A nasogastric tube is inserted through the nose and down the throat into the stomach or small intestine. This is used when enteral nutrition is only needed for a few weeks.

- A gastrostomy tube is inserted into the stomach or a jejunostomy tube is inserted into the small intestine through an opening made on the outside of the abdomen. This is usually used for long-term enteral feeding or for patients who cannot use a tube in the nose and throat.

The type of formula used is based on the specific needs of the patient. There are formulas for patients who have special health conditions, such as diabetes, or other needs, such as religious or cultural diets.

Parenteral Nutrition

Parenteral nutrition carries nutrients directly into the bloodstream. It is used when the patient cannot take food by mouth or by enteral feeding. Parenteral feeding does not use the stomach or intestines to digest food. Nutrients are given to the patient directly into the blood, through a catheter inserted into a vein. These nutrients include proteins, fats, vitamins, and minerals.

The catheter may be placed into a vein in the chest or in the arm. A central venous access catheter is placed beneath the skin and into a large vein in the upper chest. The catheter is put in place by a surgeon. This type of catheter is used for long-term parenteral feeding. A peripheral venous catheter is placed into a vein in the arm. A peripheral venous catheter is put in place by trained medical staff. This type of catheter is usually used for short-term parenteral feeding for patients who do not have a central venous access catheter. The patient is checked often for infection or bleeding at the place where the catheter enters the body.

Nutrition Trends in Cancer

Some cancer patients try special diets to improve their prognosis. Cancer patients may try special diets to make their treatment work better, prevent side effects from treatment, or to treat the cancer itself. However, for most of these special diets, there is no evidence that shows they work.

Vegetarian or Vegan Diet

It is not known if following a vegetarian or vegan diet can help side effects from cancer treatment or the patient's prognosis. If the patient already follows a vegetarian or vegan diet, there is no evidence that shows they should switch to a different diet.

Macrobiotic Diet

A macrobiotic diet is a high-carbohydrate, low-fat, plant-based diet. No studies have shown that this diet will help cancer patients.

Ketogenic Diet

A ketogenic diet limits carbohydrates and increases fat intake. The purpose of the diet is to decrease the amount of glucose (sugar) the tumor cells can use to grow and reproduce. It is a hard diet to follow because exact amounts of fats, carbohydrates, and proteins are needed. However, the diet is safe.

Several clinical trials are recruiting glioblastoma patients to study whether a ketogenic diet affects glioblastoma tumor activity. Patients with glioblastoma who want to start a ketogenic diet should talk to their doctor and work with a registered dietitian. However, it is not yet known how the diet will affect the tumor or its symptoms.

Dietary Supplements

Some cancer patients may take dietary supplements. A dietary supplement is a product that is added to the diet. It is usually taken by mouth, and usually has one or more dietary ingredients. Cancer patients may take dietary supplements to improve their symptoms or treat their cancer.

Vitamin C

Vitamin C is a nutrient that the body needs in small amounts to function and stay healthy. It helps fight infection, heal wounds, and keep tissues healthy. Vitamin C is found in fruits and vegetables. It can also be taken as a dietary supplement.

Probiotics

Probiotics are live microorganisms used as dietary supplements to help with digestion and normal bowel function. They may also help keep the gastrointestinal tract healthy. Studies have shown that taking probiotics during radiation therapy and chemotherapy can help prevent diarrhea caused by those treatments. This is especially true for patients receiving radiation therapy to the abdomen. Cancer patients who are receiving radiation therapy to the abdomen or chemotherapy that is known to cause diarrhea may be helped by probiotics.

Melatonin

Melatonin is a hormone made by the pineal gland (tiny organ near the center of the brain). Melatonin helps control the body's sleep cycle. It can also be made in a laboratory and taken as a dietary supplement.

Several small studies have shown that taking a melatonin supplement with chemotherapy and/or radiation therapy for treatment of solid tumors may be helpful. It may help reduce side effects of treatment. Melatonin does not appear to have side effects.

Oral Glutamine

Oral glutamine is an amino acid that is being studied for the treatment of diarrhea and mucositis (inflammation of the lining of the digestive system, often seen as mouth sores) caused by chemotherapy or radiation therapy. Oral glutamine may help prevent mucositis or make it less severe.

Cancer patients who are receiving radiation therapy to the abdomen may benefit from oral glutamine. Oral glutamine may reduce the severity of diarrhea. This can help the patients continue with their treatment plan.

Nutrition Needs at End of Life

For patients at the end of life, the goals of nutrition therapy are focused on relieving symptoms rather than getting enough nutrients.

Common symptoms that can occur at the end of life include the following:

- Anorexia (loss of appetite)

- Dry mouth

- Swallowing problems

- Nausea

- Vomiting

Patients who have problems swallowing may find it easier to swallow thick liquids than thin liquids. Patients often do not feel much hunger at all and may want very little food. Sips of water, ice chips, and mouth care can decrease thirst in the last few days of life. Good communication with the healthcare team is important to understand the patient's changes in nutrition needs.

Patients and families decide how much nutrition and fluids will be given at the end of life. Cancer patients and their caregivers have the right to make informed decisions. The patient's religious and cultural preferences may affect their decisions. The healthcare team may work with the patient's religious and cultural leaders when making decisions. The healthcare team and a registered dietitian can explain the benefits and risks of using nutrition support for patients at the end of life. In most cases, there are more harms than benefits.

Chapter 55

Exercising during Cancer Treatment and Beyond

What Is Physical Activity?

Physical activity is defined as any movement that uses skeletal muscles and requires more energy than does resting. Physical activity can include working, exercising, performing household chores, and leisure-time activities such as walking, tennis, hiking, bicycling, and swimming. Physical activity is essential for people to maintain a balance between the number of calories consumed and the number of calories used. Consistently expending fewer calories than are consumed leads to obesity, which scientists have convincingly linked to increased risks of 13 different cancers. Additionally, evidence indicates that physical activity may reduce the risks of several cancers through other mechanisms, independent of its effect on obesity.

This chapter contains text excerpted from the following sources: Text beginning with the heading "What Is Physical Activity?" is excerpted from "Physical Activity and Cancer Fact Sheet," National Cancer Institute (NCI), January 27, 2017; Text under the heading "So What Should Cancer Patients and Survivors Do?" is excerpted from "Physical Activity for Cancer Patients," Office of Disease Prevention and Health Promotion (ODPHP), U.S. Department of Health and Human Services (HHS), January 30, 2014. Reviewed May 2018.

What Is Known about the Relationship between Physical Activity and Reduced Risks of Cancer?

There is substantial evidence that higher levels of physical activity are linked to lower risks of several cancers.

- **Colon cancer:** Colon cancer is one of the most extensively studied cancers in relation to physical activity. A 2009 meta-analysis of 52 epidemiologic studies that examined the association between physical activity and colon cancer risk found that the most physically active individuals had a 24 percent lower risk of colon cancer than those who were the least physically active. A pooled analysis of data on leisure-time physical activity (activities done at an individual's discretion generally to improve or maintain fitness or health) from 12 prospective U.S. and European cohort studies reported a risk reduction of 16 percent, when comparing individuals who were most active to those where least active. Incidence of both distal colon and proximal colon cancers is lower in people who are more physically active than in those who are less physically active. Physical activity is also associated with a decreased risk of colon adenomas (polyps), a type of colon polyp that may develop into colon cancer. However, it is less clear whether physical activity is associated with lower risks that polyps that have been removed will come back.

- **Breast cancer:** Many studies show that physically active women have a lower risk of breast cancer than inactive women; in a 2013 meta-analysis of 31 prospective studies, the average breast cancer risk reduction associated with physical activity was 12 percent. Physical activity has been associated with a reduced risk of breast cancer in both premenopausal and postmenopausal women; however, the evidence for an association is stronger for postmenopausal breast cancer. Women who increase their physical activity after menopause may also have a lower risk of breast cancer than women who do not.

- **Endometrial cancer:** Many studies have examined the relationship between physical activity and the risk of endometrial cancer (cancer of the lining of the uterus). In a meta-analysis of 33 studies, the average endometrial cancer risk reduction associated with high versus low physical activity was 20 percent. There is some evidence that the association between physical activity and endometrial cancer risk may reflect the effect of physical activity on obesity, a known risk factor for endometrial cancer.

For a number of other cancers, there is more limited evidence of a relationship with physical activity. In a study of over 1 million individuals, leisure-time physical activity was linked to reduced risks of esophageal adenocarcinoma, liver cancer, gastric cardia cancer (a type of stomach cancer), kidney cancer, myeloid leukemia, myeloma, and cancers of the head and neck, rectum, and bladder.

Is Physical Activity Beneficial for Cancer Survivors?

Research indicates that physical activity may have beneficial effects for several aspects of cancer survivorship—specifically, weight gain, quality of life, cancer recurrence or progression, and prognosis (likelihood of survival). Most of the evidence for the potential benefits of physical activity in cancer survivors comes from people diagnosed with breast or colorectal cancer.

- **Weight gain.** Both reduced physical activity and the side effects of cancer treatment can contribute to weight gain after a cancer diagnosis. In a cohort study (a type of epidemiologic study), weight gain after breast cancer diagnosis was linked to worse survival. In a meta-analysis of randomized controlled clinical trials examining physical activity in cancer survivors, physical activity was found to reduce both body mass index and body weight.

- **Quality of life.** A Cochrane Collaboration systematic review of controlled clinical trials of exercise interventions in cancer survivors indicated that physical activity may have beneficial effects on overall health-related quality of life and on specific quality-of-life issues, including body image/self-esteem, emotional well-being, sexuality, sleep disturbance, social functioning, anxiety, fatigue, and pain. In a 2012 meta-analysis of randomized controlled trials examining physical activity in cancer survivors, physical activity was found to reduce fatigue and depression and to improve physical functioning, social functioning, and mental health.

- **Recurrence, progression, and survival.** Being physically active after a cancer diagnosis is linked to better cancer-specific outcomes for several cancer types.

- **Breast cancer:** Consistent evidence from epidemiologic studies links physical activity after diagnosis with better breast cancer outcomes. For example, a large cohort study found that women who exercised moderately (the equivalent of walking 3–5 hours per week at an average pace) after a breast cancer diagnosis had approximately 40–50 percent lower risks of breast cancer recurrence, death from breast cancer, and death from any cause compared with more sedentary women. The potential physical activity benefit with regard to death from breast cancer was most apparent in women with hormone receptor-positive tumors. Another prospective cohort study found that women who had breast cancer and who engaged in recreational physical activity roughly equivalent to walking at an average pace of 2–2.9 mph for 1 hour per week had a 35–49 percent lower risk of death from breast cancer compared with women who engaged in less physical activity.

- **Colorectal cancer:** Evidence from multiple epidemiologic studies suggests that physical activity after a colorectal cancer diagnosis is associated with reduced risks of dying from colorectal cancer. In a large prospective cohort of patients with colorectal cancer, those who engaged in leisure-time physical activity had a 31 percent lower risk of death than those who did not, independent of their leisure-time physical activity before diagnosis.

Findings from epidemiologic studies cannot completely exclude reverse causation as a possible explanation of the link between physical activity and better cancer outcomes. That is, people who feel good are more likely to exercise and be physically active than people who do not feel good.

So What Should Cancer Patients and Survivors Do?

The best advice is to start a new physical activity program with the help of a trained specialist. The Cancer Exercise Training Institute (CETI) provides scientifically-based information on exercise therapy as a critical component of cancer recovery. Cancer exercise specialists, or CES, are specifically trained at the institute to treat the range of conditions common to those undergoing cancer treatment. Many cancer patients present with limited range of motion, poor posture, neck and back pain and with lymphedema (or at a high risk for developing it). A cancer exercise specialist also is well versed in the specific problems caused by different kinds of cancer (and their treatment) and can help guide the patient back to his or her best normal.

Chapter 56

Coping with the Emotions of Cancer

Just as cancer affects your physical health, it can bring up a wide range of feelings you're not used to dealing with. It can also make existing feelings seem more intense. They may change daily, hourly, or even minute to minute. This is true whether you're currently in treatment, done with treatment, or a friend or family member. These feelings are all normal. Often the values you grew up with affect how you think about and deal with cancer. For example some people:

- Feel they have to be strong and protect their friends and families

- Seek support and turn to loved ones or other cancer survivors

- Ask for help from counselors or other professionals

- Turn to their faith to help them cope

Whatever you decide, it's important to do what's right for you and not to compare yourself with others. Your friends and family members may share some of the same feelings. If you feel comfortable, share this information with them.

This chapter includes text excerpted from "Coping with Cancer—Feelings and Cancer," National Cancer Institute (NCI), November 6, 2017.

Overwhelmed

When you first learn that you have cancer, you may feel as if your life is out of control. This could be because:

- You wonder if you're going to live

- Your normal routine is disrupted by doctor visits and treatments

- People use medical terms that you don't understand

- You feel like you can't do the things you enjoy

- You feel helpless and lonely

Even if you feel out of control, there are ways you can take charge. Try to learn as much as you can about your cancer. Ask your doctor questions and don't be afraid to say when you don't understand. Also, many people feel better if they stay busy. You can take part in activities such as music, crafts, reading, or learning something new.

Denial

When you were first diagnosed, you may have had trouble believing or accepting the fact that you have cancer. This is called denial. It can be helpful because it can give you time to adjust to your diagnosis. It can also give you time to feel hopeful and better about the future. Sometimes, denial is a serious problem. If it lasts too long, it can keep you from getting the treatment you need. The good news is that most people work through denial. Usually by the time treatment begins, most people accept the fact that they have cancer and move forward. This is true for those with cancer as well as the people they love and care about.

Anger

People with cancer often feel angry. It's normal to ask, "Why me?" and be angry at the cancer. You may also feel anger or resentment towards your healthcare providers, your healthy friends and your loved ones. And if you're religious, you may even feel angry with God. Anger often comes from feelings that are hard to show, such as fear, panic, frustration, anxiety, or helplessness. If you feel angry, you don't have to pretend that everything is okay. Anger can be helpful in that it may motivate you to take action. Talk with your family and friends about your anger. Or, ask your doctor to refer you to a counselor.

Fear and Worry

It's scary to hear that you have cancer. You may be afraid or worried about:

- Being in pain, either from the cancer or the treatment
- Feeling sick or looking different as a result of your treatment
- Taking care of your family
- Paying your bills
- Keeping your job
- Dying

Some fears about cancer are based on stories, rumors, or wrong information. To cope with fears and worries, it often helps to be informed. Most people feel better when they learn the facts. They feel less afraid and know what to expect. Learn about your cancer and understand what you can do to be an active partner in your care. Some studies even suggest that people who are well-informed about their illness and treatment are more likely to follow their treatment plans and recover from cancer more quickly than those who are not.

Hope

Once people accept that they have cancer, they often feel a sense of hope. There are many reasons to feel hopeful. Millions of people who have had cancer are alive today. Your chances of living with cancer—and living beyond it—are better now than they have ever been before. And people with cancer can lead active lives, even during treatment. Some doctors think that hope may help your body deal with cancer. So, scientists are studying whether a hopeful outlook and positive attitude helps people feel better. Here are some ways you can build your sense of hope:

- Plan your days as you've always done.
- Don't limit the things you like to do just because you have cancer.
- Look for reasons to have hope. If it helps, write them down or talk to others about them.
- Spend time in nature.

- Reflect on your religious or spiritual beliefs.

- Listen to stories about people with cancer who are leading active lives.

Stress and Anxiety

Both during and after treatment, it's normal to have stress over all the life changes you are going through. Anxiety means you have extra worry, can't relax, and feel tense. You may notice that:

- Your heart beats faster

- You have headaches or muscle pains

- You don't feel like eating, or you eat more.

- You feel sick to your stomach or have diarrhea

- You feel shaky, weak, or dizzy

- You have a tight feeling in your throat and chest

- You sleep too much or too little

- You find it hard to concentrate

If you have any of these feelings, talk to your doctor. Though they are common signs of stress, you will want to make sure they aren't due to medicines or treatment.

Stress can keep your body from healing as well as it should. If you're worried about your stress, ask your doctor to suggest a counselor for you to talk to. You could also take a class that teaches ways to deal with stress. The key is to find ways to control your stress and not to let it control you.

Sadness and Depression

Many people with cancer feel sad. They feel a sense of loss of their health, and the life they had before they learned they had the disease. Even when you're done with treatment, you may still feel sad. This is a normal response to any serious illness. It may take time to work through and accept all the changes that are taking place.

When you're sad, you may have very little energy, feel tired, or not want to eat. For some, these feelings go away or lessen over time. But for others, these emotions can become stronger. The painful feelings don't get any better, and they get in the way of daily life. This may be a medical condition called depression. For some, cancer treatment may have added to this problem by changing the way the brain works.

Getting Help for Depression

Depression can be treated. Below are common signs of depression. If you have any of the following signs for more than two weeks, talk to your doctor about treatment. Be aware that some of these symptoms could be due to physical problems, so it's important to talk about them with your doctor.

Emotional signs:

- Feelings of sadness that don't go away
- Feeling emotionally numb
- Feeling nervous or shaky
- Having a sense of guilt or feeling unworthy
- Feeling helpless or hopeless, as if life has no meaning
- Feeling short-tempered, moody
- Having a hard time concentrating, feeling scatterbrained
- Crying for long periods of time or many times each day
- Focusing on worries and problems
- No interest in the hobbies and activities you used to enjoy
- Finding it hard to enjoy everyday things, such as food or being with family and friends
- Thinking about hurting yourself
- Thoughts about killing yourself

Body changes:

- Unintended weight gain or loss not due to illness or treatment
- Sleep problems, such as not being able to sleep, having nightmares, or sleeping too much
- Racing heart, dry mouth, increased perspiration, upset stomach, diarrhea
- Changes in energy level
- Fatigue that doesn't go away
- Headaches, other aches and pains

If your doctor thinks that you suffer from depression, he or she may give you medicine to help you feel less tense. Or, he or she may refer you to other experts. Don't feel that you should have to control these feelings on your own. Getting the help you need is important for your life and your health.

Guilt

If you feel guilty, know that many people with cancer feel this way. You may blame yourself for upsetting the people you love, or worry that you're a burden in some way. Or, you may envy other people's good health and be ashamed of this feeling. You might even blame yourself for lifestyle choices that you think could have led to your cancer. These feelings are all very common. It may help you to share them with someone. Let your doctor know if you would like to talk with a counselor or go to a support group.

Loneliness

People with cancer often feel lonely or distant from others. This may be for a number of reasons:

- Friends sometimes have a hard time dealing with cancer and may not visit or call you.

- You may feel too sick to take part in the hobbies and activities you used to enjoy.

- Sometimes, even when you're with people you care about, you may feel that no one understands what you're going through.

It's also normal to feel alone after treatment. You may miss the support you got from your healthcare team. Many people have a sense that their safety net has been pulled away, and they get less attention. It's common to still feel cut off from certain friends or family members. Some of them may think that now that treatment is over, you will be back to normal soon, even though this may not be true. Others may want to help but don't know how. Look for emotional support in different ways. It could help you to talk to other people who have cancer or to join a support group. Or, you may feel better talking only to a close friend or family member, or counselor, or a member of your faith or spiritual community. Do what feels right for you.

Gratitude

Some people see their cancer as a "wake-up call." They realize the importance of enjoying the little things in life. They go places they've never been. They finish projects they had started but put aside. They spend more time with friends and family. They mend broken relationships. It may be hard at first, but you can find joy in your life if you have cancer. Pay attention to the things you do each day that make you smile. They can be as simple as drinking a good cup of coffee or talking to a friend.

You can also do things that are more special to you, like being in nature or praying in a place that has meaning for you. Or, it could be playing a sport you love or cooking a good meal. Whatever you choose, embrace the things that bring you joy when you can.

Ways to Cope with Your Emotions

Express Your Feelings

People have found that when they express strong feelings like anger or sadness, they're more able to let go of them. Some sort out their feelings by talking to friends or family, other cancer survivors, a support group, or a counselor. But even if you prefer not to discuss your cancer with others, you can still sort out your feelings by thinking about them or writing them down.

Look for the Positive

Sometimes this means looking for the good even in a bad time or trying to be hopeful instead of thinking the worst. Try to use your energy to focus on wellness and what you can do now to stay as healthy as possible.

Don't Blame Yourself for Your Cancer

Some people believe that they got cancer because of something they did or did not do. Remember, cancer can happen to anyone.

Don't Try to Be Upbeat If You're Not

Many people say they want to have the freedom to give in to their feelings sometimes. As one woman said, "When it gets really bad, I just tell my family I'm having a bad cancer day and go upstairs and crawl into bed."

You Choose When to Talk about Your Cancer

It can be hard for people to know how to talk to you about your cancer. Often loved ones mean well, but they don't know what to say or how to act. You can make them feel more at ease by asking them what they think or how they feel.

Find Ways to Help Yourself Relax

Whatever activity helps you unwind, you should take some time to do it. Meditation, guided imagery, and relaxation exercises are just a few ways that have been shown to help others; these may help you relax when you feel worried.

Be as Active as You Can

Getting out of the house and doing something can help you focus on other things besides cancer and the worries it brings. Exercise or gentle yoga and stretching can help too.

Look for Things You Enjoy

You may like hobbies such as woodworking, photography, reading, or crafts. Or find creative outlets such as art, music, or dance.

Look at What You Can Control

Some people say that putting their lives in order helps. Being involved in your healthcare, keeping your appointments, and making changes in your lifestyle are among the things you can control. Even setting a daily schedule can give you a sense of control. And while no one can control every thought, some say that they try not to dwell on the fearful ones, but instead, do what they can to enjoy the positive parts of life.

Chapter 57

Talking to Children about Your Cancer

Even though your children will be upset when they learn about your cancer, don't pretend that everything is okay. Even very young children can sense when something is wrong. They will see that you don't feel well, are away from home more often, or can't spend as much time with them as you used to. Children as young as 18 months old begin to notice what's going on around them. It's important to be honest. Telling the truth is better than letting them imagine the worst. Give your kids time to ask questions and express their feelings.

What Children of All Ages Need to Know

About Cancer

- Nothing your child did, thought, or said caused you to get cancer.

- Just because you have cancer doesn't mean you'll die from it. In fact, many people live with cancer for a long time.

This chapter includes text excerpted from "Coping with Cancer—Talking to Children about Your Cancer" National Cancer Institute (NCI), December 2, 2014. Reviewed May 2018.

- Your child can't make you well. But there are ways he or she can make you feel better.

- Scientists are finding many new ways to treat cancer.

About Living with Cancer in the Family

- Your child is not alone. Other children have parents who have cancer.

- It's okay to be upset, angry, or scared.

- Your child can't do anything to change the fact that you have cancer.

- Family members may act differently because they're worried about you.

- You will make sure that your children are taken care of, no matter what happens to you.

About What They Can Do

- They can help you by doing nice things like washing dishes or drawing you a picture.

- They should still go to school and take part in sports and other fun activities.

- They can talk to other adults for support, such as teachers, family members, and religious or spiritual leaders.

How Kids May Act When You Have Cancer

Children can react to cancer in many different ways. For example, they may:

- Be confused, scared, lonely, or overwhelmed

- Feel guilty and think that something they did or said caused your cancer

- Feel angry when they are asked to be quiet or to do more chores around the house

- Miss the amount of attention they're used to getting

- Regress and behave as they did when they were much younger

- Get into trouble at school or at home
- Be clingy and afraid to leave the house

Teens

If you have a teenager, know that they're at a time in their lives when they're trying to break away and be independent from their parents. Try to get them to talk about their feelings and ask questions. Tell them as much as they want to know about your cancer. Ask them for their opinions and, if possible, let them help you make decisions. Teens may want to talk with other people in their lives. Friends can be a great source of support for them, especially those who also have a serious illness in their family. Other family members, teachers, coaches, and spiritual leaders can also help. Encourage your teenage children to talk about their fears and feelings with people they trust.

Adult Children

If you have adult children, your relationship with them may change now that you have cancer. You may:

- Ask them to help with making healthcare decisions, paying bills, or taking care of the house
- Ask them to explain medical information
- Need them to go to the doctor with you or pick up medicines
- Rely on them for emotional support
- Feel awkward when they help with your physical care

For some parents, it may be hard to ask for comfort and care from their grown children. But it's important to talk about cancer with your family members, even if they get upset or worry about you. Try to include them when talking about your treatment. Let them know the choices you would like them to make about your care, in case you're too sick to make the choices yourself. Recognize that it may be hard for your children to have this talk and that, like you, they're trying to adjust to your illness.

Chapter 58

Sexuality and Reproductive Issues among Women with Cancer

Chapter Contents

Section 58.1

Renewing Intimacy and Sexuality after Gynecologic Cancer

This section includes text excerpted from "Sexual Health
Issues in Women with Cancer," National Cancer
Institute (NCI), September 22, 2017.

Women being treated for cancer may experience changes that affect
their sexual life during, and sometimes after, treatment. While you
may not have the energy or interest in sexual activity that you did
before treatment, feeling close to and being intimate with your spouse
or partner is probably still important.

Your doctor or nurse may talk with you about how cancer treatment
might affect your sexual life, or you may need to be proactive and ask
questions such as:

- What sexual changes or problems are common among women
  receiving this type of treatment?

- What methods of birth control or protection are recommended
  during treatment?

Whether or not your sexual health will be affected by treatment
depends on factors such as:

- The type of cancer

- The type of treatment(s)

- The amount (dose) of treatment

- The length (duration) of treatment

- Your age at the time of treatment

- The amount of time that has passed since treatment

- Other personal health factors

Cancer Treatments May Cause Sexual Problems in Women

Some problems that affect a woman's sexual health during treatment are temporary and improve once treatment has ended. Other side effects may be long term or may start after treatment. Your doctor will talk with you about side effects you may have based on your treatment(s):

- Chemotherapy can lower estrogen levels and cause primary ovarian insufficiency. This means the ovaries aren't producing hormones and releasing eggs. Symptoms may include hot flashes, irregular or no periods, and vaginal dryness, which can make sexual intercourse difficult or painful. Chemotherapy can also affect vaginal tissue, which may cause sores.

- Hormone therapy (also called endocrine therapy) may cause low estrogen levels which can lead to symptoms such as hot flashes, irregular or no periods, and vaginal dryness.

- Radiation therapy to the pelvis (such as to the bladder, cervix, colon, ovaries, rectum, uterus, or vagina) can cause low estrogen levels and, therefore, vaginal dryness. Vaginal stenosis (less elastic, narrow, shorter vagina), vaginal atrophy (weak vaginal muscles and thin vaginal wall), and vaginal itching, burning, and inflammation can also cause pain and discomfort during sex.

- Surgery for gynecologic cancers may affect your sexual life. Treatment for other cancers can also bring about physical changes that may affect the way you view your body. Your healthcare team will talk with you about what to expect and teach you how to adjust after surgery, such as after a mastectomy or an ostomy, for example.

- Medicines such as opioids and some drugs used to treat depression may lower your interest in sex.

Ways to Manage Sexual Health Issues

People on your healthcare team have helped others to cope during this difficult time and can offer valuable suggestions. You may also want to talk with a sexual health expert to get answers to any questions or concerns. Most women can be sexually active during treatment, but

657

you'll want to confirm this with your doctor. For example, there may be times during treatment when you are at increased risk of infection or bleeding and may be advised to abstain from sexual intercourse.

Your healthcare team can help you:

- Learn about medicine and exercises to make sex more comfortable, including:

  - Vaginal gels or creams to stop a dry, itchy, or burning feeling

  - Vaginal lubricants or moisturizers

  - Vaginal estrogen cream that may be appropriate for some types of cancer

  - A dilator to help prevent or reverse scarring, if radiation therapy or graft-versus-host disease (GvHD) has affected your vagina

  - Exercises for pelvic muscles to lower pain, improve bladder retention, improve bowel function, and increase the flow of blood to the area, which can improve your sexual health

- **Manage related side effects:** Talk with your doctor or nurse about problems such as pain, fatigue, hair loss, loss of interest in activities, sadness, or trouble sleeping, that may affect your sex life. Speaking up about side effects can help you get the treatment and support you need to feel better.

- **Learn about condoms and/or contraceptives:** Condoms may be advised to prevent your partner's exposure to some types of chemotherapy that may remain in vaginal secretions. If you are of childbearing age, contraceptives may be advised to prevent pregnancy while you are receiving treatment and for a period of time following treatment.

- **Get support and counseling:** During this time, you can gain strength and support by sharing your concerns with people you are close to. You may also benefit from participating in a professionally moderated or led support group. Your nurse or social worker can recommend support groups and counselors in your area.

Talking with Your Healthcare Team about Sexual Health Issues

As you think about the changes that treatment has brought into your life, make a list of questions to discuss with your doctor, nurse, or social worker. Consider adding these to your list:

- What sexual problems are common among women receiving this treatment?

- What sexual problems might I have during treatment?

- When might these changes occur?

- How long might these problems last? Will any of these problems be permanent?

- How can these problems be prevented, treated, or managed?

- What specialist(s) would you suggest that I talk with to learn more?

- Is there a support group that you recommend?

- What method(s) of birth control are advised?

- What precautions do I need to take during treatment? For example, should my partner use a condom? Are there times when I should avoid sexual activity?

Section 58.2

Cancer and Fertility Preservation

This section contains text excerpted from the following sources: Text in this section begins with excerpts from "Fertility Issues in Girls and Women with Cancer," National Cancer Institute (NCI), September 22, 2017; Text beginning with the heading "Questions from Women Getting Radiation Therapy" is excerpted from "What Women Can Do about Changes in Sexuality and Fertility," National Cancer Institute (NCI), April 2007. Reviewed May 2018.

Many cancer treatments can affect a girl's or woman's fertility. Most likely, your doctor will talk with you about whether or not cancer treatment may increase the risk of, or cause, infertility. However, not all doctors bring up this topic. Sometimes you, a family member, or parents of a child being treated for cancer may need to initiate this conversation.

Whether or not fertility is affected depends on factors such as:

- Your baseline fertility
- Your age at the time of treatment
- The type of cancer and treatment(s)
- The amount (dose) of treatment
- The length (duration) of treatment
- The amount of time that has passed since cancer treatment
- Other personal health factors

It's important to learn how the recommended cancer treatment may affect fertility before starting treatment, whenever possible. Consider asking questions such as:

- Could treatment increase the risk of, or cause, infertility? Could treatment make it difficult to become pregnant or carry a pregnancy in the future?
- Are there other recommended cancer treatments that might not cause fertility problems?
- Which fertility option(s) would you advise for me?
- What fertility preservation options are available at this hospital? At a fertility clinic?
- Would you recommend a fertility specialist (such as a reproductive endocrinologist) who I could talk with to learn more?
- Is condom use advised, based on the treatment I'm receiving?
- Is birth control recommended?
- After treatment, what are the chances that my fertility will return? How long might it take for my fertility to return?

Cancer Treatments May Affect Your Fertility

Cancer treatments are important for your future health, but they may harm reproductive organs and glands that control fertility. Changes to your fertility may be temporary or permanent. Talk with your healthcare team to learn what to expect, based on your treatment(s):

- Chemotherapy (especially alkylating agents) can affect the ovaries, causing them to stop releasing eggs and estrogen. This is called primary ovarian insufficiency (POI). Sometimes POI is temporary and your menstrual periods and fertility return after treatment. Other times, damage to your ovaries is permanent and fertility doesn't return. You may have hot flashes, night sweats, irritability, vaginal dryness, and irregular or no menstrual periods. Chemotherapy can also lower the number of healthy eggs in the ovaries. Women who are closer to the age of natural menopause may have a greater risk of infertility.

- Radiation therapy to or near the abdomen, pelvis, or spine can harm nearby reproductive organs. Some organs, such as the ovaries, can often be protected by ovarian shielding or by oophoropexy—a procedure that surgically moves the ovaries away from the radiation area. Radiation therapy to the brain can also harm the pituitary gland. This gland is important because it sends signals to the ovaries to make hormones such as estrogen that are needed for ovulation. The amount of radiation given and the part of your body being treated both play a role in whether or not fertility is affected.

- Surgery for cancers of the reproductive system and for cancers in the pelvis region can harm nearby reproductive tissues and cause scarring, which can affect your fertility. The size and location of the tumor are important factors in whether or not fertility is affected.

- Hormone therapy (also called endocrine therapy) used to treat cancer can disrupt the menstrual cycle, which may affect your fertility. Side effects depend on the specific hormones used and may include hot flashes, night sweats, and vaginal dryness.

- Bone marrow transplants, peripheral blood stem cell transplants, and other stem cell transplants involve receiving high doses of chemotherapy and/or radiation. These treatments can damage the ovaries and may cause infertility.

- Other treatments: Talk with your doctor to learn whether or not other types of treatment such as immunotherapy and targeted cancer therapy may affect your fertility.

Emotional Considerations and Support for Fertility Issues

For some women, infertility can be one of the most difficult and upsetting long-term effects of cancer treatment. While it might feel overwhelming to think about your fertility right now, most people benefit from having talked with their doctor (or their child's doctor, when a child is being treated for cancer) about how treatment may affect their fertility and about options to preserve fertility. Although most people want to have children at some point in their life, families can come together in many ways. For extra support during this time, reach out to your healthcare team with questions or concerns, as well as to professionally led support groups.

Fertility Preservation Options for Girls and Women

Women and girls with cancer have options to preserve their fertility. These procedures may be available at the hospital where you are receiving cancer treatment or at a fertility preservation clinic. Talk with your doctor about the best option(s) for you based on your age, the type of cancer you have, and the specific treatment(s) you will be receiving. The success rate, financial cost, and availability of these procedures varies.

- Egg freezing (also called egg or oocyte cryopreservation) is a procedure in which eggs are removed from the ovary and frozen. Later the eggs can be thawed, fertilized with sperm in the lab to form embryos, and placed in a woman's uterus. Egg freezing is a newer procedure than embryo freezing.

- Embryo freezing (also called embryo banking or embryo cryopreservation) is a procedure in which eggs are removed from the ovary. They are then fertilized with sperm in the lab to form embryos and frozen for future use.

- Ovarian shielding (also called gonadal shielding) is a procedure in which a protective cover is placed on the outside of the body, over the ovaries and other parts of the reproductive system, to shield them from scatter radiation.

- Ovarian tissue freezing (also called ovarian tissue cryopreservation) is still considered an experimental procedure, for young girls who haven't gone through puberty and don't have mature eggs. It involves surgically removing part or all of an ovary and then freezing the ovarian tissue, which contains eggs. Later, the tissue is thawed and placed back in a woman. Although pregnancies have occurred as a result of this procedure, it's only an option for some types of cancer.

- Ovarian transposition (also called oophoropexy) is an operation to move the ovaries away from the part of the body receiving radiation. This procedure may be done during surgery to remove the cancer or through laparoscopic surgery.

- Radical trachelectomy (also called radical cervicectomy) is surgery used to treat women with early-stage cervical cancer who would like to have children. This operation removes the cervix, nearby lymph nodes, and the upper part of the vagina. The uterus is then attached to the remaining part of the vagina, with a special band that serves as the cervix.

- Treatment with gonadotropin-releasing hormone agonist (also called GnRHa), a substance that causes the ovaries to stop making estrogen and progesterone. Research is ongoing to assess the effectiveness of giving GnRHa to protect the ovaries.

If you choose to take steps to preserve your fertility, your doctor and a fertility specialist will work together to develop a treatment plan that includes fertility preservation, whenever possible.

Questions from Women Getting Radiation Therapy

What If I Think I May Be Pregnant Now?

Make sure to tell your doctor or nurse if you think you may be pregnant now. Radiation therapy can harm your unborn baby.

I Just Started Treatment. Will I Be Able to Have Sex? Do I Need to Use Birth Control?

Talk with your doctor to find out if it is okay for you to have sex. Make sure to use a birth control method during treatment. It is very important that you don't get pregnant during radiation therapy.

I Just Don't Feel in the Mood for Sex These Days. Is This Normal?

Yes. The side effects of radiation therapy, such as being tired or in pain, can lower your sexual desire. Be easy on yourself. You are going through a lot. Talk with your partner about what you are feeling. There are many ways for you to stay close to each other during this time.

Questions from Women Getting Radiation to the Pelvis

A Woman in My Support Group Said She's Having Signs of Menopause. Will That Happen to Me?

Some women get hot flashes or stop having their periods during treatment. Tell your doctor if you notice these or other changes.

What Are Some Other Changes I Might Notice?

Radiation therapy to the pelvis can cause changes in the vagina. Many women notice pain when they have sex because the treatment can make the vagina more narrow. Or you may have a dry, itchy, or burning feeling. Talk with your doctor or nurse to get the best advice for you. For some women:

- Gels or creams may help stop a dry, itchy, or burning feeling.

- Products such as Replens®, Astroglide®, or K-Y® Liquid can help make the vagina moist.

- A device called a dilator can also help. It stretches the vagina. Talk with your nurse to learn if this would be helpful for you.

Women who want to get pregnant after treatment ends should talk with their doctor. There are things you can do now to plan for the future.

Questions to Ask Your Doctor or Nurse

1. How long will these problems last?

2. What products or treatments could help me with these problems?

3. What are all my options now if I would like to have children in the future?

4. Is there a support group for women that I could go to?

Section 58.3

Breast Cancer Treatment during Pregnancy

This section includes text excerpted from "Breast Cancer Treatment during Pregnancy (PDQ®)—Health Professional Version," National Cancer Institute (NCI), December 22, 2017.

Generally, pregnant women with stage I or stage II breast cancer are treated in the same way as nonpregnant patients, with some modifications to protect the fetus.

Treatment options for early/localized/operable breast cancer in pregnant women include the following:

1. Surgery. Postpartum radiation therapy may also be given to women diagnosed with breast cancer late in pregnancy.

2. Chemotherapy (after the first trimester)

3. Endocrine therapy (after delivery)

The use of trastuzumab during pregnancy is contraindicated.

Surgery

Surgery is recommended as the primary treatment of breast cancer in pregnant women. The data regarding safety of sentinel lymph node biopsy in pregnant patients are limited to several retrospective case series. One study examined sentinel lymph node biopsy in eight patients in the first trimester, nine patients in the second trimester, and eight patients in the third trimester. Technetium Tc 99m alone was used in 16 patients, methylene blue dye alone was used in seven patients, and two patients had unknown mapping methods. All 25 patients had live-born infants, of whom 24 were healthy, and one had a cleft palate (in the setting of other maternal risk factors).

Because radiation in therapeutic doses may expose the fetus to potentially harmful scatter radiation, modified radical mastectomy is the treatment of choice if the breast cancer was diagnosed early in

665

pregnancy. If diagnosed late in pregnancy, breast-conserving surgery with postpartum radiation therapy has been used for breast preservation. An analysis has been performed that helps to predict the risk of waiting to have radiation.

Chemotherapy

Data suggest that it is safe to administer certain chemotherapeutic drugs after the first trimester, with most pregnancies resulting in live births with low rates of morbidity in the newborns.

Anthracycline-based chemotherapy (doxorubicin plus cyclophosphamide or fluorouracil, doxorubicin, and cyclophosphamide (FAC)) appears to be safe to administer during the second and/or third trimester on the basis of limited prospective data. Safety data on the use of taxanes during pregnancy are limited.

Evidence (use of chemotherapy during the second and/or third trimester of pregnancy):

1. A multicenter case-control study compared pediatric outcomes of 129 children whose mothers had breast cancer with matched children of women without cancer. In the pregnancy study group, 96 children (74.4%) were exposed to chemotherapy, 11 (8.5%) to radiation therapy, 13 (10.1%) to surgery alone, 2 (1.7%) to other drug treatments, and 14 (10.9%) to no treatment.

   - The study showed that there was no significant difference in birth weight per ref below the 10th percentile (22% in the breast cancer treatment-exposed group versus 15.2 percent in the control group, $P = .16$) or in cognitive development based on the Bayley score ($P = .08$). The gestational age at birth was correlated with cognitive outcome in the two study groups.

   - Evaluation of cardiac function among 47 children, who were age 36 months in the study group, showed normal cardiac findings.

2. In a prospective single-arm study, 57 pregnant breast cancer patients were treated with FAC in the adjuvant or neoadjuvant setting.

   - Survey data collected when the children were aged 2 months to 157 months revealed that no stillbirths, miscarriages, or perinatal deaths occurred.

- One child born vaginally at a gestational age of 38 weeks had a subarachnoid hemorrhage (SAH) on day 2 postpartum, one child had Down syndrome, and two children had congenital anomalies (club foot and bilateral ureteral reflux).

3. The findings of the prospective single-arm study above were consistent with other smaller retrospective series of anthracycline-based chemotherapy.

4. A systematic review studied 40 case reports of taxane administration during the second or third trimesters of pregnancy.

- Minimal maternal, fetal, or neonatal toxicity was observed.

Endocrine Therapy

Endocrine therapy is generally avoided until after delivery. Case reports and a literature review of tamoxifen during pregnancy show that tamoxifen administration during pregnancy is associated with vaginal bleeding, miscarriage, congenital abnormalities such as Goldenhar syndrome (GS), and fetal death. Breastfeeding is also not recommended concurrently with endocrine therapy.

Targeted Therapy

The use of trastuzumab during pregnancy is contraindicated based on results of a systematic review of 17 studies (18 pregnancies, 19 newborns). Of the fetal complications noted, occurrence of oligohydramnios/anhydramnios was the most common (61.1%) adverse event. Of the pregnancies exposed to trastuzumab during the second or third trimester, 73.3 percent of the pregnancies were complicated with oligohydramnios/anhydramnios. Of the pregnancies exposed to trastuzumab exclusively during the first trimester, 0 percent ($P = 0.043$) of the pregnancies were complicated with oligohydramnios/anhydramnios. The mean gestational age at delivery was 33.8 weeks, and the mean weight of newborns at delivery was 2,261 grams or 4.984 pounds. In 52.6 percent of cases, a healthy neonate was born. At the long-term evaluation, all children who were without problems at birth were healthy, with a median follow-up of 9 months, and four of nine children who faced troubles at birth had died within an interval ranging from birth to 5.25 months. All children exposed to trastuzumab in utero exclusively in the first trimester were completely healthy at birth. The data suggest that for women who become pregnant during trastuzumab administration and wish to continue pregnancy, trastuzumab should be stopped and pregnancy would be allowed to continue.

Special Considerations for Pregnancy and Breast Cancer

Lactation

Suppression of lactation does not improve prognosis. If surgery is planned, however, lactation is suppressed to decrease the size and vascularity of the breasts. If chemotherapy is to be given, lactation is also suppressed because many antineoplastic agents (i.e., cyclophosphamide and methotrexate), when given systemically, may occur in high levels in breast milk and would affect the nursing baby. Women receiving chemotherapy should not breastfeed.

Fetal Consequences of Maternal Breast Cancer

No damaging effects on the fetus from maternal breast cancer have been demonstrated, and there are no reported cases of maternal-fetal transfer of breast cancer cells.

Pregnancy in Patients with a History of Breast Cancer

Based on limited retrospective data, pregnancy does not appear to compromise the survival of women with a previous history of breast cancer, and no deleterious effects have been demonstrated in the fetus. Some physicians recommend that patients wait 2 years after diagnosis before attempting to conceive. This allows early recurrence to become manifest, which may influence the decision to become a parent. Little is known about pregnancy after bone marrow transplantation and high-dose chemotherapy with or without total-body irradiation. In one report of pregnancies after bone marrow transplantation for hematologic disorders, a 25 percent incidence of preterm labor and low birth weight for gestational age infants was noted.

Chapter 59

Taking Charge of Your Follow-Up Care

All cancer survivors should have follow-up care. Follow-up care for cancer means seeing a healthcare provider for regular medical checkups once you're finished with treatment. These checkups may include blood work, as well as other tests and procedures that look for any changes in your health, or any problems that may occur due to your cancer treatment. These visits are also a time to check for physical and emotional problems that may develop months or years after treatment ends.

Your follow-up care plan, along with a summary of your cancer treatment, is part of what is called a survivorship care plan. This plan will have all the information for you and your doctor to discuss to ensure that you get regular and thorough care after your treatment ends. Note that the information in this chapter focuses on follow-up care for your cancer treatment. But it's important that you continue to receive your routine care from your primary care provider in addition to follow-up cancer care.

Getting a Follow-Up Care Plan

Once your cancer treatment ends, you should receive a follow-up cancer care plan from your oncologist or someone on your treatment

This chapter includes text excerpted from "Coping with Cancer—Follow-Up Medical Care," National Cancer Institute (NCI), July 18, 2017.

team. A follow-up care plan is a set of recommendations for your cancer care after treatment ends. Many cancer organizations recommend the use of such a document. For follow-up cancer care, you may see the same doctor who treated you for cancer, or you may see another healthcare provider, such as one who specializes in follow-up care for cancer survivors. Or you may decide to go to your primary care doctor. You can discuss which doctor(s) to see with your healthcare team. Follow-up care for childhood cancer survivors is very similar to the steps for adults.

Common Questions after Treatment Ends

When you receive your follow-up care plan from your doctor or other healthcare provider, answers to the questions below should be provided. Make sure to ask any other questions you may have:

- How long will it take for me to get better and feel more like myself?

- Which doctor(s) should I see for my follow-up care? How often?

- What symptoms should I watch out for?

- What tests do I need after treatment is over? How often will I have them?

- What are long-term health issues I might expect as a result of my cancer treatment?

- What is the chance that my cancer will return?

- What records do I need to keep about my treatment?

- What can I do to take care of myself and be as healthy as possible?

- Can you suggest a support group that might help me?

You might find it helpful to write these questions down. When you meet with the doctor or follow-up care specialist, you can take notes or record your talks to refer to later. Talk about any concerns you have related to your follow-up care plan.

Your Follow-Up Care Schedule

Each patient has a different follow-up care schedule. How often you return for follow-up visits is based on:

- The type of cancer you had

- The treatment you received
- Your overall health, including possible treatment-related problems

In general, people return to the doctor for follow-up appointments every 3–4 months during the first 2–3 years after treatment, and once or twice a year after that.

At these visits, you may have a physical exam along with blood tests and other necessary tests and procedures. Which tests you receive and how often you receive them will be based on what your doctor thinks is best for you when creating your follow-up care plan.

What to Tell Your Doctor during Follow-Up Visits

When you meet with your doctor for follow-up visits, it's important to talk openly about any physical or emotional problems you're having. Always mention any symptoms, pain, or concerns that are new or that won't go away. But keep in mind that just because you have new symptoms, it doesn't necessarily mean the cancer has come back. It's normal to have fears about every ache and pain that arises, but they may just be problems that your doctor can easily address.

Other things you should tell your doctor:

- Any physical problems that interfere with your daily life, such as fatigue; problems with bladder, bowel, or sexual function; having a hard time concentrating; memory changes; trouble sleeping; or weight gain or loss
- Any new medicines, vitamins, herbs, or supplements you're taking
- Changes in your family medical history
- Any emotional problems you're having, such as anxiety or depression

It's important to be aware of any changes in your health between scheduled visits. Report any problems to your doctor immediately. They can decide whether the problems are related to the cancer, the treatment you received, or an unrelated health issue.

Your Treatment Summary

Your oncologist or a member of your treatment team should give you a written summary of the treatment you received. Keep this with you to share with your primary care doctor and any other doctors you see. Many people keep their treatment summary in a binder or folder, along with their medical records. This way, key facts about your treatment will always be in the same place.

Types of Health Information in the Treatment Summary

- The date you were diagnosed

- The type of cancer you had

- Pathology report(s) that describe the type and stage of cancer in detail

- Places and dates of each treatment, such as the details of all surgeries; the sites and total amounts of radiation therapy; and the names and doses of chemotherapy and all other drugs

- Key lab reports, X-ray reports, computed tomography (CT) scans, and magnetic resonance imaging (MRI) reports

- List of signs and symptoms to watch for and possible long-term effects of treatment

- Contact information for all health professionals involved in your treatment

- Any problems that occurred during or after treatment

- Any supportive care you received during treatment (such as medicines for depression or anxiety, emotional support, and nutritional supplements)

Many cancer survivors say that getting involved with their follow-up care was a good way for them to regain some of the control they felt they lost during cancer treatment. Being an active partner with your doctor and asking for help from other members of the healthcare team is the first step. Knowing what to expect after cancer treatment can help you and your family make plans, lifestyle changes, and important decisions about the future.

Guidelines for Follow-Up Care

The following programs or organizations provide helpful follow-up care guidelines for some cancers. You can use them to help you talk with your doctor, but they aren't meant to take the place of your doctor's knowledge or judgment.

- The American Society of Clinical Oncology (ASCO) provides care plans and follow-up care guidelines for cancer survivors.

- The Children's Oncology Group (COG), an National Cancer Institute (NCI)-supported clinical trials group, offers long-term follow-up guidelines for survivors of childhood, adolescent, and young adult cancers. It also has a series of fact sheets called Health Links, which provide information for healthy living after childhood cancer.

- The Journey Forward, a program created by a group of cancer-related organizations, provides a set of easy-to-use tools to help patients create a survivorship care plan. Its online "Cancer Care Plan Builder" allows your oncologist (or other cancer follow-up care specialist) to create a full medical summary and recommendations for follow-up care for you and your healthcare providers.

- The OncoLife Survivorship Care Plan was developed by Livestrong and the University of Pennsylvania. It provides survivors of adult cancers with a personalized survivorship care plan, based on the information they enter into an online program.

- The National Comprehensive Cancer Network (NCCN) includes information about follow-up care for cancer, along with guidance on making a follow-up care plan.

Guidelines for a Healthy Lifestyle after Cancer Treatment

After cancer treatment, many survivors want to find ways to reduce the chances of their cancer coming back. Some worry that the way they eat, the stress in their lives, or their exposure to chemicals may put them at risk for recurrence. Cancer survivors find that this is a time when they take a good look at how they take care of themselves and how they might live a healthier life.

Ask your doctor about developing a survivorship care plan that includes ways you can take care of your physical, emotional, social, and spiritual needs. If you find that it's hard to talk about these issues, it may be helpful to know that the more you do it, the easier it becomes. Your doctor may also suggest another member of the healthcare team for you to talk with about wellness, such as a social worker, nutritionist, clergy member, or nurse.

673

Some general tips for all cancer survivors include:

Quit smoking. Smoking after cancer treatment can increase the chances of getting cancer at the same or a different site.

Cut down on how much alcohol you drink. Drinking alcohol increases the risk of certain cancers.

Maintain a healthy weight. Eating well and staying active can help you reach a healthy weight and stay there. Eat well. A healthy and balanced diet is important for overall wellness. This includes eating fruits, vegetables, whole grains, and protein. Talk with your doctor or a dietitian to find out about any special dietary needs that you may have. You could also ask if you should talk to a nutritionist for guidance on eating a healthy diet.

Eat well. A healthy and balanced diet is important for overall wellness. This includes eating fruits, vegetables, whole grains, and protein. Talk with your doctor or a dietitian to find out about any special dietary needs that you may have. You could also ask if you should talk to a nutritionist for guidance on eating a healthy diet.

Exercise and stay active. Research suggests that staying active after cancer may help lower the risk of recurrence and lead to longer survival. In addition, moderate exercise (walking, biking, swimming) for about 30 minutes every—or almost every—day can:

- Reduce anxiety and depression
- Improve mood and boost self-esteem
- Reduce fatigue, nausea, pain, and diarrhea

It's important to start an exercise program slowly and increase activity over time. Some people may need to take special care in exercising. Talk with your doctor before you begin any exercise program, and work with your doctor or a specialist (such as a physical therapist) if needed. If you need to stay in bed during your recovery, even doing small activities can help. Stretching or moving your arms or legs can help you stay flexible, and relieve muscle tension.

Part Eight

Additional Help and Information

Chapter 60

A Glossary of Cancer-Related Terms

adjuvant therapy: Additional cancer treatment given after the primary treatment to lower the risk that the cancer will come back. Adjuvant therapy may include chemotherapy, radiation therapy, hormone therapy, targeted therapy, or biological therapy.

alopecia: The lack or loss of hair from areas of the body where hair is usually found. Alopecia can be a side effect of some cancer treatments.

angiogenesis inhibitor: A substance that may prevent the formation of blood vessels. In anticancer therapy, an angiogenesis inhibitor may prevent the growth of new blood vessels that tumors need to grow.

basal cell carcinoma: Cancer that begins in the lower part of the epidermis (the outer layer of the skin). It may appear as a small white or flesh-colored bump that grows slowly and may bleed. Basal cell carcinomas are usually found on areas of the body exposed to the sun. Basal cell carcinomas rarely metastasize (spread) to other parts of the body. They are the most common form of skin cancer. Also called basal cell cancer.

benign: Not cancerous. Benign tumors may grow larger but do not spread to other parts of the body. Also called nonmalignant.

This glossary contains terms excerpted from documents produced by several sources deemed reliable.

bilateral salpingo-oophorectomy: Surgery to remove both ovaries and both fallopian tubes.

biological therapy: Treatment to boost or restore the ability of the immune system to fight cancer, infections, and other diseases. Also used to lessen certain side effects that may be caused by some cancer treatments. Agents used in biological therapy include monoclonal antibodies, growth factors, and vaccines. These agents may also have a direct anti tumor effect. Also called biological response modifier therapy, biotherapy, BRM therapy, and immunotherapy.

biopsy: The removal of cells or tissues for examination by a pathologist. The pathologist may study the tissue under a microscope or perform other tests on the cells or tissue. There are many different types of biopsy procedures. When a wide needle is used, the procedure is called a core biopsy. When a thin needle is used, the procedure is called a fine-needle aspiration biopsy.

bone marrow: The soft, sponge-like tissue in the center of most bones. It produces white blood cells, red blood cells, and platelets.

BRCA1: A gene on chromosome 17 that normally helps to suppress cell growth. A person who inherits certain mutations (changes) in a *BRCA1* gene has a higher risk of getting breast, ovarian, and other types of cancer.

BRCA2: A gene on chromosome 13 that normally helps to suppress cell growth. A person who inherits certain mutations (changes) in a *BRCA2* gene has a higher risk of getting breast, ovarian, and other types of cancer.

breast-conserving surgery: An operation to remove the breast cancer but not the breast itself. Types of breast-conserving surgery include lumpectomy (removal of the lump), quadrantectomy (removal of one quarter, or quadrant, of the breast), and segmental mastectomy (removal of the cancer as well as some of the breast tissue around the tumor and the lining over the chest muscles below the tumor). Also called breast-sparing surgery.

CA-125: A substance that may be found in high amounts in the blood of patients with certain types of cancer, including ovarian cancer. CA-125 levels may also help monitor how well cancer treatments are working or if cancer has come back. Also called cancer antigen 125.

carcinoma: Cancer that begins in the skin or in tissues that line or cover internal organs.

carcinoma in situ: A group of abnormal cells that remain in the place where they first formed. They have not spread. These abnormal cells may become cancer and spread into nearby normal tissue. Also called stage 0 disease.

cervical intraepithelial neoplasia: Growth of abnormal cells on the surface of the cervix. Numbers from 1 to 3 may be used to describe how abnormal the cells are and how much of the cervical tissue is involved. Also called CIN.

cervix: The lower, narrow end of the uterus that forms a canal between the uterus and vagina.

chemotherapy: Treatment with drugs that kill cancer cells.

clinical breast exam: A physical exam of the breast performed by a healthcare provider to check for lumps or other changes. Also called CBE.

clinical trial: A type of research study that tests how well new medical approaches work in people. These studies test new methods of screening, prevention, diagnosis, or treatment of a disease. Also called clinical study.

colon: The longest part of the large intestine, which is a tube-like organ connected to the small intestine at one end and the anus at the other. The colon removes water and some nutrients and electrolytes from partially digested food. The remaining material, solid waste called stool, moves through the colon to the rectum and leaves the body through the anus.

colonoscopy: Examination of the inside of the colon using a colonoscope, inserted into the rectum. A colonoscope is a thin, tube-like instrument with a light and a lens for viewing. It may also have a tool to remove tissue to be checked under a microscope for signs of disease.

colostomy: An opening into the colon from the outside of the body. A colostomy provides a new path for waste material to leave the body after part of the colon has been removed.

colposcopy: Examination of the vagina and cervix using a lighted magnifying instrument called a colposcope.

complementary and alternative medicine (CAM): Forms of treatment that are used in addition to (complementary) or instead of (alternative) standard treatments. These practices generally are not considered standard medical approaches.

computed tomography (CT) scan: A series of detailed pictures of areas inside the body taken from different angles. The pictures are created by a computer linked to an X-ray machine. Also called CAT scan, computerized axial tomography scan, computerized tomography, and CT scan.

conization: Surgery to remove a cone-shaped piece of tissue from the cervix and cervical canal. Conization may be used to diagnose or treat a cervical condition. Also called cone biopsy.

cryosurgery: A procedure in which tissue is frozen to destroy abnormal cells. Liquid nitrogen or liquid carbon dioxide is used to freeze the tissue. Also called cryoablation and cryosurgical ablation.

cyst: A sac or capsule in the body. It may be filled with fluid or other material.

diethylstilbestrol (DES): A synthetic form of the hormone estrogen that was prescribed to pregnant women between about 1940 and 1971 because it was thought to prevent miscarriages. DES may increase the risk of uterine, ovarian, or breast cancer in women who took it. It also has been linked to an increased risk of clear cell carcinoma of the vagina or cervix in daughters exposed to diethylstilbestrol before birth.

dilation and curettage (D&C): A procedure to remove tissue from the cervical canal or the inner lining of the uterus. The cervix is dilated (made larger) and a curette (spoon-shaped instrument) is inserted into the uterus to remove tissue. Also called D&C and dilatation and curettage.

dilator: A device used to stretch or enlarge an opening.

ductal carcinoma in situ (DCIS): A noninvasive condition in which abnormal cells are found in the lining of a breast duct. The abnormal cells have not spread outside the duct to other tissues in the breast. In some cases, DCIS may become invasive cancer and spread to other tissues, although it is not known at this time how to predict which lesions will become invasive. Also called intraductal carcinoma.

dysplasia: Cells that look abnormal under a microscope but are not cancer.

dysplastic nevus: A type of nevus (mole) that looks different from a common mole. A dysplastic nevus is often larger with borders that are not easy to see. Its color is usually uneven and can range from pink to dark brown. Parts of the mole may be raised above the skin surface.

A dysplastic nevus may develop into malignant melanoma (a type of skin cancer).

early-stage breast cancer: Breast cancer that has not spread beyond the breast or the axillary lymph nodes. This includes ductal carcinoma in situ (DCIS) and stage I, stage IIA, stage IIB, and stage IIIA breast cancers.

endometriosis: A benign condition in which tissue that looks like endometrial tissue grows in abnormal places in the abdomen.

endometrium: The layer of tissue that lines the uterus.

estrogen: A type of hormone made by the body that helps develop and maintain female sex characteristics and the growth of long bones. Estrogens can also be made in the laboratory. They may be used as a type of birth control and to treat symptoms of menopause, menstrual disorders, osteoporosis, and other conditions.

excisional biopsy: A surgical procedure in which an entire lump or suspicious area is removed for diagnosis. The tissue is then examined under a microscope.

fallopian tube: A slender tube through which eggs pass from an ovary to the uterus. In the female reproductive tract, there is one ovary and one fallopian tube on each side of the uterus.

fine-needle aspiration: The removal of tissue or fluid with a thin needle for examination under a microscope. Also called FNA biopsy.

gestational trophoblastic tumor: Any of a group of tumors that develops from trophoblastic cells (cells that help an embryo attach to the uterus and help form the placenta) after fertilization of an egg by a sperm. The two main types of gestational trophoblastic tumors are hydatidiform mole and choriocarcinoma. Also called gestational trophoblastic disease (GTD).

grade: A description of a tumor based on how abnormal the cancer cells look under a microscope and how quickly the tumor is likely to grow and spread. Grading systems are different for each type of cancer.

graft: Healthy skin, bone, or other tissue taken from one part of the body and used to replace diseased or injured tissue removed from another part of the body.

gynecologic cancer: Cancer of the female reproductive tract, including the cervix, endometrium, fallopian tubes, ovaries, uterus, and vagina.

gynecologic oncologist: A doctor who specializes in treating cancers of the female reproductive organs.

hormone: One of many chemicals made by glands in the body. Hormones circulate in the bloodstream and control the actions of certain cells or organs. Some hormones can also be made in the laboratory.

hormone replacement therapy (HRT): Hormones (estrogen, progesterone, or both) given to women after menopause to replace the hormones no longer produced by the ovaries. Also called HRT and menopausal hormone therapy (MHT).

human papillomavirus (HPV): A type of virus that can cause abnormal tissue growth (for example, warts) and other changes to cells. Infection for a long time with certain types of HPV can cause cervical cancer. HPV can also play a role in some other types of cancer, such as anal, vaginal, vulvar, penile, and oropharyngeal cancers.

hysterectomy: Surgery to remove the uterus and, sometimes, the cervix. When the uterus and the cervix are removed, it is called a total hysterectomy. When only the uterus is removed, it is called a partial hysterectomy.

immunotherapy: Treatment to boost or restore the ability of the immune system to fight cancer, infections, and other diseases. Also used to lessen certain side effects that may be caused by some cancer treatments. Agents used in immunotherapy include monoclonal antibodies, growth factors, and vaccines. These agents may also have a direct anti tumor effect. Also called biological response modifier therapy, biological therapy, biotherapy, and BRM therapy.

intraepithelial: Within the layer of cells that form the surface or lining of an organ.

invasive cancer: Cancer that has spread beyond the layer of tissue in which it developed and is growing into surrounding, healthy tissues. Also called infiltrating cancer.

laser therapy: Treatment that uses intense, narrow beams of light to cut and destroy tissue, such as cancer tissue. Laser therapy may also be used to reduce lymphedema (swelling caused by a buildup of lymph fluid in tissue) after breast cancer surgery.

lobular carcinoma in situ (LCIS): A condition in which abnormal cells are found in the lobules of the breast. Lobular carcinoma in situ seldom becomes invasive cancer; however, having it in one breast increases the risk of developing breast cancer in either breast. Also called LCIS.

loop electrosurgical excision procedure: A technique that uses electric current passed through a thin wire loop to remove abnormal tissue. Also called LEEP and loop excision.

lumpectomy: Surgery to remove abnormal tissue or cancer from the breast and a small amount of normal tissue around it. It is a type of breast-sparing surgery.

lymph node: A rounded mass of lymphatic tissue that is surrounded by a capsule of connective tissue. Lymph nodes filter lymph (lymphatic fluid), and they store lymphocytes (white blood cells). They are located along lymphatic vessels. Also called lymph gland.

lymphatic system: The tissues and organs that produce, store, and carry white blood cells that fight infections and other diseases. This system includes the bone marrow, spleen, thymus, lymph nodes, and lymphatic vessels (a network of thin tubes that carry lymph and white blood cells). Lymphatic vessels branch, like blood vessels, into all the tissues of the body.

lymphedema: A condition in which extra lymph fluid builds up in tissues and causes swelling. It may occur in an arm or leg if lymph vessels are blocked, damaged, or removed by surgery.

magnetic resonance imaging (MRI): A procedure in which radio waves and a powerful magnet linked to a computer are used to create detailed pictures of areas inside the body. These pictures can show the difference between normal and diseased tissue. Magnetic resonance imaging makes better images of organs and soft tissue than other scanning techniques, such as computed tomography (CT) or X-ray. Magnetic resonance imaging is especially useful for imaging the brain, the spine, the soft tissue of joints, and the inside of bones. Also called NMRI and nuclear magnetic resonance imaging.

malignant: Cancerous. Malignant tumors can invade and destroy nearby tissue and spread to other parts of the body.

mammography: The use of film or a computer to create a picture of the breast.

mastectomy: Surgery to remove the breast (or as much of the breast tissue as possible).

menopause: The time of life when a woman's ovaries stop producing hormones and menstrual periods stop. Natural menopause usually occurs around age 50. A woman is said to be in menopause when she hasn't had a period for 12 months in a row. Symptoms of menopause include hot flashes, mood swings, night sweats, vaginal dryness, trouble concentrating, and infertility.

metastasis: The spread of cancer from one part of the body to another. A tumor formed by cells that have spread is called a metastatic tumor or a metastasis. The metastatic tumor contains cells that are like those in the original (primary) tumor. The plural form of metastasis is metastases.

mutation: Any change in the deoxyribonucleic acid (DNA) of a cell. Mutations may be caused by mistakes during cell division, or they may be caused by exposure to DNA-damaging agents in the environment. Mutations can be harmful, beneficial, or have no effect. If they occur in cells that make eggs or sperm, they can be inherited; if mutations occur in other types of cells, they are not inherited. Certain mutations may lead to cancer or other diseases.

neoadjuvant therapy: Treatment given as a first step to shrink a tumor before the main treatment, which is usually surgery, is given. Examples of neoadjuvant therapy include chemotherapy, radiation therapy, and hormone therapy. It is a type of induction therapy.

oncologist: A doctor who specializes in treating cancer. Some oncologists specialize in a particular type of cancer treatment. For example, a radiation oncologist specializes in treating cancer with radiation.

oophorectomy: Surgery to remove one or both ovaries.

ostomy: An operation to create an opening (a stoma) from an area inside the body to the outside. Colostomy and urostomy are types of ostomies.

ovary: One of a pair of female reproductive glands in which the ova, or eggs, are formed. The ovaries are located in the pelvis, one on each side of the uterus.

palliative care: Care given to improve the quality of life of patients who have a serious or life-threatening disease. The goal of palliative care is to prevent or treat as early as possible the symptoms of a disease, side effects caused by treatment of a disease, and psychological, social, and spiritual problems related to a disease or its treatment. Also called comfort care, supportive care, and symptom management.

Pap (Papanicolaou) test: A procedure in which cells are scraped from the cervix for examination under a microscope. It is used to detect cancer and changes that may lead to cancer. A Pap test can also show conditions, such as infection or inflammation, that are not cancer. Also called Pap smear and Papanicolaou test.

pathologist: A doctor who identifies diseases by studying cells and tissues under a microscope.

polyp: A growth that protrudes from a mucous membrane.

positron emission tomography (PET) scan: A procedure in which a small amount of radioactive glucose (sugar) is injected into a vein, and a scanner is used to make detailed, computerized pictures of areas inside the body where the glucose is used. Because cancer cells often use more glucose than normal cells, the pictures can be used to find cancer cells in the body.

precancerous: A term used to describe a condition that may (or is likely to) become cancer. Also called premalignant.

progesterone: A type of hormone made by the body that plays a role in the menstrual cycle and pregnancy. Progesterone can also be made in the laboratory. It may be used as a type of birth control and to treat menstrual disorders, infertility, symptoms of menopause, and other conditions.

progestin: Any natural or laboratory-made substance that has some or all of the biologic effects of progesterone, a female hormone.

prophylactic mastectomy: Surgery to reduce the risk of developing breast cancer by removing one or both breasts before disease develops. Also called preventive mastectomy.

radiation therapy: The use of high-energy radiation from X-rays, gamma rays, neutrons, protons, and other sources to kill cancer cells and shrink tumors. Radiation may come from a machine outside the body (external-beam radiation therapy (EBRT)), or it may come from radioactive material placed in the body near cancer cells (internal radiation therapy). Systemic radiation therapy uses a radioactive substance, such as a radio-labeled monoclonal antibody, that travels in the blood to tissues throughout the body. Also called irradiation and radiotherapy.

radical mastectomy: Surgery for breast cancer in which the breast, chest muscles, and all of the lymph nodes under the arm are removed. For many years, this was the breast cancer operation used most often, but it is used rarely now. Doctors consider radical mastectomy only when the tumor has spread to the chest muscles. Also called Halsted radical mastectomy.

raloxifene: The active ingredient in a drug used to reduce the risk of invasive breast cancer in postmenopausal women who are at high risk of the disease or who have osteoporosis. It is also used to prevent and treat osteoporosis in postmenopausal women. It is also being studied in the prevention of breast cancer in certain premenopausal women and in the prevention and treatment of other conditions. Raloxifene blocks the effects of the hormone estrogen in the breast and increases the amount of calcium in bone. It is a type of selective estrogen receptor modulator (SERM).

sarcoma: A cancer of the bone, cartilage, fat, muscle, blood vessels, or other connective or supportive tissue.

speculum: An instrument used to widen an opening of the body to make it easier to look inside.

squamous cell: Flat cell that looks like a fish scale under a microscope. These cells cover inside and outside surfaces of the body. They are found in the tissues that form the surface of the skin, the lining of the hollow organs of the body (such as the bladder, kidney, and uterus), and the passages of the respiratory and digestive tracts.

stage: The extent of a cancer in the body. Staging is usually based on the size of the tumor, whether lymph nodes contain cancer, and whether the cancer has spread from the original site to other parts of the body.

stem cell transplant: A method of replacing immature blood-forming cells in the bone marrow that have been destroyed by drugs, radiation, or disease. Stem cells are injected into the patient and make healthy blood cells. A stem cell transplant may be autologous (using a patient's own stem cells that were saved before treatment), allogeneic (using stem cells donated by someone who is not an identical twin), or syngeneic (using stem cells donated by an identical twin).

tamoxifen: A drug used to treat certain types of breast cancer in women and men. Also called tamoxifen citrate.

tumor: An abnormal mass of tissue that results when cells divide more than they should or do not die when they should. Tumors may be benign (not cancer), or malignant (cancer). Also called neoplasm.

ultrasound: A procedure in which high-energy sound waves are bounced off internal tissues or organs and make echoes. The echo patterns are shown on the screen of an ultrasound machine, forming a picture of body tissues called a sonogram. Also called ultrasonography.

unresectable: Unable to be removed with surgery.

uterus: The small, hollow, pear-shaped organ in a woman's pelvis. This is the organ in which a fetus develops. Also called womb.

vagina: The muscular canal extending from the uterus to the exterior of the body. Also called birth canal.

vulva: The external female genital organs, including the clitoris, vaginal lips, and the opening to the vagina.

vulvar cancer: Cancer of the vulva (the external female genital organs, including the clitoris, vaginal lips, and the opening to the vagina).

wound: A break in the skin or other body tissues caused by injury or surgical incision (cut).

X-ray: A type of high-energy radiation. In low doses, X-rays are used to diagnose diseases by making pictures of the inside of the body. In high doses, X-rays are used to treat cancer.

Chapter 61

Resources for More Information about Cancer in Women

General Cancer Information

Agency for Healthcare Research and Quality (AHRQ)
5600 Fishers Ln.
Rockville, MD 20857
Phone: 301-427-1364
Website: www.ahrq.gov

American Association for Cancer Research (AACR)
615 Chestnut St.
17th Fl.
Philadelphia, PA 19106-4404
Phone: 215-440-9300
Fax: 215-440-9313
Website: www.aacr.org
E-mail: aacr@aacr.org

American Cancer Society (ACS)
250 Williams St. N.W.
Atlanta, GA 30303
Toll-Free: 800-ACS-2345
(800-227-2345)
Toll-Free Fax: 800-279-2018
Website: www.cancer.org

American Childhood Cancer Organization (ACCO)
P.O. Box 498
Kensington, MD 20895-0498
Toll-Free: 855-858-2226
Phone: 301-962-3520
Fax: 301-962-3521
Website: www.acco.org

Resources in this chapter were compiled from several sources deemed reliable; all contact information was verified and updated in May 2018.

689

American Institute for Cancer Research (AICR)
1560 Wilson Blvd.
Ste. 1000
Arlington, VA 22209
Toll-Free: 800-843-8114
Fax: 202-328-7226
Website: www.aicr.org
E-mail: aicrweb@aicr.org

Angel Flight Mid-Atlantic
Air Charity Network (ACN)
4620 Haygood Rd.
Ste. 2
Virginia Beach, VA 23455
Toll-Free: 877-621-7177
Phone: 757-318-9174
Fax: 757-464-1284
Website: www.
angelflightmidatlantic.org

Association of Community Cancer Centers (ACCC)
1801 Research Blvd., Ste. 400
Rockville, MD 20850
Phone: 301-984-9496
Fax: 301-770-1949
Website: www.accc-cancer.org

Be The Match®
National Marrow Donor
Program (NMDP)
500 N. Fifth St.
Minneapolis, MN 55401
Toll-Free: 800-MARROW2
(800-627-7692)
Website: bethematch.org

Benefits.gov
Toll-Free: 800-FED-INFO
(800-333-4636)
Website: www.benefits.gov

Camp Kesem
10586 W. Pico Blvd.
Ste. 196
Los Angeles, CA 90064
Phone: 260-22-KESEM
(260-225-3736)
Website: www.campkesem.org

Canadian Cancer Society (CCS)
565 W. 10th Ave.
Vancouver, BC V5Z 4J4
Toll-Free: 800-663-2524
Phone: 604-872-4400
Website: www.cancer.ca/
fr-ca/?region=bc
E-mail: inquiries@bc.cancer.ca

Cancer and Careers
CEW Foundation
159 W. 25th St.
Eighth Fl.
Phone: 646-929-8032
Fax: 212-685-3334
Website: www.cancerandcareers.
org

Cancer Financial Assistance Coalition (CFAC)
Website: www.cancerfac.org

Cancer Hope Network (CHN)
2 N. Rd.
Ste. A
Chester, NJ 07930
Toll-Free: 877-HOPENET
(877-467-3638)
Fax: 908-879-6518
Website: www.
cancerhopenetwork.org
E-mail: info@
cancerhopenetwork.org

CancerCare
275 Seventh Ave.
New York, NY 10001
Toll-Free: 800-813-HOPE
(800-813-4673)
Website: www.cancercare.org
E-mail: info@cancercare.org

Centers for Disease Control and Prevention (CDC)
1600 Clifton Rd.
Atlanta, GA 30329-4027
Toll-Free: 800-CDC-4636
(800-232-4636)
Toll-Free TTY: 888-232-6348
Website: www.cdc.gov
E-mail: cdcinfo@cdc.gov

Cleaning for a Reason
211 S. Stemmons
Ste. G
Lewisville, TX 75067
Toll-Free: 877-337-7233
Fax: 972-316-4138
Website: cleaningforareason.org
E-mail: info@cleaningforareason.org

Colorectal Cancer Control Program (CRCCP)
4770 Buford Hwy N.E.
Atlanta, GA 30341
Toll-Free: 800-CDC-4636
(800-232-4636)
Toll-Free TTY: 888-232-6348
Website: www.cdc.gov/cancer/crccp/index.htm
E-mail: cdcinfo@cdc.gov

Colorectal CareLine
Patient Advocate Foundation (PAF)
421 Butler Farm Rd.
Hampton, VA 23666
Toll-Free: 866-657-8634
Website: www.colorectalcareline.org

Co-Pay Relief Program (CPR)
Patient Advocate Foundation (PAF)
421 Butler Farm Rd.
Hampton, VA 23666
Toll-Free: 866-512-3861
Phone: 757-952-0118
Fax: 757-952-0119
Website: www.copays.org

Corporate Angel Network (CAN)
Westchester County Airport
One Loop Rd.
White Plains, NY 10604-1215
Toll-Free: 866-328-1313
Phone: 914-328-1313
Fax: 914-328-3938
Website: www.corpangelnetwork.org
E-mail: info@corpangelnetwork.org

Dana-Farber Cancer Institute
450 Brookline Ave.
Boston, MA 02215
Toll-Free: 866-408-DFCI
(866-408-3324)
Phone: 617-632-3000
Website: www.dana-farber.org

Eldercare Locator
Administration for Community
Living (ACL)
330 C St. S.W.
Washington, DC 20201
Toll-Free: 800-677-1116
Phone: 202-401-4634
Website: eldercare.acl.gov/
Public/Index.aspx
E-mail: eldercarelocator@n4a.
org

*Facing Our Risk of Cancer
Empowered (FORCE)*
16057 Tampa Palms Blvd. W.
PMB Ste. 373
Tampa, FL 33647
Toll-Free: 866-824-RISK
(866-824-7475)
Fax: 954-827-2200
Website: www.facingourrisk.org
E-mail: info@facingourrisk.org

Good Days
6900 Dallas Pkwy
Ste. 200
Plano, TX 75024
Toll-Free: 877-968-7233
Phone: 972-608-7141
Fax: 214-570-3621
Website: www.mygooddays.org
E-mail: info@mygooddays.org

Health Well Foundation
20440 Century Blvd., Ste. 250
Germantown, MD 20874
Toll-Free: 800-675-8416
Toll-Free Fax: 800-282-7692
Website: www.
healthwellfoundation.org
E-mail: grants@
healthwellfoundation.org

Healthcare.gov
Centers for Medicare &
Medicaid Services (CMS)
7500 Security Blvd.
Baltimore, MD 21244
Toll-Free: 800-318-2596
Toll-Free TTY: 855-889-4325
Website: www.healthcare.gov

Hill-Burton Program
U.S. Department of Health and
Human Services (HHS)
5600 Fishers Ln.
Rockville, MD 20857
Toll-Free: 800-221-9393
Phone: 301-443-3376
Toll-Free TTY: 877-897-9910
Toll-Free Fax: 877-489-4772
Website: www.hrsa.gov/get-
health-care/affordable/hill-
burton/index.html

*Hope for Two... The Pregnant
with Cancer Network*
P.O. Box 253
Amherst, NY 14226
Toll-Free: 800-743-4471
Website: www.hopefortwo.org
E-mail: info@hopefortwo.org

*Intercultural Cancer Council
(ICC)*
Website: agable.net

*International Cancer
Information Service Group
(ICISG)*
Website: www.icisg.org

Joe's House
505 E. 79th St.
Ste. 17E
New York, NY 10075
Toll-Free: 877-JOESHOU
(877-563-7468)
Website: www.joeshouse.org
E-mail: info@joeshouse.org

Leukemia & Lymphoma Society (LLS)
3 International Dr.
Ste. 200
Rye Brook, NY 10573
Toll-Free: 800-955-4572;
888-557-7177
Website: www.lls.org
E-mail: infocenter@lls.org

LIVESTRONG
2201 E. Sixth St.
Austin, TX 78702
Toll-Free: 877-236-8820
Website: www.livestrong.org
E-mail: livestrong@livestrong.org

Lymphoma Research Foundation (LRF)
115 Bdwy.
Ste. 1301
New York, NY 10006
Toll-Free: 800-500-9976
Fax: 212-349-2886
Website: www.lymphoma.org
E-mail: LRF@lymphoma.org

Mayo Foundation for Medical Education and Research
200 First St. S.W.
Rochester, MN 55905
Toll-Free: 800-660-4582
Phone: 507-284-2511
Website: www.mayoclinic.org

M.D. Anderson Cancer Center
1515 Holcombe Blvd.
Houston, TX 77030
Toll-Free: 877-982-6532
Website: www.mdanderson.org

Melanoma International Foundation (MIF)
250 Mapleflower Rd.
Glenmoore, PA 19343
Toll-Free: 866-463-6663
Phone: 610-942-3432
Website:
melanomainternational.org

Memorial Sloan-Kettering Cancer Center (MSKCC)
1275 York Ave.
New York, NY 10065
Toll-Free: 800-525-2225
Phone: 212-639-2000
Website: www.mskcc.org
E-mail: international@mskcc.org

Mesothelioma Applied Research Foundation (MARF)
641 S. St. N.W.
Washington, DC 20001
Toll-Free: 877-363-6376
Fax: 571-363-2784
Website: www.curemeso.org
E-mail: info@curemeso.org

Moores Cancer Center (MCC)
UC San Diego Health
3855 Health Sciences Dr.
La Jolla, CA 92037
Phone: 858-657-7000
Website: health.ucsd.edu/
specialties/cancer/Pages/default.
aspx

**National Association for
Proton Therapy (NAPT)**
8400 Westpark Dr.
Second Fl.
McLean, VA 22102
Phone: 202-495-3133
Fax: 202-530-0659
Website: www.proton-therapy.
org
E-mail: info@proton-therapy.org

**National Association of
Insurance Commissioners
(NAIC)**
1100 Walnut St.
Ste. 1500
Kansas City, MO 64106-2197
Toll-Free: 866-470-6242
Phone: 816-842-3600
Fax: 816-783-8175
Website: www.naic.org
E-mail: education@naic.org

**National Breast and Cervical
Cancer Early Detection
Program (NBCCEDP)**
Centers for Disease Control and
Prevention (CDC)
4770 Buford Hwy N.E.
MS-F76
Atlanta, GA 30341
Toll-Free: 800-CDC-INFO
(800-232-4636)
Website: www.cdc.gov/cancer/
nbccedp/index.htm
E-mail: cdcinfo@cdc.gov

**National Cancer Institute
(NCI)**
9609 Medical Center Dr.
BG 9609 MSC 9760
Bethesda, MD 20892-9760
Toll-Free: 800-4-CANCER
(800-422-6237)
Website: www.cancer.gov

**National Center for
Complementary and
Integrative Health (NCCIH)**
9000 Rockville Pike
Bethesda, MD 20892
Toll-Free: 888-644-6226
Toll-Free TTY: 866-464-3615
Website: nccih.nih.gov

**National Coalition for
Cancer Survivorship (NCCS)**
8455 Colesville Rd.
Ste. 930
Silver Spring, MD 20910
Toll-Free: 877-NCCS-YES
(877-622-7937)
Website: www.canceradvocacy.
org
E-mail: info@canceradvocacy.org

*National Comprehensive
Cancer Network (NCCN)*
275 Commerce Dr.
Ste. 300
Fort Washington, PA 19034
Phone: 215-690-0300
Fax: 215-690-0280
Website: www.nccn.org

*National Foundation for
Cancer Research (NFCR)*
5515 Security Ln.
Ste. 1105
Rockville, MD 20852
Toll-Free: 800-321-CURE
(800-321-2873)
Fax: 301-654-5824
Website: www.nfcr.org

*National Heart, Lung, and
Blood Institute (NHLBI)*
31 Center Dr.
Bldg. 31
Bethesda, MD 20892
Phone: 301-592-8573
Website: www.nhlbi.nih.gov
E-mail: nhlbiInfo@nhlbi.nih.gov

*National Hospice and
Palliative Care Organization
(NHPCO)*
1731 King St.
Alexandria, VA 22314
Toll-Free: 800-658-8898
Phone: 703-837-1500
Fax: 703-837-1233
Website: www.nhpco.org
E-mail: nhpco_info@nhpco.org

*National Institute on Aging
(NIA)*
31 Center Dr. MSC 2292
Bldg. 31 Rm. 5C27
Bethesda, MD 20892
Toll-Free: 800-222-2225
Toll-Free TTY: 800-222-4225
Website: www.nia.nih.gov
E-mail: niaic@nia.nih.gov

*National Institute on Alcohol
Abuse and Alcoholism
(NIAAA)*
5635 Fishers Ln.
Rm. 2005 MSC 9304
Bethesda, MD 20892-9304
Toll-Free: 888-MY-NIAAA
(888-696-4222)
Phone: 301-443-3860
Website: www.niaaa.nih.gov
E-mail: niaaaweb-r@exchange.
nih.gov

*National Institutes of Health
(NIH)*
9000 Rockville Pike
Bethesda, MD 20892
Phone: 301-496-4000
TTY: 301-402-9612
Website: www.nih.gov
E-mail: NIHinfo@od.nih.gov

*National Lymphedema
Network (NLN)*
411 Lafayette St.
Sixth Fl.
New York, NY 10003
Phone: 646-722-7410
Fax: 415-908-3813
Website: www.lymphnet.org
E-mail: nln@lymphnet.org

Native American Cancer Research (NACR)
3022 S. Nova Rd.
Pine, CO 80470
Toll-Free: 800-537-8295
Phone: 303-838-9359
Website: natamcancer.org

NeedyMeds.org
P.O. Box 219
Gloucester, MA 01931
Toll-Free: 800-503-6897
Fax: 206-260-8850
Website: www.needymeds.org
E-mail: info@needymeds.org

Novartis AG
Phone: 862-778-5388
Fax: 732-673-5262
Website: www.novartis.com

Office On Women's Health (OWH)
U.S. Department of Health and Human Services (HHS)
200 Independence Ave. S.W.
Rm. 712E
Washington, DC 20201
Toll-Free: 800-994-9662
Phone: 202-690-7650
Fax: 202-205-2631
Website: www.womenshealth.gov

OncoLink
The Perelman Center for Advanced Medicine
3400 Civic Center Blvd., Ste. 2338
Philadelphia, PA 19104
Phone: 215-349-8895
Fax: 215-349-5445
Website: www.oncolink.org
E-mail: hampshire@uphs.upenn.edu

Patient Advocate Foundation (PAF)
421 Butler Farm Rd.
Hampton, VA 23666
Toll-Free: 800-532-5274
Fax: 757-873-8999
Website: www.patientadvocate.org
E-mail: help@patientadvocate.org

Physicians Committee
5100 Wisconsin Ave.
Ste. 400
Washington, DC 20016
Phone: 202-686-2210
Website: www.pcrm.org
E-mail: pcrm@pcrm.org

Prevent Cancer Foundation
1600 Duke St.
Ste. 500
Alexandria, VA 22314
Toll-Free: 800-227-2732
Phone: 703-836-4412
Fax: 703-836-4413
Website: www.preventcancer.org

R.A. Bloch Cancer Foundation
Bloch Cancer Hotline
One H&R Block Way
Kansas City, MO 64105
Toll-Free: 800-433-0464
Phone: 816-854-5050
Fax: 816-854-8024
Website: www.blochcancer.org
E-mail: hotline@blochcancer.org

Ronald McDonald House Charities (RMHC)
One Kroc Dr.
Oak Brook, IL 60523
Phone: 630-623-7048
Fax: 630-623-7488
Website: www.rmhc.org
E-mail: info@rmhc.org

The Salvation Army
National Headquarters
615 Slaters Ln.
P.O. Box 269
Alexandria, VA 22313
Toll-Free: 800-SAL-ARMY
(800-725-2769)
Phone: 703-684-5500
Fax: 703-684-5500
Website: www.
salvationarmyusa.org

The Samfund
89 S. St.
Ste. LL02
Boston, MA 02211
Phone: 617-938-3484
Toll-Free Fax: 866-496-8070
Website: www.thesamfund.org
E-mail: info@thesamfund.org

Sarcoma Alliance
775 E. Blithedale
Ste. 334
Mill Valley, CA 94941
Phone: 415-381-7236
Fax: 415-381-7235
Website: www.sarcomaalliance.
org
E-mail: info@sarcomaalliance.
org

Sisters Network, Inc. (SNI)
9668 Westheimer Rd.
Ste. 200-132
Houston, TX 77063
Toll-Free: 866-781-1808
Phone: 713-781-0255
Website: www.
sistersnetworkinc.org
E-mail: infonet@
sistersnetworkinc.org

Society of Laparoendoscopic Surgeons (SLS)
7330 S.W. 62nd Pl.
Ste. 410
Miami, FL 33143
Phone: 305-665-9959
Website: www.sls.org
E-mail: info@sls.org

Society of Surgical Oncology (SSO)
9525 W. Bryn Mawr Ave.
Ste. 870
Rosemont, IL 60018
Phone: 847-427-1400
Fax: 847-427-1411
Website: www.surgonc.org
E-mail: info@surgonc.org

State Health Insurance Assistance Program (SHIP)
Centers for Medicare &
Medicaid Services (CMS)
7500 Security Blvd.
Baltimore, MD 21244
Toll-Free: 877-402-8219
Phone: 410-767-6860
Toll-Free TTY: 800-735-2258
Website: www.medicare.gov/
contacts

Susan G. Komen
5005 LBJ Fwy
Ste. 526
Dallas, TX 75244
Toll-Free: 877-GOKOMEN
(877-465-6636)
Website: ww5.komen.org
E-mail: helpline@komen.org

The Ulman Cancer Fund for Young Adults
1215 E. Fort Ave.
Ste. 104
Baltimore, MD 21230
Toll-Free: 888-393-FUND
(888-393-3863)
Phone: 410-964-0202
Toll-Free Fax: 888-964-0402
Website: www.ulmanfund.org
E-mail: info@ulmanfund.org

United Healthcare Children's Foundation (UHCCF)
P.O. Box 41
MN017-W400
Minneapolis, MN 55440
Toll-Free: 855-MY-UHCCF
(855-698-4223)
Website: www.uhccf.org
E-mail: customerservice@uhccf.org

United Way Worldwide
701 N. Fairfax St.
Alexandria, VA 22314
Phone: 703-836-7112
Website: www.unitedway.org

U.S. Food and Drug Administration (FDA)
10903 New Hampshire Ave.
Silver Spring, MD 20993
Toll-Free: 888-INFO-FDA
(888-463-6332)
Website: www.fda.gov

U.S. Social Security Administration (SSA)
Office of Public Inquiries
6401 Security Blvd.
1100 W. High Rise
Baltimore, MD 21235
Toll-Free: 800-772-1213
Toll-Free TTY: 800-325-0778
Website: www.ssa.gov

Us TOO International, Inc.
2720 S. River Rd.
Ste. 112
Des Plaines, IL 60018
Toll-Free: 800-80-USTOO
(800-808-7866)
Phone: 630-795-1002
Fax: 630-795-1602
Website: www.ustoo.org
E-mail: ustoo@ustoo.org

Women's Cancer Resource Center (WCRC)
2908 Ellsworth St.
Berkeley, CA 94705
Toll-Free: 888-421-7900
Phone: 510-420-7900
Fax: 510-809-0240
Website: www.wcrc.org
E-mail: wcrc@wcrc.org

Breast Cancer Resources

African American Breast Cancer Alliance (AABCA)
P.O. Box 8981
Minneapolis, MN 55408
Phone: 612-462-6813
Website: aabcainc.org
E-mail: aabca@aabcainc.org

American Breast Cancer Foundation (ABCF)
10400 Little Patuxent Pkwy
Ste. 480
Columbia, MD 21044
Phone: 410-730-5105
Website: www.abcf.org
E-mail: info@abcf.org

Breast Cancer Action (BCAction)
275 Fifth St.
Ste. 307
San Francisco, CA 94103
Toll-Free: 877-2STOPBC
(877-278-6722)
Phone: 415-243-9301
Fax: 415-243-3996
Website: www.bcaction.org
E-mail: info@bcaction.org

Breast Cancer Research Foundation (BCRF)
28 W. 44th St.
Ste. 609
New York, NY 10036
Toll-Free: 866-FIND-A-CURE
(888-346-3228)
Fax: 646-497-0890
Website: www.bcrf.org
E-mail: bcrf@bcrfcure.org

HealthyWomen
P.O. Box 430
Red Bank, NJ 07701
Toll-Free: 877-986-9472
Phone: 732-530-3425
Website: www.healthywomen.org
E-mail: info@healthywomen.org

Imaginis®
25 E. Ct. St.
Ste. 301
Greenville, SC 29601
Phone: 864-209-1139
Website: www.imaginis.com
E-mail: learnmore@imaginis.com

Johns Hopkins Breast Cancer Center
601 N. Caroline St.
Baltimore, MD 21287
Phone: 410-955-5000
Website: www.hopkinsmedicine.org

Living Beyond Breast Cancer (LBBC)
40 Monument Rd.
Ste. 104
Bala Cynwyd, PA 19004
Toll-Free: 855-807-6386
Phone: 610-645-4567
Fax: 610-645-4573
Website: www.lbbc.org
E-mail: mail@lbbc.org

National Breast and Cervical Cancer Early Detection Program (NBCCEDP)
Website: www.cdc.gov/cancer/
nbccedp/index.htm

National Breast Cancer Coalition (NBCC)
1010 Vermont Ave. N.W.
Ste. 900
Washington, DC 20005
Toll-Free: 800-622-2838
Phone: 202-296-7477
Fax: 202-265-6854
Website: www.
breastcancerdeadline2020.org
E-mail: info@
breastcancerdeadline2020.org

National Breast Cancer Foundation (NBCF)
2600 Network Blvd.
Ste. 300
Frisco, TX 75034
Website: www.
nationalbreastcancer.org

SHARE Cancer Support
165 W. 46th St.
Ste. 712
New York, NY 10036
Toll-Free: 844-ASK-SHARE
(844-275-7427)
Phone: 212-719-0364
Website: www.
sharecancersupport.org
E-mail: info@
sharecancersupport.org

Gynecologic Cancer Resources

American College of Obstetricians and Gynecologists (ACOG)
409 12th St. S.W.
Washington, DC 20024-2188
Toll-Free: 800-673-8444
Phone: 202-638-5577
Website: www.acog.org
E-mail: international@acog.org

American Society for Colposcopy and Cervical Pathology (ASCCP)
1530 Tilco Dr., Ste. C
Frederick, MD 21704
Toll-Free: 800-787-7227
Phone: 301-733-3640
Fax: 240-575-9880
Website: www.asccp.org
E-mail: info@asccp.org

Foundation for Women's Cancer (FWC)
230 W. Monroe
Ste. 710
Chicago, IL 60606
Phone: 312-578-1439
Fax: 312-235-4059
Website: www.
foundationforwomenscancer.org
E-mail: FWCinfo@sgo.org

International Gynecologic Cancer Society (IGCS)
P.O. Box 6387
Louisville, KY 40206
Phone: 707-732-4427
Website: www.igcs.org
E-mail: info@igcs.org

National Cervical Cancer Coalition (NCCC)

American Sexual Health
Association (ASHA)
P.O. Box 13827
Research Triangle Park, NC
27709
Toll-Free: 800-685-5531
Website: www.nccc-online.org
E-mail: nccc@ashasexualhealth.
org

National HPV and Cervical Cancer Prevention Resource Center

American Sexual Health
Association (ASHA)
P.O. Box 13827
Research Triangle Park, NC
27709
Phone: 919-361-8400
Website: www.ashasexualhealth.
org/stdsstis/hpv

National Ovarian Cancer Coalition (NOCC)

3800 Maple Ave., Ste. 435
Dallas, TX 75219
Toll-Free: 888-OVARIAN
(888-682-7426)
Phone: 214-273-4200
Website: ovarian.org

Ovarian Cancer Research Fund Alliance (OCRFA)

1101 14th St. N.W., Ste. 850
Washington, DC 20005
Toll-Free: 866-399-6262
Phone: 202-331-1332
Fax: 212-947-5652
Website: ocrfa.org
E-mail: info@ocrf.org

Resources for Other Types of Cancer

American Gastroenterological Association (AGA)

4930 Del Ray Ave.
Bethesda, MD 20814
Phone: 301-654-2055
Fax: 301-654-5920
Website: www.gastro.org
E-mail: member@gastro.org

American Liver Foundation (ALF)

39 Bdwy.
Ste. 2700
New York, NY 10006
Toll-Free: 800-465-4837
Phone: 212-668-1000
Fax: 212-483-8179
Website: www.liverfoundation.
org

American Lung Association (ALA)
55 W. Wacker Dr.
Ste. 1150
Chicago, IL 60601
Toll-Free: 800-LUNGUSA
(800-586-4872)
Website: www.lung.org
E-mail: info@lung.org

American Melanoma Foundation (AMF)
Phone: 858-412-3271
Website: www.myamf.org

American Society for Gastrointestinal Endoscopy (ASGE)
3300 Woodcreek Dr.
Downers Grove, IL 60515
Toll-Free: 866-353-ASGE
(866-353-2743)
Phone: 630-573-0600
Fax: 630-963-8332
Website: www.asge.org
E-mail: info@asge.org

American Society of Colon and Rectal Surgeons (ASCRS)
85 W. Algonquin Rd.
Ste. 550
Arlington Heights, IL 60005
Phone: 847-290-9184
Fax: 847-427-9656
Website: www.fascrs.org
E-mail: ascrs@fascrs.org

Colon Cancer Alliance
1025 Vermont Ave. N.W.
Ste. 1066
Washington, DC 20005
Toll-Free: 877-422-2030
Toll-Free Fax: 866-304-9075
Website: www.ccalliance.org

Kidney Cancer Association (KCA)
9450 S.W. Gemini Dr. #38269
Beaverton, OR 97008-7105
Toll-Free: 800-850-9132
Fax: 847-332-2978
Website: www.kidneycancer.org
E-mail: office@kidneycancer.org

Leukemia & Lymphoma Society (LLS)
3 International Dr.
Ste. 200
Rye Brook, NY 10573
Toll-Free: 800-955-4572
Website: www.lls.org
E-mail: customersupport@lls.org

Lung Cancer Alliance (LCA)
1700 K St. N.W.
Ste. 660
Washington, DC 20006
Toll-Free: 800-298-2436
Phone: 202-463-2080
Website: www.
lungcanceralliance.org
E-mail: info@lungcanceralliance.
org

Lung Cancer Online Foundation (LCOF)
Website: www.lungcanceronline.
org

Lymphoma Research Foundation (LRF)
115 Bdwy.
Ste. 1301
New York, NY 10006
Toll-Free: 800-500-9976
Phone: 212-349-2910
Fax: 212-349-2886
Website: www.lymphoma.org
E-mail: helpline@lymphoma.org

Melanoma Education Foundation (MEF)
P.O. Box 2023
Peabody, MA 01960
Phone: 978-535-3080
Fax: 978-535-5602
Website: www.skincheck.org
E-mail: mef@skincheck.org

Multiple Myeloma Research Foundation (MMRF)
383 Main Ave.
Fifth Fl.
Norwalk, CT 06851
Phone: 203-972-0464
Fax: 203-972-1259
Website: www.themmrf.org
E-mail: info@themmrf.org

National Brain Tumor Foundation (NBTF)
55 Chapel St.
Ste. 200
Newton, MA 02458
Phone: 617-924-9997
Fax: 617-924-9998
Website: www.braintumor.org

National Lymphedema Network (NLN)
411 Lafayette St.
Sixth Fl.
New York, NY 10003
Phone: 646-722-7410
Fax: 510-208-3110
Website: www.lymphnet.org
E-mail: nln@lymphnet.org

Pancreatic Cancer Action Network (PanCAN)
1500 Rosecrans Ave.
Ste. 200
Manhattan Beach, CA 90266
Toll-Free: 877-435-8650
Phone: 310-725-0025
Fax: 310-725-0029
Website: www.pancan.org
E-mail: info@pancan.org

The Skin Cancer Foundation
205 Lexington Ave.
11th Fl.
New York, NY 10016
Phone: 212-725-5176
Fax: 212-725-5751
Website: www.skincancer.org
E-mail: info@skincancer.org

ThyCa: Thyroid Cancer Survivors' Association, Inc.
P.O. Box 1102
Olney, MD 20830-1102
Toll-Free: 877-588-7904
Fax: 630-604-6078
Website: www.thyca.org
E-mail: thyca@thyca.org

Chapter 62

How to Find a Cancer Support Group

Cancer Support Groups

Cancer support groups are meetings for people with cancer and those touched by the disease. They can have many benefits. Even though a lot of people receive support from friends and family, the number one reason they join a support group is to be with others with similar cancer experiences. Some research shows that joining a support group improves both quality of life and survival.

Support groups can:

- Help you feel better, more hopeful, and not so alone

- Give you a chance to talk about your feelings and work through them

- Help you deal with practical problems, such as problems at work or school

- Help you cope with side effects of treatment

This chapter includes text excerpted from "Coping—Cancer Support Groups," National Cancer Institute (NCI), December 2, 2014. Reviewed May 2018. The appended list of additional resources in this chapter were compiled from several sources deemed reliable; all contact information was verified and updated in May 2018.

Types of Support Groups

Some groups focus on all kinds of cancer. Others talk about just one kind, such as a group for women with breast cancer or one for men with prostate cancer. Some can be open to everyone or just for people of a certain age, sex, culture, or religion. For instance, some groups are just for teens or young children.

Support groups can also be helpful for children or family members. These groups focus on family concerns such as role changes, relationship changes, financial worries, and how to support the person with cancer. Some groups include both cancer survivors and family members.

Telephone support groups are when everyone dials in to a phone line that is linked together, like a conference call. They can share and talk to others with similar experiences from all over the country. There is usually little or no charge.

Online support groups are "meetings" that take place online. People meet through chat rooms, listservs, or moderated discussion groups and talk with each other over email. People often like online support groups because they can take part in them any time of the day or night. They're also good for people who can't travel to meetings. But always talk with your doctor about cancer information you learn from the Internet.

Where to Find a Support Group

Many hospitals, cancer centers, community groups, and schools offer cancer support groups. Here are some ways to find groups near you:

- Call your local hospital and ask about its cancer support programs

- Ask your social worker to suggest groups

- Do an online search for groups. Or go to the Association of Cancer Online Resources (ACOR), which offers access to mailing lists that provide support and information to those affected by cancer and related disorders.

Is a Support Group Right for Me?

A support group may not be right for everyone. For some people, hearing about others' problems can make them feel worse. Or you may find that your need for a support group changes over time.

If you have a choice of support groups, visit a few and see what they are like. See which ones make sense for you. Although many groups are free, some charge a small fee. Find out if your health insurance pays for support groups.

If you're thinking about joining a support group, here are some questions you may want to ask the group's contact person:

- How large is the group?

- Who attends (survivors, family members, types of cancer, age range)?

- How long are the meetings?

- How often does the group meet?

- How long has the group been together?

- Who leads the meetings—a professional or a survivor?

- What is the format of the meetings?

- Is the main purpose to share feelings, or do people also offer tips to solve common problems?

- If I go, can I just sit and listen?

- Before joining a group, here are questions you may want to ask yourself:

- Am I comfortable talking about personal issues?

- Do I have something to offer to the group?

- What do I hope to gain by joining a group?

Support groups vary greatly, and if you have one bad experience, it doesn't mean these groups aren't a good option for you. You may also want to find another cancer survivor with whom you can discuss your cancer experience. Many organizations can pair you with someone who had your type of cancer and is close to your age and background.

Online Support

Cancer Survivors Network
American Cancer Society (ACS)
Website: csn.cancer.org

OncoChat
Website: www.oncochat.org

LiveHelp
National Cancer Institute (NCI)
Website: www.cancer.gov/
livehelp

Support Helplines

*American Cancer Society
(ACS)*
Toll-Free: 800-ACS-2345
(800-227-2345)

CancerCare
Toll-Free: 800-813-HOPE
(800-813-4673)
Phone: 212-302-2400

*Cancer Information and
Counseling Line (CICL)*
Toll-Free: 800-525-3777

Cancer Research Foundation
Toll-Free: 800-227-2732

Susan G. Komen
Toll-Free: 877-GO KOMEN
(877-465-6636)

*Living Beyond Breast Cancer
(LBBC)*
Toll-Free: 888-753-5222

*National Cancer Institute's
Cancer Information Service*
Toll-Free: 800-422-6237

*SHARE: Self Help for
Women with Breast or
Ovarian Cancer*
Toll-Free: 866-891-2392

Support Organizations

*American Society of Clinical
Oncology (ASCO)*
2318 Mill Rd., Ste. 800
Alexandria, VA 22314
Toll-Free: 888-282-2552
Phone: 703-299-0158
Fax: 703-299-0255
Website: www.asco.org
E-mail: customerservice@asco.
org

Avon Breast Cancer Crusade
P.O. Box 3535
New York, NY 10163
Toll-Free: 800-510-9255
Website: avonbcc.org

Black Women's Health Imperative (BWHI)
55 M St. S.E.
Ste. 940
Washington, DC 20003
Phone: 202-787-5930
Website: www.bwhi.org
E-mail: info@bwhi.org

Cancer Support Community (CSC)
734 15th St. N.W.
Ste. 300
Washington, DC 20005
Toll-Free: 888-793-9355
Phone: 202-659-9709
Fax: 202-974-7999
Website: www.
cancersupportcommunity.org
E-mail: help@
cancersupportcommunity.org

Celebrating Life Foundation (CLF)
1121 E. Spring Creek Pkwy
Ste. 110-118
Plano, TX 75074
Phone: 214-475-0661
Website: celebratinglife.org
E-mail: Clf@airmail.net

Reach to Recovery
American Cancer Society (ACS)
250 Williams St. N.W.
Atlanta, GA 30303
Toll-Free: 800-ACS-2345
(800-227-2345)
Website: www.cancer.org/
treatment/support-programs-
and-services/reach-to-recovery.
html

Look Good Feel Better® (LGFB)
Toll-Free: 800-395-LOOK
(800-395-5665)
Website: www.
lookgoodfeelbetter.org

TLC Tender Loving Care
American Cancer Society (ACS)
P.O. Box 395
Louisiana, MO 63353-0395
Toll-Free: 800-850-9445
Toll-Free Fax: 800-279-2018
Website: www.tlcdirect.org
E-mail: customerservice@
tlccatalog.org

Vital Options International: Generating Global Cancer Conversations
Phone: 818-508-5657
Website: www.vitaloptions.org
E-mail: info@vitaloptions.org

Young Survival Coalition (YSC)
80 Broad St.
Ste. 1700
New York, NY 10004
Toll-Free: 877-972-1011
Fax: 646-257-3030
Website: www.youngsurvival.org

Index

Index

Page numbers followed by 'n' indicate a footnote. Page numbers in *italics* indicate a table or illustration.

A

abdominoperineal resection, radiation therapy 262

acetaminophen
cancer treatment 517
neutropenia 588
ovarian cancer 229

"Across Many Health Behaviors, Long-Term Oral Contraceptive Use Lowers Risk for Ovarian and Endometrial Cancers" (NCI) 222n

acupuncture
cancer pain treatment 555
hot flash treatment 594
integrative medicine practices 488
pruritus 607

acute myeloid leukemia
BRCA1 114
lung cancer 305
smoking 36

addiction
nicotine 40
pain relievers 599

adenocarcinoma
cancer staging 402
smoking 43
tumor markers 393
vaginal cancer 239

adjuvant therapy
breast cancer 150
chemotherapy 136
colorectal cancer 272
defined 677
endometrial cancer 185
gallbladder cancer 299
gestational trophoblastic disease (GTD) 195
lung cancer 311
ovarian cancer 207
skin cancer 342
uterine sarcoma cancer 236
vaginal cancer 245
vulvar cancer 253

African American Breast Cancer Alliance (AABCA), contact 699

Agency for Healthcare Research and Quality (AHRQ)
contact 689
publication
robotic surgery 429n

air pollution
cancer risk 88